SUPER NUTRITION GARDENING

HOW TO GROW YOUR OWN POWERCHARGED FOODS

DR. WILLIAM S. PEAVY

WARREN PEARY

AVERY PUBLISHING GROUP INC.
Garden City Park, New York

Cover Design: Ann Vestal
Cover Photography: J. Michael Dombroski
Typesetting: Widget Design; Mount Marion, New York
Original Artwork: Widget Design (and others)

Library of Congress Cataloging-in-Publication Data

Peavy, William S.
Super nutrition gardening : how to grow your own PowerCharged food / by William S. Peavy, Warren Peary.
p. cm.
Includes bibliographical references (p.) and index.
ISBN 0-89529-532-6 (softcover)
1. Vegetable gardening. 2. Organic gardening. 3. Vegetables. 4. Food. I. Peary, Warren. II. Title. III. Title: PowerCharged food.
SB324.3.P42 1992
635—dc20 92-25950
CIP

Printed in the United States of America

10 9 8 7 6 5 4 3 2

Contents

Acknowledgments v
Foreword vii
Preface ix

1. Why You Need PowerCharged Food 1

Which minerals and vitamins are widely deficient in our diets? • How does this affect our health? • How will your own PowerCharged food garden ensure you against deficiencies? • And why is food, rather than supplements, the best source of minerals and vitamins?

2. Why Our Food Is Deficient 13

Why is the nutritional quality of our food today far less than it was for our grandparents? • Why does it continue to decline? • Why are big harvests no indication of nutrition? • Which minerals and vitamins are most deficient in our soils, and how does this affect our food?

3. The Fountain of Youth 25

Learn how to grow a special kind of PowerCharged food year-round on your kitchen counter. • Learn why food enzymes are the best-kept health secret and why sprouts are the fountain of youth. • Which sprouts are the best? • How exactly do you create your own sprout garden?

4. The Pesticide Menace 39

Are pesticides really dangerous? • Are they something we should try to avoid, or are the doses so small in food that it really doesn't matter? • And doesn't the government protect our safety anyway?

5. Site Selection and Layout 49

If you are a new gardener, what are the things you look for in picking a suitable spot for your garden? • What is the best type of layout and shape? • What do you need to do to prepare your garden spot for soil charging?

6. Charging Your Soil 63

What is charging the soil? • How does it produce food that is high in nutrition? • Why do chemical fertilizers, as they're currently used, result in low-nutrition food? • What is a good soil charging program for growing spray-free food that is PowerCharged with nutrition?

7. The Planting Plan 81

How can you avoid being overflowing with vegetables one month and without any at all the next month? • How do you know what to plant, how much of each kind of vegetable to plant, what spacing to use, which varieties to get, and when to plant?

8. Planting With Ease 95

Why should bedding plants be conditioned before setting them outdoors? • What is the difference between planting large seeds and small seeds? • What is the secret way to get perfect stands of small seeds every planting? • Why is thinning important, and how do you do it?

Acknowledgments

THE great scientist Sir Isaac Newton said, "If I have seen farther than others, it is because I have stood upon the shoulders of giants."

In writing *Super Nutrition Gardening,* we also have stood upon the shoulders of giants. Julius Hensel, in his book *Bread From Stones,* pointed out the importance of soil mineralization using powdered rock. Sir Albert Howard, a British agricultural scientist, in his classic book, *An Agricultural Testament,* described in detail how the recycling of organic wastes results in a superior organic fertilizer called compost.

In the United States a few years later, J.I. Rodale, inspired by Howard's work, began publishing *Organic Gardening Magazine,* urging gardeners and farmers to return to the basics—to build up the soil's organic matter. About the same time, a man with impeccable credentials added to the works of Hensel, Howard, and Rodale. This man was Dr. William Albrecht, head of the Soils Department of the University of Missouri, who in the 1950s urged growers to mineralize and balance their soils. He pointed out that insects tend to attack crops grown on infertile soils and that hybridization of seeds lowered the quality of food crops even though it increased the yields. He also stated a basic law of eco-agriculture when he wrote, "To grow plants, you must first feed the soil and then let the soil feed the plants," rather than feeding plants by applying fertilizer to them.

Now, as we are nearing the year 2000, there are other voices that are natural extensions of the old pioneers. These voices urge us to recycle, to save the planet, to simplify our lifestyles, and to move toward a plant-based diet. One of these voices belongs to Dr. Paul Erlich, population biologist at Stanford University, who foretells the diet of the future in his book *Population Bomb.*

Another farsighted leader is John Robbins, who gave up a fortune to pursue basic truth, detailed in his unusual book *Diet for a New America.*

Foreword

DR. William Peavy is a Ph.D. research scientist who has done extensive research on how to grow food of maximum nutrition while preserving the environment. As a former Professor of Horticulture for Texas A&M University, and as a private consultant in agriculture, he has seen the damage done to our health and the health of the Earth by our agribusiness-dominated food production system. He has seen the inner sanctums of the petrochemical industry that produces our food without regard for the environment.

Central to his forty years of study has been the question: How can people grow food with the highest possible nutrition in harmony with the planet's life-support systems? What is the optimum balance of soil nutrients which plants can assimilate and convert into the vitamins, minerals, enzymes, and proteins that nourish us? His search has been to find how people can grow food which keeps their health at its highest level.

Super Nutrition Gardening represents the culmination of Dr. Peavy's work. It shows in easy-to-follow steps how everyone living in cities or towns, with little or no land, can grow food that will keep their immune systems strong because it is charged with all the elements of optimum nutrition—and do so without using pesticides or other poisons!

Many people who want to shift to a better diet today recognize that meats, with their high saturated fat and cholesterol levels, and their absence of fiber, vitamin C, and many other essential nutrients, are anything but the cornerstones of sound nutrition that the Beef Council would like us to believe they are. Yet, when we picture our dinner plates and remove the meat dish, we are left with the sorry sight of perhaps some boiled peas that were pretty tasteless to begin with. The answer as to how to move in a more healthy and vegetarian direction is to be found in consuming grains, beans, vegetables, fruits, seeds, sprouts, and nuts that have not been overcooked, oversalted, overprocessed, or oversweetened, and have been grown with respect for the soil from which they arise. Nothing tastes as good as home-grown vegetables, and nothing is as healthy for us either, especially if we have the benefit of Dr. Peavy's impressive research.

It is a liberating step to grow some of our own food, not only because it improves our health but because it brings us into contact with the miracle of life and the wonders of the living Earth. Reconnecting with the Earth is healing and connects us to the sources of our lives.

Even if we only grow some sprouts in a small kitchen garden, we are taking a step toward survival. During these times of environmental deterioration, when the planet's ecosystems are so wounded, nothing could be more important than for us to have direct contact in our own lives with the life force and living spirit of the Earth and its incredible ability to nourish us when we live in harmony with the laws of nature.

Unfortunately, the Great American Food Machine violates these laws and does irreparable damage to the soil, to the animals and plants, and to our bodies and those of our children. Dr. Peavy's work points toward a way out of this disaster, toward a lifestyle that is healthy, independent, and worthy of the name human.

—John Robbins, author
Diet for a New America

Preface

I grew up on a small farm in the 1930s, when there was no money to buy anything, but we always had plenty of home-grown food, fresh in the summer and home-canned or home-dried in the winter. Our diet was simple but wholesome and nourishing. I didn't have a single cavity until after leaving the farm for college.

We had to grow a big food garden for survival, but I realize now it not only meant survival but good health as well. That green thumb my Mom and Dad had came from doing, not dreaming. Their love for nature and growing food has stayed with me all these years through four university degrees. Today, more than ever before, growing some of your own food is important.

Your own backyard garden is the greatest health insurance policy you have. Did you know that eating a diet high in fresh vegetables and fruits and low in fat will protect you from practically every disease known to man, including heart disease and most types of cancer? It's true! The National Cancer Institute, the American Heart Association, the National Institutes of Health, and the Surgeon General of the United States have documented this.

In fact, eating large servings of home-grown vegetables every day may be the most important thing you can do for your health. Vegetables are wonder foods. They are packed with vitamins and minerals, contain virtually no fat and no cholesterol, and provide more nutrition, calorie for calorie, than any other food on Earth. And in the case of legumes, they are loaded with protein and high-energy complex carbohydrates. Notable among vegetables are vitamins C, carotenoid A, E, B-6, and folacin, and the minerals calcium, potassium, magnesium, iron, zinc, copper, selenium, and manganese.Vegetables even contain substances known as phytochemicals, such as flavonoids, indoles, and isoflavones, which have special cancer-protecting properties. Vegetables are the most important disease-preventing weapon we have in our arsenal. And your backyard garden is the greatest source of health on Earth!

Why not buy everything from the store? Most food today is grown in nutrient-depleted soil, is lacking in essential minerals, trace elements, and vitamins, and is polluted with spray residues. Even food advertised as "organic" at twice the cost may be low in essential minerals and vitamins. The fact is that none of the food we eat today has the level of nutrition that our grandparents enjoyed. And this greatly affects the status of our health. If you really want to get super-healthy, high-nutrition food, you need to grow it yourself. But exactly how do you grow food for maximum nutrition?

All the old gardening books leave you hanging when it comes to showing you how to grow food for maximum nutrition. But now, by following the principles of soil science, you can learn exactly how to grow spray-free PowerCharged food that is 100 percent to 1,200 percent higher in nutrition than anything you can buy anywhere! This is proven with independent laboratory analysis. This is the first time these special methods have been revealed. You will not find them anywhere else.

Best of all, PowerCharged methods are designed to work with nature, not against it. And that means your gardening will be simplified. Forget about poisonous sprays. Plants grown in properly balanced soil are healthy and less subject to insect attack, so poisonous sprays are not needed. Forget about weeds. Weeds are no problem when nature's way is followed. Forget about plowing up your soil all the time with heavy equipment. Soil does not need constant tillage once it is treated properly. By following PowerCharged methods, you can sit back and enjoy the bounty of your own health-promoting, high-nutrition food garden.

PowerCharged food, loaded with minerals, will also taste better than anything you've ever had in your life. You will even learn (in Chapter 3) how to start growing PowerCharged food right away in your kitchen in only five minutes a day.

Everything you'll learn in this book is the result of forty years of scientific research and practical experience growing successful gardens from the East Coast to the West and everywhere in between. There is no guesswork or vague generalities. You will learn exactly what works wherever you are.

I have blazed the trail that leads to saving money on your grocery and health care bills. I have drawn the road map for you. You are now holding this map in your hands. I sincerely believe that if you make PowerCharged food a large part of your diet, you will experience greater health and vitality than you ever thought possible. Your immune system will become stronger, your aging will slow, your body will be able to cleanse itself of toxins, and disease will be prevented.

Good luck and happy gardening!

—Dr. William S. Peavy

1. *Why You Need PowerCharged Food*

POWERCHARGED food is food that contains the highest level of minerals and vitamins possible. Any vegetable, legume, fruit, nut, seed, or grain that is grown using the special PowerCharged methods given in this book is PowerCharged food. Imagine for a minute going back in time 250 years, when you could eat food grown in the most fertile, virgin soil possible, with just the right balance of acidity-alkalinity, organic matter, and the optimal concentration of minerals producing the healthiest high-nutrition food imaginable. That is exactly what PowerCharged food duplicates.

This is important because our food today is not delivering the nutrients it should. Many dietary studies show that most of us are deficient in several or more key minerals and vitamins. These deficiencies occur with the minerals calcium, magnesium, iron, zinc, copper, selenium, and manganese and the vitamins C, carotenoid A, B-6, and folacin.[1] Most of us could also use more potassium and vitamin E in our diets.

These deficiencies are contributing factors to many of the diseases that plague us today, including heart disease, cancer, diabetes, atherosclerosis, osteoporosis, and dozens more. Even if you look and feel fine right now, if you have minor deficiencies your body will be slowly breaking down although you won't feel a thing until some illness or disease manifests in twenty years or more. PowerCharged food is specifically grown to provide the highest level possible of the minerals and vitamins that are most likely to be deficient in our diets so we can enjoy super health.

WHAT GOES INTO POWERCHARGED FOOD

There are twenty-three mineral nutrients that a plant needs to absorb to make PowerCharged food. When plants are grown properly, their absorption of those twenty-three mineral nutrients can be maximized, boosting the nutrition of the food. Of those twenty-three nutrients, seventeen are needed by both plants and humans for life. The big six nutrients are nitrogen, phosphorus, potassium, calcium, magnesium, and sulfur. The eleven remaining elements needed by both plants and humans are considered trace minerals. They are iron, zinc, copper, manganese, boron, molybdenum, chlorine, sodium, cobalt, vanadium, and silicon.

Bet you didn't know that plants and humans need so many elements. But we humans need six trace elements that plants don't need at all for their life processes. The six are iodine, selenium, chromium, lithium, nickel, and arsenic. Arsenic? That's right. According to the latest research, trace amounts are actually needed in our body. That comes to twenty-three mineral nutrients that we need in our food.

Those twenty-three mineral nutrients, along with carbon, hydrogen, and oxygen, are all the elements known to be essential for human life.[2] (See Figure 1.1.) Plants incorporate all those elements into their tissues and turn them into nutrients for our bodies. Plants take the minerals and incorporate them into enzymes. They take nitrogen and turn it into amino acids. All the essential amino acids that animals are not able to synthesize must be gotten from plants. A given amino acid is exactly the same in a plant as in an animal.

A deficiency of even one element in our food will eventually lead to health problems in our bodies. We would actually die of a deficiency disease if any of those elements were missing from our bodies. The problem we face is not getting enough of some of those minerals from our diets, notably calcium, magnesium, iron, zinc, copper, selenium, and manganese along with vitamins C, A, B-6, and folacin. (See "What the Minerals and Vitamins Do and Where You Get Them" inset beginning on page 4.)

WHY WE NEED MINERALS AND VITAMINS

The minerals and vitamins in food are essential to our bodies' enzymes. Enzymes are special types of substances upon which all metabolic life processes depend. Our bodies are like machines in which the moving parts are chemicals. Enzymes are the tiny sparkplugs that keep the huge engine of metabolism in motion. Without enzymes we would be dead.

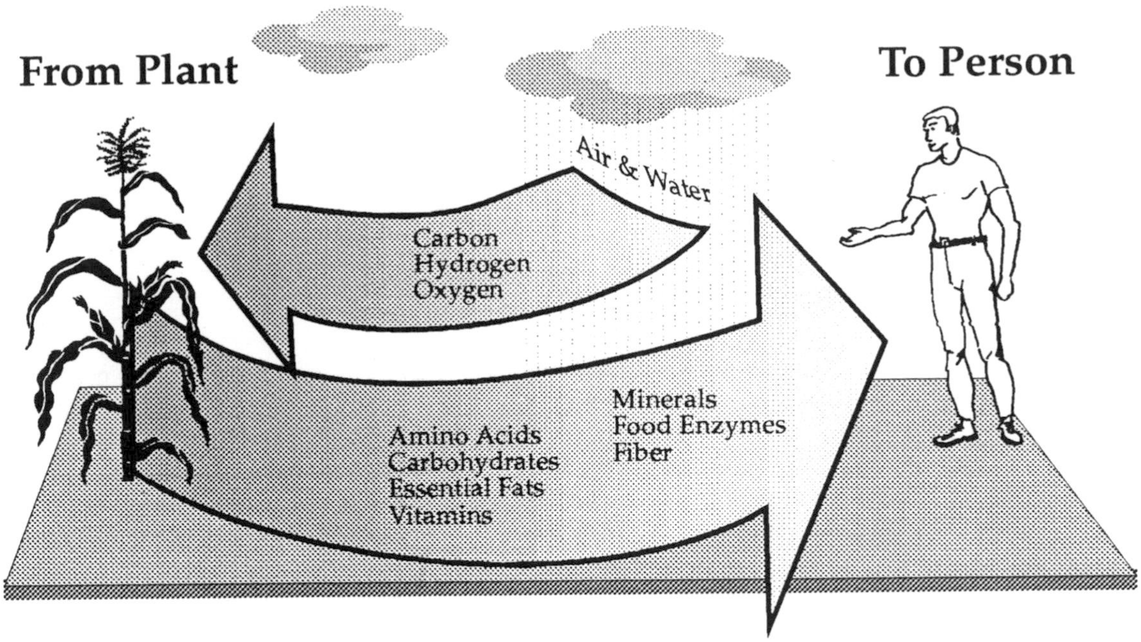

Essential Elements		Who Needs What
1. Nitrogen 2. Phosphorus 3. Potassium	4. Calcium 5. Magnesium 6. Sulfur	The Mineral Nutrients Needed by Humans and Plants in the Greatest Amount.
7. Iron 8. Zinc 9. Copper 10. Manganese 11. Boron 12. Molybdenum	13. Chlorine 14. Sodium 15. Cobalt 16. Vanadium + 17. Silicon	The Trace Mineral Nutrients Needed by Humans and Plants.
18. Iodine 19. Selenium 20. Chromium 21. Lithium+	22. Nickel 23. Arsenic Fluorine ++	The Trace Minerals Needed Only by Humans.

\+ Vanadium and Lithium considered to be probably essential as of this writing.
++ Fluorine is considered non-essential but has some beneficial pharmacological properties.

Figure 1.1 Twenty-Three Essential Elements From the Soil

There are twenty-three elements needed for human health that come from the soil. Plants convert these elements, along with carbon, hydrogen, and oxygen, into food nutrients—amino acids, carbohydrates, essential fats, vitamins, minerals, enzymes, and fiber. A deficiency or absence of even one element produces deficient food, which can result in health problems in the body.

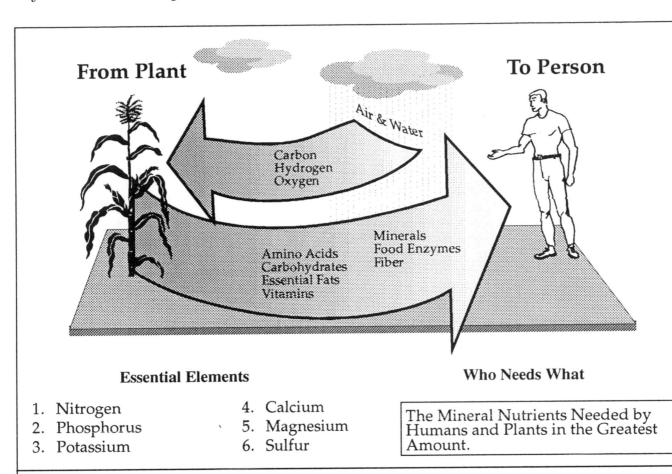

What the Minerals and Vitamins Do and Where You Get Them

Mineral or Vitamin	Function	Best Garden Sources In Descending Order
CALCIUM	Needed for strong bones and maintaining the acid-base balance of the blood. Vital to functioning of heart, muscles, and nerves. Should always have a dietary calcium-to-phosphorus ratio of 1:1 or calcium is withdrawn from bone to preserve proper blood pH. Excess dietary protein also causes a loss of calcium from bone. Deficiency causes loss of bone density, tooth decay, periodontal disease, and osteoporosis.	Bok choy cabbage, Turnip greens, Collard greens, Mustard greens, Beet greens, Parsley, Broccoli, Looseleaf lettuce (all higher than milk, calorie for calorie). Also high: Celery, Romaine lettuce, Kale, Okra, regular Cabbage, Summer squash, Green beans, Cauliflower.
MAGNESIUM	Key element in central nervous system. Essential for heart, nerves, and muscle function. Regulates heartbeat and electrical activity throughout the body. Needed for amino acid synthesis, cell division, and the release of energy in cells. Essential for synthesis of immune cells. Deficiencies related to nervous afflictions, weakened immunity, heart dysfunction, kidney stones, cancer, and epilepsy. Plant foods are the major source.	Spinach, Beet greens, Broccoli, Parsley, Summer squash, Beets, Turnip greens, Mustard greens, Bok choy cabbage, Celery, Asparagus, Cucumber, Green beans, Bean sprouts, Kohlrabi, regular Cabbage, Sunflower seeds, Black-eyed peas, Looseleaf lettuce, Tomato, Sweet pepper, Eggplant, Beans in general (Black-eyed, Black, Garbanzo, Kidney, Lima, Navy, Pinto, Soy, etc.).
IRON	Carries oxygen to every cell as part of hemoglobin in red blood cells. Enables cells to generate energy. Required for making new cells, amino acids, hormones, and immunity. Needs the co-nutrients copper, folacin, and B-6 to be made into hemoglobin. Deficiency of iron or co-nutrients causes chronic tiredness, weakness, regular headaches, anemia, fatigue, and heart enlargement due to lack of oxygen in the blood. Absorption of iron from plant foods is boosted higher than from meat by having vitamin C in the meal.	Parsley, Spinach, Butterhead lettuce, Swiss chard, Bok choy cabbage, Mustard greens, Looseleaf lettuce, Beet greens, Green peas, Jerusalem artichoke, Kale, Broccoli, Green beans, Collard greens, Asparagus, Cabbage, Tomato, Cauliflower, Beans in general. (All these foods have more iron, calorie for calorie, than lean steak.)

ZINC	Essential for DNA synthesis, cell division, growth, healing, immune function, tooth development, and male fertility. Works in seventy enzymes throughout the body. Needed for protein and fat metabolism. Detoxifies heavy metals. Zinc-to-copper ratio should be around 5:1 and never more than 10:1. Excess zinc causes copper deficiency leading to degeneration of the heart muscle. Zinc deficiency causes poor healing, poor appetite, lethargy, impaired immunity, and other disruptions in metabolism.	Collard greens, Spinach, Mushrooms, Alfalfa sprouts, Dandelion greens, Parsley, Bok choy cabbage, Romaine lettuce, Summer squash, Asparagus, Beet greens, Looseleaf lettuce, Black-eyed peas, Mustard greens, Beans in general. (Calorie for calorie, all compare favorably with meat as a source of zinc.)
COPPER	Works in enzymes needed for the elasticity of blood vessels and the aorta, for the strength of connective tissue, and for the health of the entire cardiovascular system. Protects nervous system from free radical damage. Needed for normal bone and lung development. Needed for iron to be made into hemoglobin and for lymphocyte function. Deficiencies cause aortic aneurysms, lesions, degeneration of the heart muscle, and promotes heart disease and stroke. Too much zinc in the diet causes copper deficiency.	Nuts and seeds tend to be high, followed by legumes (beans, peas, lentils), whole grains, and most vegetables and fruits grown in properly mineralized soil. Plant foods are the major source of copper. Most animal foods contain little.
SELENIUM	A major anti-oxidant. Main biological role in the enzyme glutathione peroxidase. Protects against the oxidation of cellular material by free radicals. Strengthens immunity. Protects against cancer by protecting cells from oxidation. Helps slow aging process. Protects against heavy metal intoxication. Deficiencies allow free radicals to damage cells, promoting cancer, vascular disease, heart enlargement (Keshan disease), infertility, and reduced resistance to heavy metal intoxication.	When grown in proper soil, whole grains, including corn, contain high amounts with high availability. Highest biological value in the form of seleno-amino acids. This is the primary form found in plant foods. Animal foods have comparatively low availability. Legumes, vegetables, nuts and seeds are also good sources when grown in proper soil.
MANGANESE	Needed to metabolize proteins and fats. Activator of enzymes needed for health of nerves, muscles, and normal brain function. Protects against free radical damage. Needed for the body to use glucose properly. Needed to make acetylcholine in nerve endings. Deficiency causes poor muscular strength and coordination, weakens immunity, promotes diabetes, and is linked to multiple sclerosis.	Whole grains, beans, peas, lentils, nuts, seeds, and some vegetables and fruits, particularly berries, if grown in properly mineralized soil. Plant foods are the major source of manganese.

VITAMIN C	A major anti-oxidant. Scavanges free radicals throughout the body. This protects against cells being oxidized and so protects against cancer, cardiovascular disease, and inflammatory diseases such as arthritis. Helps slow the aging process and greatly strengthens immune function. Is a major component of immune cells. Used by T-cells in fighting and destroying tumors, bacteria, and other pathogens. Cleanses the body of toxic heavy metals. Makes collagen (connective tissue that holds the cells together). Produces the "fight or flight" adrenal hormones. Deficiencies greatly weaken immunity and allow free radicals to damage cells, promoting cancer and many other diseases. Is very heat sensitive and destroyed by cooking.	Red sweet pepper, Green pepper, Parsley, Cauliflower, Bok choy cabbage, Broccoli, regular Cabbage, Strawberries, Kohlrabi, Mustard greens, Brussels sprouts, Romaine lettuce, Turnip greens, Cantaloupe, Asparagus, Spinach, Tomato, Honeydew melon, Raspberries, Celery, Bean sprouts, Butternut squash, Watermelon, Green beans. (For tropical climates, Papaya, Grapefruit, Orange, and Mango are very high in vitamin C.)
VITAMIN A	Another major anti-oxidant. Cleanses the body of free radicals, protecting against cellular damage. Strengthens the immune system. Produces mucus to protect against infection. Needed for stability of cell membranes, night vision, and many other functions. The carotenoid precursor form (such as beta-carotene) from plant foods is the only form to have substantial anti-oxidant activity and protection against cancer. Retinol form from animal foods is toxic in excess.	Carrots, Spinach, Turnip greens, Red sweet pepper, Bok choy cabbage, Sweet potato, Mustard greens, Green onions, Butternut squash, Romaine lettuce, Parsley, Looseleaf lettuce, Cantaloupe, Winter squash, Tomato, Apricots, Broccoli, Asparagus, Green pepper, Green beans, Zucchini and Summer squash, Peaches.
VITAMIN B-6	Key vitamin needed to metabolize protein. Allows amino acids to be used for DNA synthesis and cell reproduction. Needed for growth, healing, and the production of immune cells. Deficiency causes incomplete conversion of amino acids, resulting in toxic intermediates. These can accumulate and promote cancer (especially bladder), atherosclerosis, diabetes, and kidney stones. The two forms of B-6 most commonly found in food, pyridoxal and pyridoxamine, are heat sensitive and destroyed by cooking. Most plant foods provide more B-6 than does meat, which must be cooked at high temperatures to kill bacteria.	Bok choy cabbage, Spinach, Turnip greens, Cauliflower, Broccoli, Sweet pepper, Asparagus, Parsley, Zucchini squash, regular Cabbage, Tomato, Summer squash, Romaine lettuce, Potato, Beans in general, Eggplant, Collard greens, Looseleaf lettuce, Kohlrabi, Corn, Sunflower seeds. (All provide more B-6 than meat provides, even after normal cooking.)

FOLACIN	Needed for cell repair, cell reproduction, growth, and healing. Needed to metabolize protein. Needed to create red blood cells and immune cells and to repair DNA. High intake may slow aging by promoting rapid cell regeneration. Deficiencies slow healing and cell regeneration, weaken the immune system, cause anemia, and allow DNA damage to go unrepaired, which can contribute to cancer. Plant foods are the major source of folacin, which is destroyed by heat.	Spinach, Romaine lettuce, Turnip greens, Parsley, Asparagus, Collard greens, Cabbage, Dandelion greens, Broccoli, Cauliflower, Bean sprouts, Beets, Bok choy cabbage, Alfalfa sprouts, Zucchini and Summer squash, Cucumber, Green beans, Honeydew melon, Cantaloupe, Black-eyed peas, Winter squash, Sweet pepper, Celery, Eggplant, Beans in general.
VITAMIN E	Major anti-oxidant. Becomes part of the membrane structure of cells, protecting them from oxidation by free radicals. Especially important in protecting cells in lungs from oxidation by environmental pollutants such as ozone. Protects immune cells, strengthening immunity. An important protective agent from diseases like cancer. Is lost in food by heat and oxidation.	Found in all foods containing polyunsaturated fats: vegetable oils (as long as not rancid), nuts, seeds, legumes, grains, and some leafy green vegetables.
POTASSIUM	Maintains proper fluid balance in the cells. Allows cells to take in nutrients and oxygen and eliminate waste. Essential for maintenance of blood pressure. Increasing potassium in diet promotes sodium excretion, lowering blood pressure. High-potassium diet more important than cutting out sodium in control of hypertension. Needed for proper functioning of muscles, including the heart muscle. Plant foods are the major source of potassium.	Bok choy cabbage, Spinach, Celery, Romaine lettuce, Parsley, Zucchini squash, Radishes, Looseleaf lettuce, Cauliflower, Asparagus, Kohlrabi, regular Cabbage, Winter and Summer squash, Tomato, Cucumber, Beets, Eggplant, Cantaloupe, Green beans, Sweet pepper, Carrots, Butternut squash, Apricots, Jerusalem artichoke, Broccoli, Peaches, Lima beans, Bananas, Potato, Oranges, Watermelon, other Beans, Sweet Corn, Peas, Pears, Apples. (All have more potassium than meat.)

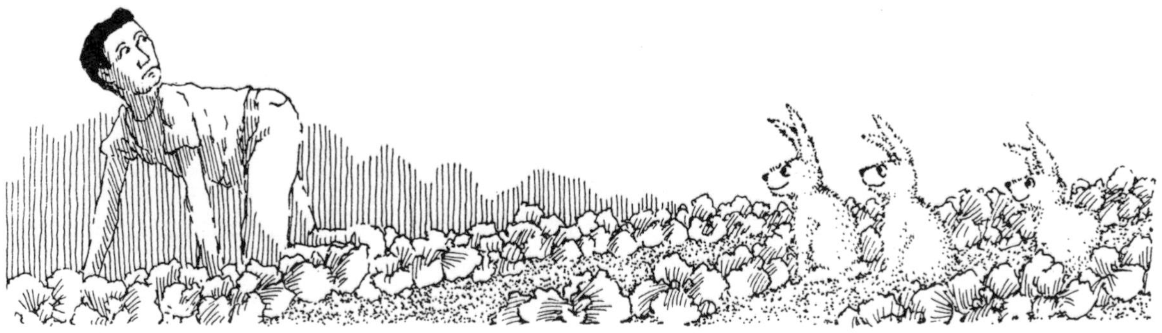

Enzymes control every vital function of the body, from the digestion of food to the production of cells to the smallest movement. Without enzymes, there would be no life. The body's enzymes, in turn, depend on small but essential amounts of trace minerals and vitamins. The non-trace minerals, such as calcium and magnesium, are also needed in enzymes.

Over a thousand enzymes have been identified; and based on estimates of metabolic functions that require enzymes, there are 30,000 or more. Enzymes work in every part of the body, from the cardiovascular system to the nervous system to the immune system to the glandular and organ system. They allow us to metabolize proteins, carbohydrates, and fats, and they release energy in the cells which allows us to move, think, and stay alive. They keep our arteries elastic so blood can flow through them; they make the organs, glands, bones, lungs, muscles, and nervous system function; they facilitate the reproduction of new cells; they give us immunity; and they constantly detoxify the body of free radicals, carcinogens, heavy metals, and anything else that could greatly damage us.

Every minute of every day the body carries on an estimated 2 million biochemical reactions, all requiring enzymes, which in turn depend on minerals and vitamins as co-enzymes. Do you see why a minor deficiency of nutrients over many years gives rise to illness? The body is slowly being deprived of the substances it needs to carry on its life processes. When enzyme activity becomes too low, those life processes break down, and illness or disease strikes.

Deficiencies in our food drastically affect the status of our health. Among the diseases influenced by deficiencies are cancer, cardiovascular disease, diabetes, degenerative arthritis, multiple sclerosis, infectious diseases, periodontal disease, and others. The book *Diet-Related Diseases: The Modern Epidemic* tells us, "Probably every disease known to mankind has some connection with diet, at least in the sense that nutritional deficiencies weaken the natural defense mechanism of the body."[3]

Nutrition and Killer Diseases tells us that "inadequate nutrition is an important contributory factor to the alarming rise in prevalence of the killer diseases, mainly, cardiovascular disease, cancer, and diabetes" and that "undiagnosed subclinical malnutrition of trace elements . . . may exist and subtly cause much physiological damage to body and brain."[4] Expanding on the relationship of deficiencies to cancer, *Nutrition and Cancer* tells us that "nutrient deficiencies may lead to biochemical abnormalities which, in turn, promote neoplastic (cancerous) processes."[5]

Deficiencies of vitamins and minerals over time deplete our body's valuable enzymes; such depletion damages the cardiovascular system and the nervous system, weakens immunity, promotes cancer and free radical damage, and accelerates aging. In the long run, even if you look and feel fine right now, these deficiencies set you up for disease years from now. This is why high-nutrition food is so important. PowerCharged food is grown specifically to provide the highest possible level of all the minerals and vitamins that are deficient in our diet. On the other hand, commercial agriculture works a little differently. . . .

Why Food Is Better Than Supplements

"Get 100% of your RDA of vitamins and minerals in one bowl of our cereal," the advertisement says. Just imagine, complete nutrition in a single bowl; you don't need any more vitamins and minerals for the rest of the day! Don't you believe this. The vitamins and minerals might be there, but it doesn't mean they're doing you much good or even any good.

Supplement makers and food fortifiers would like you to believe that our bodies can't tell the difference between synthetic vitamins and vitamins in food. The reasoning goes like this: "Synthetic vitamins are manufactured to produce the same chemicals that a vitamin is made of, so our bodies can't tell the difference." Hurray for tech-nology! We've outfoxed Mother Nature. Don't worry about what you eat, they say, just take your synthetic vitamins. If only it were that easy.

Synthetic vitamins are not the same as vitamins from food, and our bodies can tell the difference. Why is this? Let's look at vitamin C. Is vitamin C just a chemical known as ascorbic acid or more? When Svent Gyorgyi first isolated ascorbic acid as a cure for scurvy, a curious thing happened; isolated ascorbic acid would not completely cure scurvy, only delay its onset and lessen its effects; but when vitamin C concentrate from peppers was used, it would cure the scurvy completely. What was the difference? The difference was that ascorbic acid in food is always found with a class of compounds known as flavonoids, which modern researchers have confirmed are necessary to completely prevent or cure scurvy.[1]

Flavonoids are a type of phytochemical that has important recognized biological functions other than fighting scurvy. Flavonoids are natural anti-oxidants that protect us from free radical damage; they are natural protective agents against cancer; they have anti-inflammatory and anti-allergenic properties that help prevent chronic conditions like arthritis; and they boost immunity.[2] These natural substances, of which 4,000 have so far been identified, constitute the active ingredients of many folk medicines that have been used for thousands of years.

There are also needed trace element-containing enzymes (mettalo-enzymes) found with vitamin C in food. One of these is ascorbate oxidase, a copper-containing enzyme that catalyzes the oxidation of ascorbic acid at a physiological pH that makes ascorbic acid effective in the body as an anti-oxidant; another is tyrosinase, which supplies organic copper needed in the body for lymphocyte function and other pur-poses.[3] There are other co-nutrients found with vitamin C and some we probably don't even know about yet.

All those co-nutrients are needed to make vitamin C an effective protective agent against disease. Ascorbic acid alone has limited value in the body. Ascorbic acid is actually just one component of a number of nutrients that are found together in the same food and collectively known as vitamin C. They all work synergistically.

What applies to vitamin C applies to all the vitamins. Vitamins in nature are never found in pure crystalline states. They are always found in combination with proteins, mettaloenzymes, and other substances in a "complex" of nutrients.

Nature put all those nutrients together in food for a very important reason—they are all needed to work together to protect us from disease. There is a biological difference between natural and synthetic sources of vitamins.

In the case of vitamin E (tocopherol), the dextro form occurs in nature in foods such as nuts, seeds, grains, legumes, and leafy vegetables and is the form that is highly usable and biologically active in the body. Synthetic vitamin E is found as a levo form of tocopherol (listed as dl-tocopherol) and is only partially usable in the body, meaning that the unusable portion has to be eliminated.

An interesting phenomenon sometimes seen in clinical work is that treatments with high doses of synthetic vitamins, such as synthetic ascorbic acid and B-1 (thiamin), will cause adverse reactions while naturally derived vitamins at the same dose cause no such reactions. The body's biological response to synthetic vitamins can be very different from its response to the natural vitamin containing all the synergists. That is because vitamins in chemically isolated form often don't function as vitamins but more as drugs. It is the abnormally high levels of isolated chemicals in synthetic vitamins that can induce toxicity similar to the way a drug can.

ROCKS OR NAILS, ANYONE?

One of the biggest myths about food today is that we can make food healthy by enriching and fortifying it with synthetic vitamins and inorganic minerals, usually after most of the natural nutrients have been removed. In grains, mineral and vitamin losses average 75 percent or more after the germ and the bran have been removed, including losses of vitamin B-6, vitamin E, magnesium, zinc, copper, manganese, and chromium.[4] The germ and bran are the most nutrient-dense parts, and they're thrown away. Of the thirty known nutrients removed, usually only around four are added back with synthetic vitamins and inorganic minerals.

What good does all this enriching and fortifying do? Very little. Cereals and white flour are commonly enriched with iron, yet iron deficiency has been a constant problem in the American diet for fifty years! Why? The iron that the flour is enriched with is not in the same form as the iron you get from food as provided by nature. Manufacturers usually add finely powdered metallic iron, which is virtually worthless to the body.[5] That tactic enables manufacturers to say their product provides a high percentage of the recommended daily allowance for iron and other nutrients—while incurring hardly any extra cost and offering almost no value to the consumer.

The way we're supposed to get our minerals is the way they're provided to us in natural food. Living things provide minerals in organic form, biologically combined with special proteins (enzymes or amino acids) that allow our body to utilize them properly. If we could utilize minerals in any form, we could eat rocks and nails to get our minerals. But obviously we cannot. Can you imagine sprinkling rock powder over your corn flakes? Yet, that is what you're doing when you eat inorganic compounds of minerals or, even worse, elemental minerals.

Beyond proper utilization, many trace minerals are toxic, even poisonous, if we try to eat them in inorganic form. Zinc can be toxic as an inorganic chemical, such as from zinc-coated utensils or galvanized pipes. Elemental copper is considered a heavy metal; if you absorb too much, let's say from copper utensils, you can be poisoned.[6] Inorganic fluorides can be terrible poisons, but in food they're essential. Iodine can be poisonous in its elemental form but is essential in food.

It's amazing how nature converts something that's toxic to us in inorganic form into something that's a nutrient in food. You cannot get harmed from overeating trace minerals in food, only from the inorganic compounds of the mineral. You will actually never get too much of a mineral through food. Nature spreads the elements out for us and gives them to us in forms our bodies can safely use.

In the case of selenium, the organic form is selenoamino acids such as selenomethionine. In this form, it is well assimilated into the tissues for its use as an anti-oxidant and is easily tolerated at levels where inorganic forms would show toxicity.[7] Inorganic selenium compounds such as sodium selenite, while much better than elemental selenium, become toxic in much smaller amounts than with selenoamino acids and are assimilated poorly into the tissues. And what the body can't use, it has to eliminate.

The same is true of other inorganic compounds of minerals. The inorganic forms of minerals used in most supplements are "salts" of the minerals. They include calcium carbonate as a calcium source and ferrous sulfate as an iron source. They are much easier to make than organic forms and cost less. But none of those inorganic forms have the biological activity of the organic forms found in food. There are big differences between organic minerals found in living plants and the inorganic minerals found in rocks.

If you ever want to take mineral supplements, find an amino acid chelate of the mineral. But just remember that any kind of pill is only a temporary solution to whatever deficiency you might have. Why is this? Let's look at the popular multi-supplement many people rely on in place of a good diet.

First of all, any deficiency you have arose from poor food, and other deficiencies are certainly getting ready to spring up on you down the road. Multi-supplements always omit nutrients that are known to be necessary and omit nutrients that aren't yet known to be necessary but actually are, such as additional synergists still to be discovered. Secondly, look at the form in which the nutrients occur. Most use inorganic "salts" of the mineral and synthetic vitamins that have limited value in the body and end up having to be eliminated. Thirdly, many supplements don't dissolve in a period of time that would enable you to absorb whatever vitamins or minerals you're trying to get and instead will pass right through your system. And with any pill, you never really know how much you need. Because pills are concentrated, it's easy to get far too much of certain nutrients that can act like drugs.

Finally, how do you know you're getting what it says on the label? The vitamins in supplements are subject to the same losses as they are in food. If vitamins have been sitting around at room temperature for a while since manufacture, they can decompose into unusable forms. For example, when vitamin C oxidizes, it turns into dehydro C, which is useless to the body. This is even a problem with minerals in multi-supplements. Ralph Shangraw, chairman of the Department of Pharmeceutics at the University of Maryland, explains that with supplements "we haven't begun to look at whether what's on the label is in the product. The components react with each other and decompose over time."[8] The Food and Drug Administration (FDA) doesn't require any kind of stability tests, so even for supplements with expiration dates you really don't know what you're getting.

The end result of all this is that your body may have a big job eliminating the vitamins and minerals it doesn't need, because it's getting excess amounts or a form it can't utilize, and this elimination involves the use of enzymes. While it's true that vitamins and minerals are co-enzymes, they are not the enzyme itself, and the enzymes will be helped very little by the excess or unusable forms of the vitamins and minerals. The excess or unusable vitamins and minerals act in the body like drugs and have to be expelled continuously. This constant use of the body's enzymes for the elimination of unneeded or unusable nutrients taxes the body's enzyme-making machinery. And whatever depletes your body of enzymes is not good. This can actually end up hurting your health in the long run more than helping it.

All we're saying is, popping handfuls of supplements every day is not the route to good long-term health. Get your vitamins and minerals from food as much as possible. If you take a supplement, make sure it duplicates the natural food source as closely as possible. And know that it is no substitute for good food.

2. *Why Our Food Is Deficient*

YOU'VE probably heard that we are the best-fed nation in the world. That is a myth. Most of us are not getting the minerals and vitamins we really need. Why is this? Today a significant amount of our food is grown in nutrient-poor soil depleted of essential mineral elements by years of highly intensive commercial farming practices. Many of our soils are starved of important trace minerals.

Zinc depletion in soil is widespread throughout the United States and becomes more severe every year.[1] The nutritional reference *Modern Nutrition in Health and Disease* acknowledges this worsening problem. It tells us that "since the zinc content of plants is largely determined by the zinc content of the soil, this type of endemic deficiency may become common as the mineral content of the world's topsoil becomes depleted."[2]

Selenium is an essential trace element that plants don't need to grow properly but humans must have. Large areas of the United States have soil with low selenium levels.[3] In 1967, a study reported that a little less than half the soil in the United States produced crops with less than adequate selenium.[4] Selenium is easily leached out of soil, so today, a quarter century later, much more of our soils are certainly deficient.

Iron is also widely depleted or unavailable in soils throughout the United States.[5] And calcium and magnesium are depleted in many soils, particularly in eastern and southern soils. This pattern is also true for many other trace elements that are most essential to us.

WHY COMMERCIALLY GROWN FOOD IS DEFICIENT

There are many causes for the deficiencies in commercially grown food.

Soil Erosion

Topsoil is the storehouse of nutrients upon which all life depends. For many decades, nutrients have been depleted from our soils as the topsoil has been eroded away. From an average of around twenty inches of topsoil two centuries ago, most farmland has only around six inches left. Nutrients are still lost by erosion over a significant amount of our farmland every year. Despite years of government efforts to combat it, around 40 percent of our harvested cropland is still considered highly erodible and losing topsoil.[6] Most of the remaining cropland is also losing topsoil, but at a more moderate rate. Three to four billion tons of topsoil are lost in the United States each year in runoff waters or blown away by wind.[7] The National Research Council reports that $18 billion worth of nutrients are lost from our soils annually because of widespread erosion.[8] Since many farming areas have little topsoil left, this is very serious.

Nutrient Uptake

Nutrient loss doesn't stop with erosion. In addition to the erosion of nutrients, soils are being depleted as almost a billion pounds of nutrients like calcium and magnesium, and trace elements like iron, zinc, copper, manganese, and boron, are lost to nutrient removal (uptake) by crops.[9] Those nutrients will not be replaced by the 38 billion pounds of synthetic chemical fertilizers used each year.[10]

Plants remove the elements from the soil as they grow and assimilate them into their tissues. A one-acre planting that produces 35 tons of tomatoes will remove around 800 pounds of mineral nutrients from the soil.[11] The rest of the weight of the tomatoes comes from the absorption of carbon in the air and hydrogen and oxygen from water. You can easily see how decades of nutrient removal can leave a soil depleted.

Modern agriculture has become like a topsoil mining operation milking the soil of nutrients. Every year our soils become more depleted of essential nutrients because of nutrient uptake by crops and erosion. And these nutrients are not replaced by the purified forms of synthetic, chemical fertilizers that are used today. All that's usually applied to soils are highly purified forms of nitrogen, phosphorus, and potassium, through chemical fertilizers. Commercial agriculture pays virtually no attention to the presence of any of the trace elements in the soil. They are rarely applied even to depleted soils.

You might be wondering, if our soils are so depleted, then why don't farmers do something about it? It's because farmers are concerned with getting big yields, and yields have little to do with the nutritional quality of food.

Hybrid Varieties

In fact, yield is often an inverse indication of food quality. First of all, genetically altered hybrid varieties, such as hybrid corn, are made to produce big yields by producing more carbohydrates while lowering the percentage of minerals in the food.

The World Health Organization tells us that "developments in agricultural technology designed primarily to increase the yield of food crops and animal products can affect the trace element content of these foods [that] . . . can change trace element intakes by man in ways which may be hazardous to human health."[12] One example is a strain of rye developed in New Zealand to get high yields. It was found to contain only one-tenth the iodine concentration of its parents, whether grown in iodine-high or iodine-low soil.[13] It was feared the iodine content of milk produced by cows eating this grass would be so low that it would cause goiter in the children drinking it. With all hybrid varieties, yields are maximized while nutritional quality is almost always lower than with natural varieties.

Chemical-Salt Fertilizers

But even more significant than hybrid varieties is the fact that plants grown in deficient soil and fed nothing but high-nitrogen chemical fertilizers will often produce big yields without absorbing a balanced mixture of nutrients. Concentrated nitrogen, phosphorus, and potassium fertilizers—collectively known as NPK fertilizers—are applied at very high rates, causing the plants to absorb it quickly, which causes big spurts of growth and high yields. But it is not balanced, healthy growth.

Plants grown with nothing but nitrogen, phosphorus, and potassium from concentrated chemical fertilizers overconsume these nutrients at the expense of all other nutrients in the soil. Absorption of these three nutrients actually displaces or crowds out the proper absorption of other nutrients in the soil, even if the other nutrients are abundant. In soil science, this is called *luxury consumption.*

Nitrogen, for instance, is usually overapplied at rates up to seven times more than the plants can use.[14] This sudden "force-feeding" of nitrogen doesn't give the plant time to convert it all into amino acids, and much of it accumulates in the plant as nitrate nitrogen instead of protein nitrogen. That is sometimes called being "blown up" with nitrogen. Nitrate appears in crops today primarily because heavy amounts of nitrogen are supplied in concentrated chemical form, which makes excessive nitrate available for uptake.[15] Nitrate content is reduced, if not eliminated, when nitrogen is supplied in amounts a plant can utilize as organic protein compounds.[16]

This "blowing up" of crops with non-protein forms of nitrogen displaces the absorption of other elements with nitrate, which is not good to be ingesting to begin with. The displacement of trace elements reduces the amount of protein that is made from the nitrogen, because plants need iron, copper, and molybdenum to transform nitrogen into amino acids.

Excess phosphorus suppresses the uptake of zinc, copper, and iron, even if those elements are in the soil in adequate amounts, while heavy nitrogen fertilization particularly blocks the proper uptake of copper in plants.[17] NPK fertilizers can even promote deficiencies of non-trace elements. Excessive amounts of potassium fertilizer suppresses the uptake of calcium and magnesium, reducing their amounts in food where they are greatly needed.[18] A sudden infusion of chemical fertilizer also increases the carbohydrates that are formed, which accounts for the higher yields at the expense of minerals and other nutrients.

Excess chemical fertilizers create deficiencies even when the soil is not depleted. They can supress the uptake of iron, zinc, copper, calcium, and magnesium. Chemical fertilizers are absorbed in abundance at the expense of other elements. They have artificially boosted yields in the face of what would otherwise be declining productivity due to massive nutrient losses from the topsoil. Modern technology has allowed us to keep getting big yields despite depleted soils. But we have paid a price with depleted food.

Some people think soil depletion is no problem, believing that if a plant will grow then it has enough nutrients. Those people don't know what they're talking about. Plants frequently grow well without accumulating mineral nutrients in their tissues in sufficient amounts to meet the long-term health needs of humans or animals.[19] Trace elements do not increase a plant's yield by increasing its output of carbohydrates; therefore, they are ignored even though they would improve the overall health of the plant, which would reduce the need for chemical sprays.[20] Crops can even grow just fine when they're completely lacking in some of the elements needed for human nutrition.

MINERAL VARIATION IN FOOD

One of the best studies of how minerals in the soil affect the mineral nutrition of food was done by Dr. Firman Bear of Rutgers University

Table 2.1

Nutritional Variations in Tomatoes

(In Milligrams per 3.5 Ounces of Fresh Weight)

Mineral	Lowest Nutrient Value	Highest Nutrient Value
Calcium	14 mg	71 mg
Magnesium	8 mg	109 mg
Iron	.015 mg	29.8 mg
Manganese	.02 mg	1 mg
Copper	0 mg	.8 mg
Boron	0 mg	.6 mg
Cobalt	0 mg	.01 mg

Based on the research of Dr. Firman Bear.

in 1948.[21] The study compared the mineral content of produce from across the country. (At the time, many western and plains states had naturally high mineralized soils.) The results were astounding. It was found that soils with a high availability of minerals in the western and plains states produced vegetables with a nutritional quality superior to vegetables coming from the mineral-leached soils in the southern and eastern United States.

The nutritional differences were tremendous. For tomatoes, Dr. Bear found the differences listed in Table 2.1.

Samples grown in highly mineralized soil had 5 times more calcium, 13 times more magnesium, and over 1,900 times more iron than samples grown in depleted soils! What's also astounding is how some samples were completely lacking or contained extremely deficient amounts of essential trace minerals such as iron, manganese, copper, and boron. Similar patterns appeared in all the vegetables.

What's really interesting about this is when you compare the highest values in the Bear study with the values reported in standard nutrition tables. The standard nutritional reference is *Handbook of the Nutritional Contents of Foods (USDA Handbook 8)*, and it is a good measure of the average nutrition in food. The 1975 version was compiled and averaged from dozens of analyses done from the turn of the century to the late 1960s, so it's a good basis for comparison. Figure 2.1 compares the mineral content of tomatoes grown in highly mineralized soil (as shown by the Bear study) with the values for tomatoes reported in the 1975 version of *Handbook 8*.

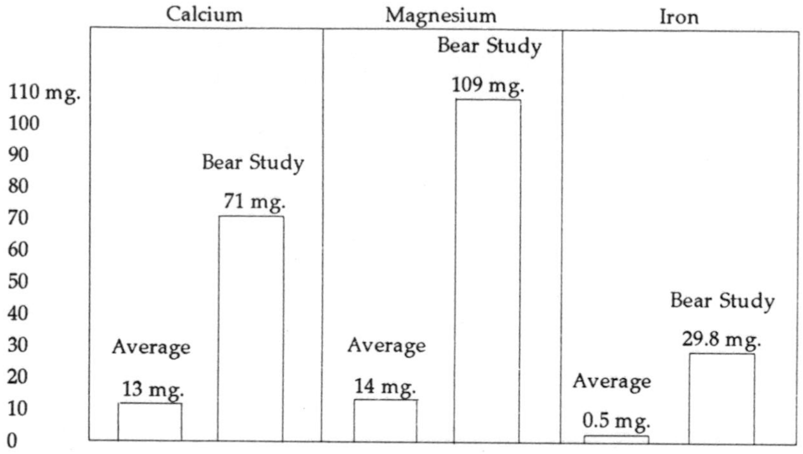

Figure 2.1. A comparison of three important nutrients shows a sharp difference between the average values reported in *Handbook 8* and the maximum values reported by Dr. Firman Bear. All data comes from an analysis of tomatoes, but Dr. Bear's samples were grown in highly mineralized soil.

The average values for minerals given in *Handbook 8* are close to or even below the lowest values found in the Bear study. This reflects the mineral-depleted condition of the majority of the soils from which the samples used in *Handbook 8* were taken. As you can see, the difference in mineral nutrition between food grown in highly mineralized vs. mineral deficient soil is enormous.

THE PROBLEM OF VITAMIN LOSS

We need a high level of vitamins in our diet, but you can't depend on the food sold in supermarkets to get it. Let's look at the reasons. Produce is harvested before it's ripe so that it will look fresh (but not actually be fresh) at the time it's sold. Most vitamins increase in concentration with the increasing ripeness of food, reaching their maximum concentration when a fruit or vegetable is fully ripe—yet, produce must be picked long before it's ripe.

The concentration of vitamins essential to cancer prevention and immune function, such as vitamin C and carotenoid A, are almost always diminished by premature picking. As an example, carrots are harvested with only one-half to one-third the vitamin A content they would have if they were left to ripen fully.[22] Green peppers would have almost twice the vitamin C content if they were left to ripen fully to red and over ten times more vitamin A (from 42 REs, or retinal equivalents, to 445 REs).[23] Vitamin E and folic acid are also lost by premature picking.[24]

Produce in the store is starting out on only half a tank of nutritional potency. But that is just the beginning. As soon as they're harvested, fruits and vegetables start losing their vitamins because of enzymatic decomposition and oxidation. Tomatoes, for example, harvested green and artificially ripened off the vine, contain around one-third less vitamin C than vine-ripened tomatoes and continue to lose vitamin C once they're red. (See Figure 2.2.)[25] A similar situation exists with other foods.

Exposure to heat and light plays a big role in the decomposition of vitamins. The longer it takes to get food from the field into your grocery bag, the more the vitamin content decreases. By the time produce is picked, taken to a packing shed, loaded onto trucks, shipped hundreds (or thousands) of miles (often under poor conditions), and finally put on the supermarket shelves, usually a week or two has passed and much of the vitamins have been lost. Just transit and holding times for produce before commercial processing can take as long as twenty hours, usually under adverse temperature conditions.[26] Then once it reaches the marketplace, it's taken to a warehouse or a supermarket where it's put out on shelves and sits until you buy it. Sometimes produce will be stored for months. During all that handling and waiting, the vitamins are being lost.

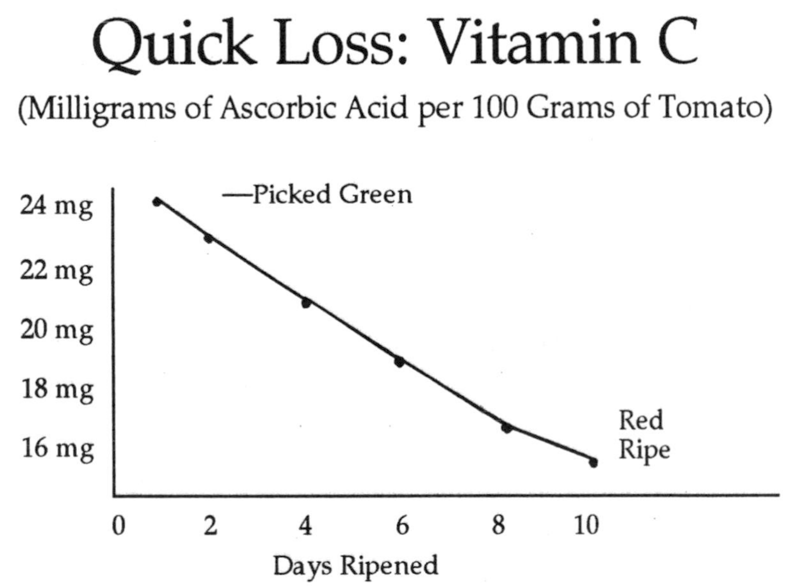

Figure 2.2. The ascorbic acid content of tomatoes starts declining as soon as they're harvested. Harvested mature-green and artificially ripened, they contain around one-third less ascorbic acid than vine-ripened tomatoes and continue to lose ascorbic acid. Ascorbic acid is a component of vitamin C and a good indicator of vitamin C content.

The Importance of Temperature

The rate of vitamin loss depends greatly on the temperature at which the food is stored. After only four days at room temperature (70°F), up to 75 percent of the vitamin A in leafy green vegetables can be gone.[27] At room temperature, vegetables lose up to 50 percent of their vitamin C only twenty-four hours after picking and up to 89 percent of their vitamin C after only two days.[28] Vegetables also lose a considerable portion of their folacin after several days at room temperature; but in refrigerator temperatures they lose little or none in two weeks.

Temperature is very important in controlling vitamin loss. Most vegetables stored for twenty-four hours at 46° to 50°F lose 10 to 30 percent of their vitamin C; but if they are immediately stored at 43°F, as in a refrigerator, in six days they lose only 10 percent of their vitamin C.[29] With most vegetables and fruits, freezing preserves the greatest amount of vitamins. The only exceptions are some of the more tropical-type vegetables and fruits, such as sweet potatoes, cucumbers, summer squash, tomatoes, bananas, citrus, and others, which hold their vitamin C best at around 59°F. With those, considerable losses occur during processing time (right after harvest), when the temperature is typically high and the food is out on display at room temperature.

You can control vitamin loss once you get vegetables and fruits into your refrigerator or a cool room, but you can't control what's happened before that time. Even if you immediately refrigerate produce from the supermarket, much of the vitamins will have already been lost during harvest, handling, holding periods, transit, and display, and there is nothing you can do about it.

Nutrition Studies

In one study, done in 1972 by the Department of Food Science and Human Nutrition of Michigan State University, it was found that tomatoes bought from local food stores contained a vitamin C content averaging 36 percent below the values reported in the USDA nutrition tables.[30] The values given by the USDA are averages of analyses done mostly at experiment stations and labs, and they often do not reflect what you actually buy at the store.

In another study, conducted by nutritional researcher Dr. Michael Colgan, it was found that the vitamin and mineral content of produce bought in stores was much lower than the levels given in nutrition tables.[31] In the most extreme example of vitamin loss ever reported, he found that one sample of oranges bought from a supermarket looked, smelled, and tasted normal but had a vitamin C content of zero. That zero was probably due to the oranges' having been stored a long time under poor conditions. In contrast, a sample of freshly picked oranges showed 116 milligrams of vitamin C per 100 grams of fruit. As a comparison, *Handbook 8* shows an average value of 50 mg/100 g. That's only 43 percent of the fresh value. Unfortunately, you might not get even *Handbook 8* values when you shop at the supermarket.

Even if some of what you buy contains nutrients at around the values given in the standard tables, that's still far below what it should be. But by growing your own vegetables and fruits, harvesting them fully ripe, and eating them fresh or putting them immediately into cold storage after harvest, you'll probably end up with a vitamin content 500 percent to 1,000 percent higher than what you get in the supermarket.

Of course, whatever you can eat fresh will have the highest vitamin content possible and taste the best. Certain vitamins, such as vitamin C, are lost even in cold storage. Potatoes, for instance, lose about half their vitamin C after only three months of cold storage and lose around two-thirds their original vitamin C after six months.[32]

Vitamin C is one of the most elusive vitamins to get because it oxidizes in heat and light so quickly, yet it is one of the most important nutrients needed to prevent disease. Many immune cells depend critically on vitamin C for their function. The activity of white blood cells, especially T-cells (T-lymphocytes) that protect the body from disease, depend on very high levels of vitamin C.[33] Vitamin C is used by and depleted from the white blood cells as they attack and kill everything from bacteria and viruses to cancer cells, so it constantly needs to be replenished. This is one reason why you need a diet that's as high as possible in fresh vegetables and fruits that will provide a high level of vitamin C and other important vitamins.

IN CONCLUSION

Bad fertilizing and man-made soil erosion have depleted large amounts of calcium and magnesium from the soil along with many trace elements such as iron, zinc, copper, selenium, and others. In addition, food loses a significant amount of vitamins in harvesting, processing, transport, and display. All of this results in deficiencies in our food.

For years, dieticians have assumed that the food we eat has the level of nutrition given in standard nutrition tables. But the fact is that none of the 300 million acres of harvested land is left with the level of nutrients it had 75 years or even 20 years ago; yet, most nutrition tables are based on foods analyzed 20 to 75, even 100 years ago. Most of these analyses do not reflect the nutritional value of food sold today. Much of what you buy at the supermarket could be below even the low values listed in the nutrition tables.

Today it's virtually impossible for you to get vitamins and minerals from food in the stores at levels needed to have optimal immune

Deficiencies in Animal Foods

Soil deficiencies affect foods of animal origin just as much as foods of plant origin. A big misconception some people have is that animal tissues and their products somehow will not be affected by nutrient-depleted plants. Not true. Minerals are depleted from the tissues in the process of an animal's metabolism and excreted. Whatever deficiencies are in plants will be passed right on to animals, just like deficiencies in plants are passed right on to humans.[1] In many cases, the essential minerals found in both plant and animal foods are found in a much higher concentration in the plant.

Differences in the level of minerals in animal foods can be just as large as the differences in plant foods. Let's look at these variations by using selenium as an example. It's often stated that meat and other animal foods are a good source of selenium but plant foods are only a good source if grown in selenium-rich soil. Nonsense! Animal foods are no better a source than the plants on which the animals feed, which in turn depend on the selenium content of the soil.

Selenium concentrations in United States wheat usually have been found to vary within the range of 0.05 microgram per gram (mcg/g) to 0.80 mcg/g, depending on the selenium content of the soil.[2] But in soils with very high levels of available selenium, wheat has been found with a selenium content in excess of 4 mcg/g.[3] Corn has been found with a selenium level as high as 2.03 mcg/g.[4]

The selenium content has been found to vary from 0.005 to 0.07 mcg/g in milk and from 0.056 to 0.50 mcg/g in eggs, depending upon whether the animals are in selenium-deficient or selenium-high areas of the country.[5] Meat shows similar variation, from 0.03 to 0.50 mcg/g, a fifteen-fold difference, with an average of 0.16 mcg/g; organ meats such as liver vary from 0.10 to 0.70 mcg/g; fish averages 0.34 mcg/g.[6]

The human body finds selenium in plant foods much more available and useful than selenium in animal foods, however. It has a much higher biological value in plant foods than in animal foods. Sixty percent of the selenium in plant foods is available for use in human tissues, but only fifteen percent of the selenium in meat is available for such use, so plant foods are a superior source.[7]

Huge variations and deficiencies occur with all the essential minerals in all foods. As with crops that still grow in deficient soil, animals with mineral deficiencies are usually still walking around and not dropping dead of a deficiency disease. Animals can survive quite a while with inadequate minerals in their tissues. It takes a long time for an animal to develop a clinical deficiency. The older an animal gets, the more likely a deficiency will worsen and manifest into a clinical deficiency.

Most deficiencies in animals never get detected, because the problem stays in a subclinical stage. Even if it becomes progressively worse, it's usually never noticed. Most animals eaten by humans are finished off in confinement facilities and slaughtered as soon as possible. The conditions in those facilities are so unhealthy to begin with that animals are routinely drugged with antibiotics and drugs to keep them from dying of disease, and as long as the animal is alive it's considered healthy.

Even if a deficiency in an animal never becomes clinical, it can still be serious, just as it is with humans. There are four stages of a deficiency as the minerals become progressively depleted from the tissues. The first three stages will progress without notice while considerable tissue depletion occurs. It isn't until the fourth stage, clinical deficiency, that a detectable deficiency disease can be observed and treated. The book *Trace Elements in Human and Animal Nutrition* tells us that "mild trace element deficiencies . . . are seldom accompanied by specific clinical signs."[8]

Many of the animals that end up becoming meat today or provide dairy products and eggs are likely to have some tissue depletion of iron, zinc, and other trace minerals because of subclinical deficiencies. Meat from deficient animals is no better a source of iron or zinc than plant foods grown on deficient soil.

functioning and enzyme activity to provide the best protection against disease. J.I. Rodale, founder of *Organic Gardening Magazine*, stated fifteen years ago that "we are a malnourished country in spite of eating more calories per person than any other country in the world" and that "it's just no longer possible to depend upon the food you buy in the stores to get all the proper nutrients."[34] He was right. Today the problem is worse because soil depletion has continued.

The problem of declining nutritional food quality is now being acknowledged by the medical community, which is recognizing that many of us are chronically deficient in certain vitamins and minerals. Medical researchers Steven Davies, M.D., and Alan Stewart, M.D., tell us that "the quality of food is often so poor that the actual nutrient intake in terms of vitamins [and] minerals . . . is inadequate and can produce disease" and that while we get plenty of calories "what we suffer from is malnutrition."[35] Supporting this, medical researcher Dr. David G. Williams reports that "as many as 58 percent of the patients hospitalized in the U.S. are thought to be malnourished" (*American Medical News* 85; 5:31) and furthermore, "many of the so-called degenerative diseases associated with aging are now being linked to nutritional deficiencies."[36]

Long-term marginal deficiencies slowly and silently disrupt the normal functioning of our body, making us vulnerable to degenerative diseases. This is exactly what is happening to most of us today—we're not getting quite enough of some of the essential minerals and vitamins over long periods of time—and the cumulative effect can be very serious.

A diet high in minerals and vitamins and the enzymes to digest them is crucial to you and your family's health. That is why you need PowerCharged food. And the fastest, easiest, and quickest way to start growing PowerCharged food is, believe it or not, right on your kitchen counter.

3. *The Fountain of Youth*

THE Spanish explorer Ponce de Leon searched off the Florida coast for a marvelous fountain he had heard could restore youth. He never found this legendary fountain, but you can. It is the eating of sprouted seeds that have not been heated over 118°F, the temperature at which enzyme destruction begins. Sprouts are freshly germinated edible seeds such as beans and grains. They are easy to grow and delicious to eat. In fact, all you need is a kitchen counter and five minutes a day. Even if you're in an apartment in the middle of a city, you can sprout!

The rejuvenating and life-giving properties of sprouts may be one of the great health secrets of our time. Sprouts provide two important things in our diet—a steady year-round source of vitamins and a high concentration of food enzymes. Both keep the body's enzyme activity high. If you recall from Chapter 1, enzymes, which are made out of vitamins and minerals, are the most vital factor that sustains our body's life processes. Without enzymes, we would be dead. And it is that very thing, enzyme depletion, that is a fundamental cause of aging. It is the loss of the body's enzymes which decreases the life processes in the cells. As the cells' life processes decrease, they are not able to replace themselves as quickly. At the same time, as enzyme activity decreases, the cells become more susceptible to damage by free radicals and other toxic substances, which further hinders cell reproduction. It is the body's inability to replace old cells with healthy new ones at a fast enough rate and the concurrent loss in the body's enzymes that is precisely responsible for aging and increased susceptibility to disease as we get older. This is why immunity tends to decrease with age—immune cells aren't being replaced at a fast enough rate to protect the body adequately from disease. Staying biologically young and healthy is a matter of keeping enzyme activity in our bodies at a maximum. That is exactly what sprouts do, which is why they can be called the fountain of youth.

YEAR-ROUND VITAMINS

To begin with, sprouts are the most reliable year-round source of vitamin C, carotenoid A, and many B vitamins (such as folacin), all of which are usually in short supply in our diet. Sprouting seeds, grains, and legumes greatly increases their content of those vitamins.[1] For example, the vitamin A content (per calorie) of sprouted mung beans is two-and-a-half times higher than the dry bean, and some beans have more than eight times more vitamin A after being sprouted.[2]

Dry seeds, grains, and legumes, while rich in protein and complex carbohydrates, contain no vitamin C. But after sprouting, they contain around 20 milligrams per 3.5 ounces, a tremendous increase.[3] Also, if grown in decent soil or taken from your own garden, seeds, grains, and legumes will be high in organic minerals—so your sprouts will be an excellent source of minerals as well as vitamins.

The great advantage in getting vitamins from sprouts you grow yourself is that you get a consistently high vitamin content without losses. In the dead of winter, when you can't grow anything or get fresh produce anywhere, sprouts will provide a consistently reliable source of fresh, high-nutrient vegetables rich in vitamin C, vitamin A, and B vitamins. This will keep your immune system strong and your health in top condition when almost everyone else is getting sick. Why do you think so many people come down with colds and flus in the winter more than any other time? Because they're not getting the vegetables and fruits that would keep their immune systems strong.

Have you ever heard of a vegetable that continues to gain vitamins after you harvest it? Sprouts do! Sprouts are living foods. Even after you harvest your sprouts and refrigerate them, they will continue to grow slowly, and their vitamin content will actually increase. Contrast that with store-bought fruits and vegetables, which start losing their vitamins as soon as they're picked and often have to be shipped a thousand miles or more in the winter.

SPROUTS SAVE OUR ENZYMES

Sprouts preserve our body's enzymes, which is extremely important. How do they do this? First of all, sprouted beans, grains, nuts, and seeds are extremely easy to digest. Sprouting essentially pre-digests the food for us by breaking down the concentrated starch into simpler carbohydrates and the protein into free amino acids, so our own enzymes don't have to work so hard.[4] If you've ever had trouble digesting beans properly, just sprout them and you'll have no trouble at all. Sprouting also removes anti-nutrients such as enzyme inhibitors, and that makes sprouts even easier to digest, further sparing enzymes.[5] Another anti-nutrient is phytates, which is what stops some people from enjoying grains such as wheat. Many people who can't eat unsprouted wheat find they can eat all the sprouted wheat they want with no problem.

THE MAGIC OF FOOD ENZYMES

Perhaps the greatest thing sprouts provide is enzymes. The enzymes in sprouts are a special protein that helps our body digest the nutrients in our food and boosts the life-giving enzyme activity in our body. Food enzymes are only found in raw foods. Cooking destroys them. While all raw foods contain enzymes, the most powerful enzyme-rich foods are sprouted seeds, grains, and legumes. Sprouting increases the enzyme content in these foods enormously, to as much as forty-three times more than non-sprouted foods.[6]

Sprouting greatly increases the content of all enzymes, including proteolytic and amylolytic enzymes.[7] These enzymes digest proteins and carbohydrates (starches). They are normally produced inside the body but are also found in great concentration in raw sprouted foods. Researchers such as Dr. Edward Howell have shown how food enzymes aid us in the digestion of all the proteins, starches, and fats eaten in the same meal through their action in both the saliva and the upper part of the stomach. These food enzymes can take the place of some of our body's own enzymes, and this is very significant.

The digestion of food takes a high priority and forces the body to produce a copious flow of concentrated digestive enzymes when there are no enzymes in our food. All of us lose our ability to produce concentrated digestive enzymes as we grow older. As this happens, we are less able to use the vitamins, minerals, and other nutrients in our food, and we lose the ability to produce adequate amounts of all the other enzymes we need.

Dr. David G. Williams explains some of the consequences of inadequate enzyme production:

"As we age, our digestive system becomes less efficient. This should be obvious when you consider that anywhere from 60 to 75 percent of all hospitalizations are related to problems concerning the digestive system. . . . ulcer and indigestion medications, both prescription and over-the-counter, are among the top sellers of any class of drugs; as we age, our stomach's ability to produce hydrochloric acid lessens

BEST SOURCES OF SEEDS FOR SPROUTING

What seeds are best for sprouting? Seeds with high germination percentages so that every seed, or nearly every seed, can be sprouted. Rye, wheat, alfalfa, and lentil seeds have the overall best germination rates. Mung beans of good quality are also good. If you desire to sprout "other beans," test a small quantity before buying in large amounts.

Heat and moisture are the enemies of seeds, so the storage conditions will affect the seeds, and so will the way they were grown. Were the seeds stored in a warehouse? For how long? Were they kept cool? If they are fresh and untreated, the life force will still be in them and they will sprout. If some beans sprout and some don't, that means the quality has been affected.

Your local health food store is generally your best source of seeds suitable for sprouting. However, we have found that lentils from the supermarket have sprouted well.

Although there's no proof of it, we believe organic seeds tend to be better, particularly if the seller can furnish you with a documented copy of the grower's specifications. If you want to use a variety of sprouted beans, experiment with it. You can prove it to yourself. But even though the claim is that the bean was organically grown, let the buyer beware.

(*New England Journal of Medicine* 85; 313: 70–74); and by age 65, almost 35 percent of us don't produce any hydrochloric acid at all."[8]

Researchers such as Dr. Edward Howell have shown that much of this breakdown in the body's ability to produce enough enzymes is due to the overproduction of concentrated digestive enzymes over many years. It should be obvious from all this that our bodies were made to eat far more raw food than we currently eat. The body has only a limited capacity to make enzymes, and this overproduction of digestive enzymes over many years is directly responsible for the body's loss of all the other enzymes.

By squandering our enzyme-making capacity on digestive enzymes, the production and activity of all the other enzymes needed in our body is reduced. This is one reason why enzymes are depleted from our cells as we age. As enzyme activity is diminished in the cells, there is an acceleration of the aging process caused by free radical damage and other things that make us increasingly susceptible to disease.

When we get enzymes from our food, it spares our body from having to make such concentrated digestive enzymes. This sparing effect increases the activity of all the other enzymes in our body. Eating enzyme-rich foods such as sprouts allows our body to maximize its production of non-digestive enzymes, and that helps us produce an adequate level of enzymes all our life. And the higher the level of enzyme activity, the healthier and biologically younger we are going to be.

Since aging is, to a large extent, caused by enzyme depletion, slowing the aging process might be a matter of eating lots of enzyme-rich food every day along with an adequate intake of vitamins and minerals. Sprouted seeds, grains, and legumes are the most powerful enzyme-rich foods that exist.

MAKE YOUR OWN SPROUTS YEAR-ROUND

While fresh fruits and vegetables provide enzymes, sprouts are far more concentrated and should be eaten in the summer with every large meal even when you have your own vegetables and fruits. In the winter and spring, when your own vegetables and fruits are not available, sprouts are doubly important. Sprouts should become an integral part of your diet year-round.

But you need to make your own sprouts for highest food value. Sprouts are living food. They need to be fresh. Freshly picked from your own sprout garden, they contain the highest level of enzymes and vitamins. If they are immediately refrigerated, the "life force" will stay in the seed as they remain fresh and slowly continue to grow.

If they are not immediately refrigerated after harvest, they will stop growing and the enzymes and vitamins will start decomposing. As that happens, the enzyme and vitamin content will decline rapidly. When you buy sprouts at the supermarket, there's no telling how long they've been out on the shelves and exposed to room temperature. Even several hours of sitting in room temperature will cause a rapid loss of enzymes and vitamins. But what's even worse is that some sprouts are treated with mold inhibitors to keep them fresh looking as they sit at room temperature. Those long, white, mung bean sprouts seen in the store or at the salad bar have probably been treated with inhibitors so they could be grown to that length and preserved at room temperature.

To really get the rejuvenating value of sprouts, you need to grow your own and eat them fresh.

HOW TO USE SPROUTS IN YOUR DIET

Super-high enzyme content, high vitamin content, ease of digestibility, and removal of anti-nutrients are all reasons to eat sprouts, but enzymes are the number one reason. To get maximum enzymes, you'll need to eat sprouts uncooked. However, you might want to cook some sprouts just to increase the digestibility of the starch in beans or to eliminate some anti-nutrients in cereal grains such as wheat.

Soaking overnight and cooking beans will eliminate most of the enzyme inhibitors so that the beans are easy to digest. (Make sure you drain the soak water and cook with new water.) Cooking grains, especially in water, will neutralize much of their anti-nutrients as well. If you have special difficulty digesting starch, sprout your beans and grains a little before cooking. This will make them easier to digest and completely eliminate anti-nutrients, as well as increase the nutritional value of the protein.

There are some seeds, grains, and legumes you'll want to eat uncooked to get the benefit of raw food enzymes. This is where you get the greatest health benefit with sprouts—from eating them uncooked. Chemistry acknowledges that the proteins in food are destroyed at 160°F because of the denaturing of the protein. Since enzymes are a type of protein, you might think the same applies to them. However, Dr. Howell has shown that food enzymes begin being destroyed at 118°F.[9] To get maximum enzyme and vitamin concentration, you'll want to eat some sprouts raw or warmed up to no higher than 118°F.

Many of the sprouted seeds, grains, and legumes are very palatable eaten raw or heated no higher than 118°F. The best sprouted seeds to be eaten this way are alfalfa and sunflower seed sprouts; the best grains are wheat and rye sprouts; the best legumes are mung bean and lentil sprouts.

Alfalfa Sprouts

Alfalfa sprouts are sweet, delicate, and easy to chew. They are wonderful in tossed green salads. They can be used in place of lettuce in sandwiches. They even taste great eaten by themselves or as the main part of the One-Minute Sprout Salad. (See recipe in inset below.)

Sunflower Seed Sprouts

Sunflower seed sprouts are great in salads. The sprouting makes them easy to chew, and they add a crispy, nutty effect to salads or cooked dishes. (Toss them into an already cooked dish so they are warmed up but not cooked.) They are so good that you can eat them right out of your hand.

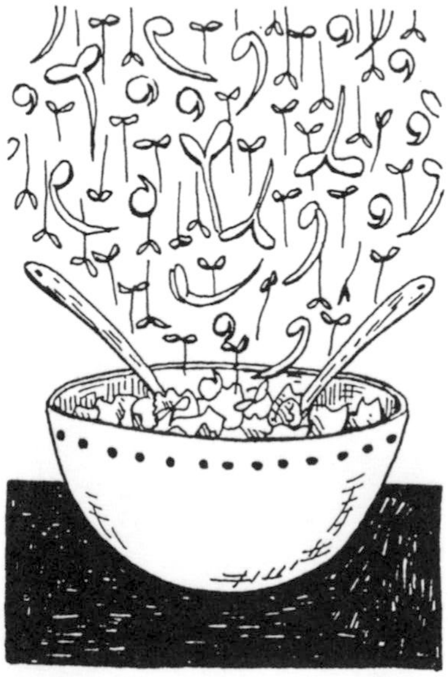

One-Minute Sprout Salad

When you are in a hurry and want to prepare something super-rich in enzymes, vitamins, and minerals to start off a meal, try this One-Minute Sprout Salad.

1 cup alfalfa sprouts
1/4 cup lentil sprouts
1/4 cup mung bean sprouts
1/4 cup rye or wheat sprouts
1/4 cup soaked sunflower seeds
1 tablespoon olive oil
1/2 teaspoon lemon juice or apple-cider vinegar
A sprinkling of onion powder
A sprinkling of garlic powder
*A few drops of soy sauce**
2 tablespoons nutritional yeast (optional)

YIELD: 1 Serving

1. Place the alfalfa sprouts in a medium-sized salad bowl. Add the remaining sprouts and the sunflower seeds.
2. Directly over the salad, dribble the olive oil and lemon juice or apple-cider vinegar, then add the onion powder, garlic powder, and soy sauce. Toss it with a fork.
3. If desired, add nutritional yeast as a tasty addition—that is, if your body can handle yeast.

* = We recommend only naturally brewed soy sauce, such as tamari or shoyu.

Wheat and Rye Sprouts

Wheat and rye sprouts are similar. Wheat sprouts are a little chewier and have a slight naturally sweet flavor. Both are high in fiber and make a great addition to many of the dishes you prepare.

Wheat and rye sprouts are excellent in tossed green salads. (Rye is a little easier to chew.) Wheat sprouts are particularly good warmed up in oatmeal, cream of wheat, or other hot cereals. You can stir rye or wheat sprouts into scrambled egg dishes or omelets for an excellent culinary effect.

Rye and wheat sprouts are excellent poured into soups, stews, or on top of main dishes after the main part of the cooking has been done. That will preserve most of the enzymes and vitamins. These sprouts are so versatile, they'll fit into any kind of cuisine. Just try them out, but cook them as little as possible to save enzymes.

Instant Sprouted-Bean Stew

Here is a way of serving sprouted beans as a warm dish that takes only a few minutes to prepare. Cooking with low heat prevents the enzymes and vitamins of the sprouts from being destroyed, while letting you enjoy a warm and nutritious main dish.

1 teaspoon olive oil
1/4 cup chopped onion
1/4 cup cooked beans (black, pinto, Northern, etc.)
1/4 cup tomato sauce or juice
1/4 cup lentil or mung bean sprouts
1/4 cup rye or wheat sprouts
Seasoning to taste: soy sauce, herbs, etc.
*2 ounces cheddar cheese, grated (optional)**

YIELD: 1 Serving

1. In a medium-sized saucepan, heat the oil over medium heat. Add the onions and sauté until soft. Add the beans and the tomato sauce or juice, and cook until warmed.
2. Reduce heat to low and toss in the sprouts and seasoning. Top with cheese, if desired. Simmer, covered, for one minute. Turn off heat, and let sit another minute.
3. Mix ingredients together and serve.

* = Alta Dena brand of raw cheese recommended. It's generally found in health food stores.

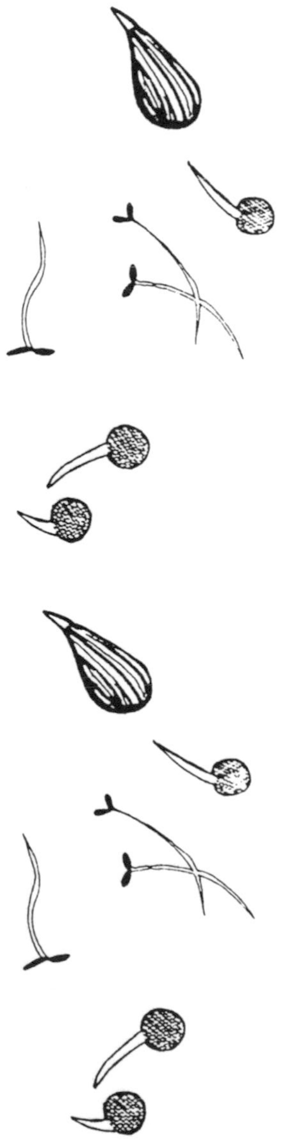

Mung Bean and Lentil Sprouts

Mung bean and lentil sprouts are the two types of legumes that taste good completely raw. Mung bean sprouts have been used in oriental cooking for thousands of years but are typically overcooked, leaving little of their enzymes or vitamins. Both mung bean and lentil sprouts are excellent in tossed green salads and are easy to chew. Mung bean sprouts in particular have a delicious sweet taste. Both

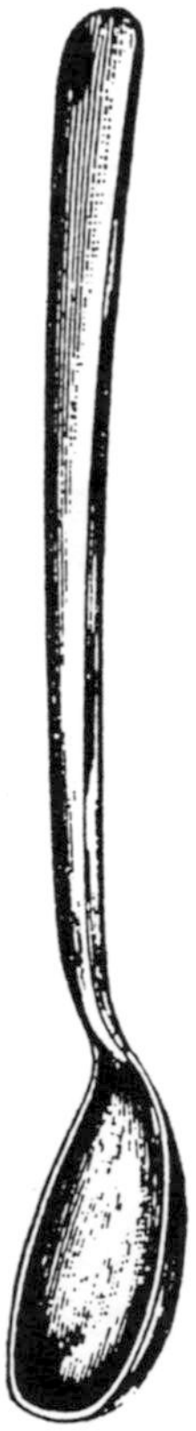

Enzyme Soup

Enzyme Soup *can be used at room temperature, chilled, or warmed up to no higher than 118°F. This soup is nutritionally equivalent to a tossed green salad without all the chewing and is great in place of a salad before a meal. This soup is an excellent way to get enzyme-rich food when you are in a hurry and don't have time to sit down and chew up a salad. It saves you from a great deal of chewing by having the blades rupture the cells of the ingredients, releasing the chlorophyll and other components.*

1/4 cup tomato juice or 1 medium-sized tomato, cut into quarters
3 large lettuce leaves, preferably romaine, green leaf, or red leaf (if the leaves are small, use more)
1 cup alfalfa sprouts
1 cup lentil sprouts
1 slice jicama and/or 1 slice sweet red pepper
1 teaspoon olive oil, or 1/4 peeled avocado
2 tablespoons nutritional yeast (optional)
1 tablespoon sesame seeds (optional)
Seasonings of your choice: soy sauce, vegetable salt, lemon juice, apple-cider vinegar, onion powder, garlic powder, etc.
1 long celery stalk
1/4 cup soaked sunflower seeds for garnish

YIELD: 1 Serving

1. In a blender or a Vita Mix container, place all the ingredients except the sunflower seeds. If using a blender, the tomato quarters must first be liquefied, and the celery stalk should be used to guide the ingredients into the blades. If using the Vita Mix machine, cut the celery into pieces.
2. Run on high speed for about 10 seconds in the Vita Mix, or for at least 20 seconds in the blender, until a thick purée forms.
3. Transfer to a soup bowl and top with soaked sunflower seeds. Mix altogether and serve.

are excellent added to soups and stews after the main cooking has been done.

You can, in fact, make a complete stew out of lightly heated mung bean sprouts, lentil sprouts, and other sprouts and still preserve some enzymes since the sprouts become cooked in a very short time. (See the Instant Sprouted-Bean Stew recipe inset on page 31.) Both mung bean and lentil sprouts are great in oriental cuisine, lightly heated, and can be used with many other cuisines.

The Richest Source of Enzymes

The most powerful enzyme-packed food you can eat is the One-Minute Sprout Salad. A large tossed green salad containing lots of sprouts is also packed with enzymes and vitamins. If you don't want to chew that much and want to save time, try the Enzyme Soup. (See "Enzyme Soup" inset on page 32.) The main meal every day should start with one of those salads to provide a dose of enzymes and boost your body's digestion and metabolic functioning.

As with enzymes, the maximum amount of vitamin C and the B vitamins from sprouts is obtained by eating them raw or not heated over 118°F. Vitamin A, a fat-soluble vitamin, is pretty much resistant to heat losses, although it does oxidize in air.

If you do only one thing for your health as a result of reading this book, it should be to eat a serving of sprouts every day.

HOW TO GROW SPROUTS

Sprouting is simple. Once you get your equipment and procedures set up, it will take you only five minutes a day to have a steady supply of sprouts. What about the sprouting time? If you start sprouting today, you will be able to harvest the most nutrition-packed, enzyme-rich food on Earth in only one to five days.

Seeds and Equipment

First, locate a good source of seeds. Your best bet is to start with alfalfa seeds. They are foolproof. Then add lentils, mung beans, rye, wheat, and sunflower seeds. Although other things can be sprouted, those six are the easiest to sprout and taste best eaten raw or only lightly heated.

A health food store should have those seeds. Make sure, especially with sunflower seeds, that they are completely raw and whole. Any roasting will destroy the germ. Your local supermarket might carry whole lentils as well. A large amount of dried seeds, grains, and legumes can be stored in a small, cool, dry space, generally for several years, and can easily be converted into fresh food.

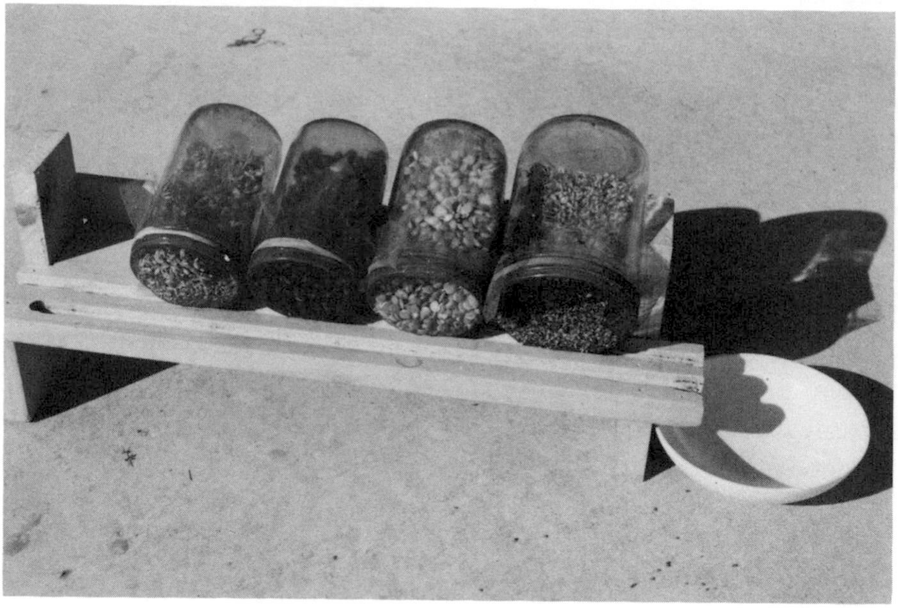

Figure 3.1 Sprouting rack.

The next thing you're going to need is some sprouting equipment. You will need jars, netting, and jar holders. For jars, use wide-mouth, straight-sided jars, one to two pints in volume. For each jar, you will need a piece of cloth netting about six to eight inches square as a cover and a strong rubber band to hold the netting in place.

The best netting is tulle (pronounced toolee), available at fabric shops. Cut the netting large enough to extend about two inches down the sides of the sprouting jar so it can be held securely by a strong rubber band. Cheesecloth can be used but has a short life compared to tulle netting. A piece of discarded pantyhose can be used if you don't have the regular netting.

The sprouting jar will need to be held at a slant, mouth side down, to drain out excess water and oxygenate the seeds. The simplest jar holder is a shallow bowl for each sprouting jar. A sprouting rack is the best jar holder of all. (See Figure 3.1.)

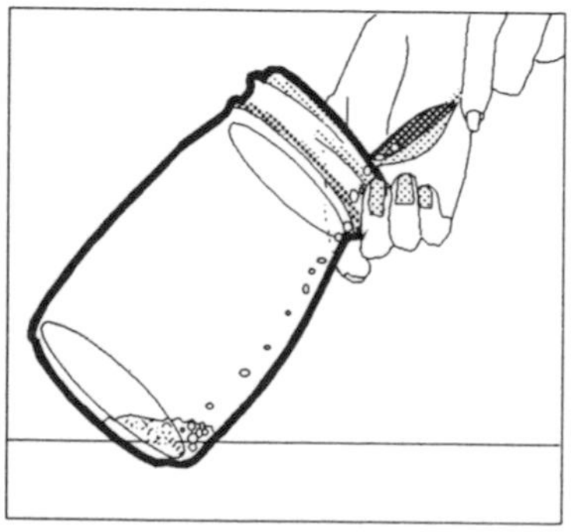

After measuring out your seeds, spoon them into your sprouting jar.

Sprouting Procedure

1. If you're starting with alfalfa seeds, measure out two level tablespoonfuls of seeds for each two-pint (one-quart) jar, as shown in Table 3.1. For other types of seeds, measure out one cup per two-pint jar. (Note: Whatever jar size you use, fill no more than one-fourth full of seeds, leaving room for expansion and oxygenation.)
2. Now you need to soak the seeds by filling the sprouting jar nearly full with plain water. This is the pre-germination stage, which

activates the very beginning of the sprouting process. Cover the mouth of the jar with a piece of cloth netting and secure it with a strong rubber band. Soak for eight to twelve hours. You can start soaking at night and begin the sprouting the next morning or start soaking in the morning and begin the sprouting when you come home in the evening. (Note: If you're soaking beans before cooking but not sprouting them, soak them in the pot you'll cook them in and drain the soak water before cooking. That will remove any anti-nutrients that could be in the soak water.)

3. After soaking, drain the water out into a sink. Place each jar, mouth down, in a bowl or on a sprouting rack at a slight slant so air and water drainage can occur.
4. From this point, start rinsing the seeds twice a day with water. Do this by filling up the jar with water and swishing the seeds around to get them thoroughly moist. Drain the water and tilt the jars back in the bowls.
5. Two to five days from the start of soaking, you'll be ready to harvest your sprouts. Seeds sprout quickly or slowly depending on the type of seed, its freshness, and the temperature. (See Table 3.1.)
6. Store your sprouts in the refrigerator until ready to use. Just leave the sprouts in the same jar where they sprouted, remove the netting, screw on the lid, and refrigerate. Or you can transfer them to Tupperware or other food storage containers and then refrigerate. Many sprouts will continue to grow while stored in the refrigerator. All sprouts in general can be stored in the refrigerator in a tight container up to seven days with no problem. Beyond that, they're not as fresh as they should be.
7. As soon as you harvest one batch of sprouts, set up another batch so you'll have a constant supply.

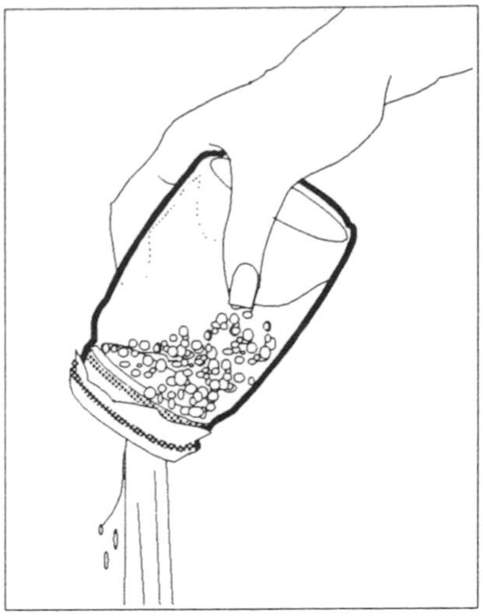

After soaking the seeds, drain the water out into a sink.

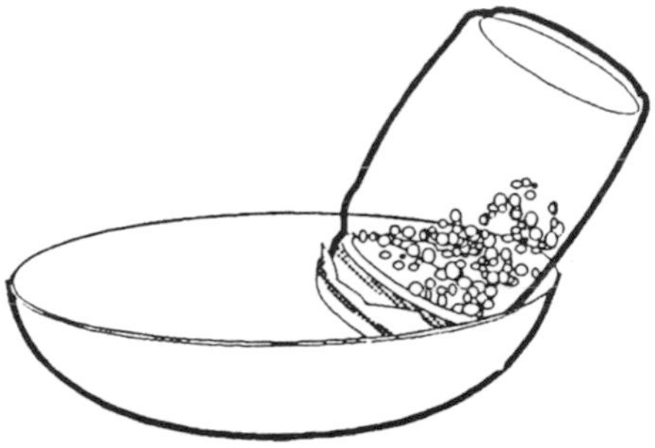

Place each jar face down in a bowl or a sprouting rack at a 30 degree to 45 degree angle.

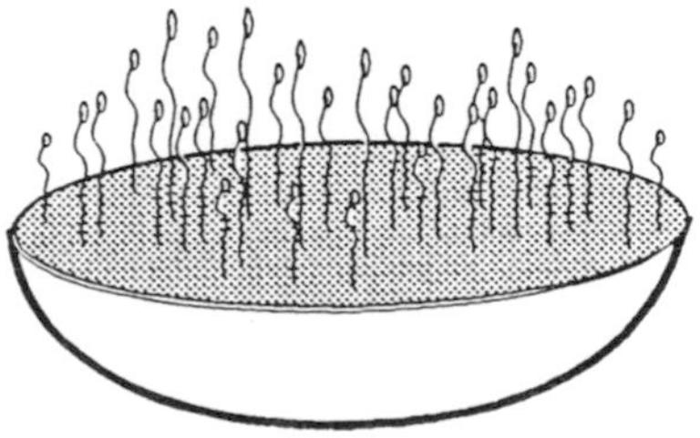

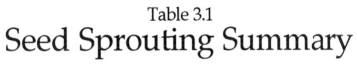

Reap the reward by eating a bowl of sprouts.

Table 3.1

Seed Sprouting Summary

Kind of Seed	Amount of Seed per Quart Jar	Sprouting Time From Start of Soak (Days)	Sprout Length at Harvest (Inches)	Yield (Cups)
Alfalfa	2 Tablespoons	4–5	1–2	4.0
Mung Bean	1 Cup	2–3	1/4–1/2	2.0
Lentil	1 Cup	2–3	1/4	3.5
Rye/Wheat	1 Cup	2–3	1/8	3.0
Sunflower	1 Cup	1–2	1/16	2.0
Other Beans	1 Cup	4–5	1/4–1/2	2.0

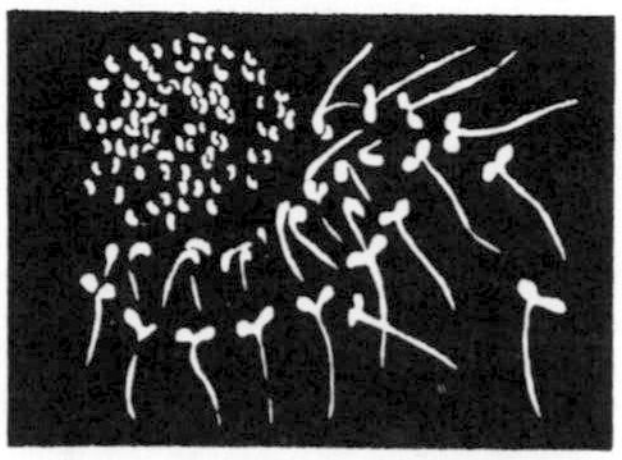

Alfalfa

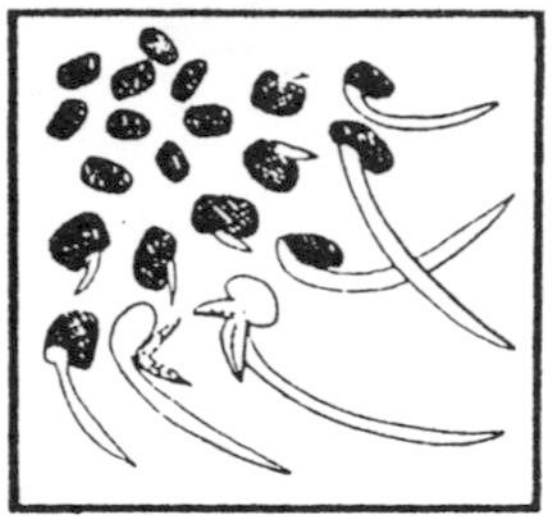

Mung Beans

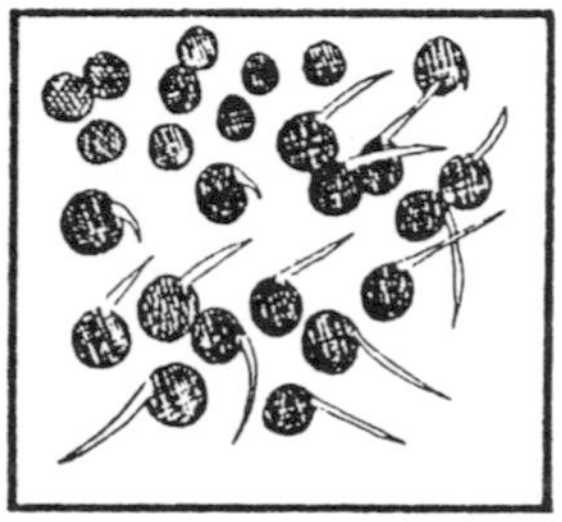

Lentils

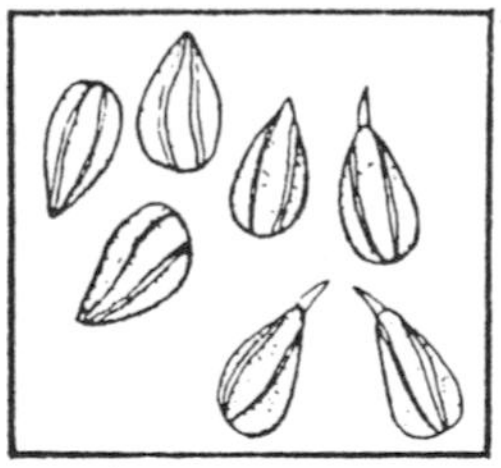

Sunflower Seeds

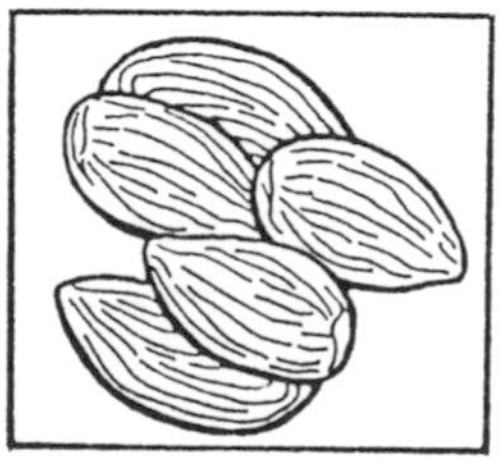

Almonds

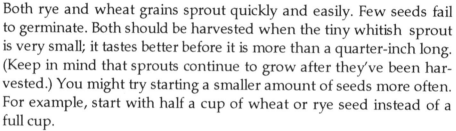

SOME SPECIAL THINGS TO KNOW ABOUT SPROUTING

Here are some additonal points for sprouting various seeds.

Alfalfa

Alfalfa seeds are the surest, most foolproof seeds to sprout. They should be placed near a windowsill or under artificial light. This makes them turn green and increases their vitamin A content. (Be sure to keep them out of direct sunlight.)

Alfalfa seeds make a tremendous amount of food for their tiny size. Alfalfa seeds sprout to twenty-four times their original volume. A single pound of alfalfa seeds contains about thirty tablespoonfuls and should keep one person in sprouts a couple of months. One tablespoonful of alfalfa seeds will yield a pint of delicious healthful sprouts in four to five days. If you eat one cup of alfalfa sprouts a day, one pound of seeds will last you about sixty days.

Rye and Wheat

Both rye and wheat grains sprout quickly and easily. Few seeds fail to germinate. Both should be harvested when the tiny whitish sprout is very small; it tastes better before it is more than a quarter-inch long. (Keep in mind that sprouts continue to grow after they've been harvested.) You might try starting a smaller amount of seeds more often. For example, start with half a cup of wheat or rye seed instead of a full cup.

Mung Beans and Lentils

Mung beans and lentils generally sprout with great ease. Occasionally, after harvest you might find a hard one that didn't soak up any water. The easiest time to look for those is just before using a portion. Spread them out on a plate. If the mung beans and lentils are of good quality, you'll rarely find a hard one.

Sunflower Seeds

Only twenty-four hours after the beginning of the sprouting process, you can start eating sunflower seed sprouts even though the sprout is barely visible. Some might not have sprouted at all by that time, but it's still okay to eat them; or you can wait the full two days for more to sprout.

Other Legumes

The ease of sprouting beans depends greatly on the quality of the bean—that is, how they've been handled and stored and for how long. Most of the beans we've tried have sprouted readily. We've had consistent success with black-eyed peas, pinto beans, garbanzo beans (chickpeas), black beans, white beans, adzuki beans, whole dried peas, and others. The only one that's given us trouble sprouting properly is soybeans, probably because they're typically stored a long time.

If seeds won't sprout or sprout poorly, the "life force" in the germ has been depleted or destroyed. That is usually due to having seeds that are too old or that have not been stored properly under cool, dry conditions. In fact, the way to see if a batch of beans has any life force left in it is to see if it will sprout. If you happen to get a batch of beans where some sprout but some start to go bad during sprouting, find another source. If you're not sure of the quality of your source, buy small amounts at first to see how reliably they sprout.

Other Seeds to Sprout

After you have mastered the art of sprouting you might want to try other kinds of seeds such as cabbage, radish, fenugreek, clover, oats, and corn. Some of those are expensive but have gourmet or other qualities that justify their use.

PRE-SPROUTED ALMONDS

Almonds are an excellent food, rich in magnesium, zinc, copper, vitamin E, and other nutrients, and should be eaten uncooked for greatest food value, as should all nuts. There are some benefits to soaking raw almonds before eating them. When soaked, they swell up, becoming tender and much easier to chew. The soaking is actually pre-sprouting, the very beginning of the sprouting process. It will activate the living germ, increasing the enzyme concentration even though you won't see any sprout. Pre-sprouting will also enhance digestion by doing away with any enzyme inhibitors that may be around the seed coat.

Soak the almonds for eight to twelve hours, like you would any other seed, until they're completely swollen. Drain the water and eat, or store them in your refrigerator. To make the almonds even easier to chew, remove the seed coat by blanching. Blanching requires heat treatment but is of such short duration it affects mostly the seed coat, leaving the blanched almonds a raw food with nearly all the enzymes intact.

To blanch, place enough water in a small pot to cover the amount of soaked almonds you have. Bring the water to a boil, shut off the heat, and dump your soaked almonds into the hot water. Swish them around about fifteen seconds, then pour the almonds into a collander and just slip off the skins.

ADVANCED SPROUTING

Sprouts for low-cost, health-giving PowerCharged food have been a well-kept secret. No other food can be stored for so long in such small spaces yet yield so much food value upon sprouting. The rejuvenating effects of a large amount of sprouts consumed daily over several weeks will show you the incredible power of raw food enzymes. You will start feeling better, have more energy, age slower, and even see an increase in your sex drive. Sprouts will promote health and well-being in your family and prevent disease in the long run. You should get sick less often, if at all, because of a stronger immune system.

You need a large and constant supply of fresh sprouts for superior health. To make that easy and even fun, get yourself a sprouting rack. (See Figure 3.1.) In a properly designed rack, you can place four or more jars all in a row. The water drains out the bottoms of the jars into grooves that lead to the end of the rack and into a saucer. Instead of emptying four or more saucers of drain water, you empty only one saucer. A good sprouting rack can be made from 1-inch by 6-inch boards.

A sprouting kit, including sprouting jars, a sprouting rack, and everything else needed for a kitchen sprout garden, will soon be available. (For sources, see Appendix A.)

4. *The Pesticide Menace*

EVERY year, 815 million pounds of pesticides are dumped onto our crops and soil. What happens to all those chemicals as they make their way through the food chain to our dinner plate? How do they affect our health? Do pesticides pose a serious threat to our health, or are the doses so small that they're insignificant? Are pesticide residues really no problem (as the FDA would like us to believe) because there are more "natural carcinogens" in food, or are pesticide residues a true menace?

To sort this out, let's look at what we do know about pesticides. There are three main types: insecticides, herbicides, and fungicides. Insecticides kill insects, herbicides kill weeds, and fungicides kill fungi that cause plant diseases. Of the total pounds of pesticides that are used every year, nearly 60 percent are known to cause tumors in laboratory animals.[1] Furthermore, two-thirds of all pesticide ingredients were in use before the Environmental Protection Agency was charged with regulating them, and those have not even been tested under current EPA standards.[2] Since older standards are laxer than today's, the health risks from those pesticides could be worse than acknowledged.

If current standards were applied, most of those older pesticides would not even be allowed on the market or would be allowed only at lower tolerances. (Tolerances specify the amount of pesticide residue that can be in food.) Most of our exposure to tumor-forming pesticides comes from those older pesticides, which are routinely present in food in levels that would not be allowed under current standards.[3]

As the EPA continues its testing program, one would hope that many of those pesticides will be banned or at least set at lower tolerances. However, it is worth noting that the EPA has not revoked a single tolerance when new information demonstrates that a pesticide has tumor-forming potential and concentrates in processed food.[4] In addition, the re-registration of older pesticides is an extremely time-consuming process that could take decades. As of 1991, only two of the 822 older pesticide ingredients in use had been re-registered under current standards.[5]

The EPA itself considers a substantial portion of all pesticides to be capable of causing tumors, yet it allows them to be used anyway. Have no doubts about it, most pesticides are dangerous poisons. With that in mind, how can the EPA allow their use at all? Our modern system of agriculture is firmly entrenched in the use of pesticides. Five billion dollars' worth of agricultural chemicals are sold in the United States each year. Even if the EPA knows that many pesticides are hazardous, it's not going to ban them outright. So it does the next best thing—it sets tolerances.

HOW A PESTICIDE IS APPROVED

The EPA establishes tolerances to cover all expected residues on food. How are tolerances determined? Does the EPA have sophisticated laboratories where they do testing? No. The makers of the pesticide supply the data needed for its registration. In other words, the EPA depends upon the chemical industry to run tests on residues in food and to do cancer studies on rats or mice. It's kind of like asking the fox to guard the chicken coop.

From the studies presented to it by the chemical industry, the EPA determines an acceptable rate of cancer that will likely result from the presence of the pesticide in food at a certain tolerance level. The EPA makes assumptions about how many extra people will experience cancer from a daily lifelong exposure to the pesticide beyond the statistical 30 percent of the population that gets cancer. That is actually very unrealistic, since we know that pesticides are likely to be a contributing factor to many cancers and not the sole cause of any single cancer. But for EPA purposes, they have to pretend that a given pesticide will be the sole cause of so many cancers.

Typically, if they determine that no more than one person in 10,000 will experience cancer from that pesticide alone, it is approved.[6] That is considered the upper bound of potential human risk, and the EPA always claims that because it employs a large safety factor the true risk is probably less than reported risk estimates.

How accurate are those assumptions about cancer risk? In reality, the whole risk assessment process is highly uncertain and arbitrary. It does not predict the actual number of cancers in which pesticides are the sole cause or a contributing factor. A 1990 text, *Chemicals in the Human Food Chain*, tells us that "risk estimates for oncogenic [tumor-forming] pesticides do not predict actual human cancer incidence."[7] The World Health Organization clearly explains that risk estimates and safety factors, which are based on extrapolating from animal models, will "always be arbitrary."[8] The National Research Council tells us the same thing about the guesswork that goes into calculating risk:

"For some types of risk, however, particularly cancer risk, there remains considerable debate about the certainty of the data and assumptions supporting calculations of acceptable risk."[9]

At best, the tolerance levels for pesticides in food are based on educated guesses. At worst, they're based on expediency. In other words, tolerances are set at large enough doses to kill the pests rather than being based on health risks. *Chemicals in the Human Food Chain* tells us, "Tolerance levels are based on the efficacy required in the field, not on health-based criteria."[10]

Of course, the EPA says the safety factor it applies to the Acceptable Daily Intake for a given pesticide is so large (typically a hundredfold) that even if you ingested the maximum acceptable amount, it would give you an intake far below a level of exposure that would produce noticeable toxicity. The Acceptable Daily Intake is the amount of a pesticide you can safely ingest from all sources throughout the day. Furthermore, the EPA says that, based on studies, the highest intake of a given pesticide throughout the population is not over 16 percent of its Acceptable Daily Intake and usually is less.[11]

UNKNOWN RISKS

So it would seem that even if tolerance levels in food are based more on industry need than on health-based criteria, we are still safe. But are we? First of all, the tolerance levels determined by current standards apply only to the newer pesticides or the older ones that have been re-registered, and the vast majority of chemical ingredients in use today fall outside that category. They were on the market before 1972, before the EPA was charged with regulating them, and are not subject to the same scrutiny as the newer ones.

So while we can make educated guesses about the adverse health effects of around one-third of the pesticides in use, the other two-thirds are being used without any real knowledge of their effects.

What about the newer pesticides that already have tolerances set under current standards? Does the EPA's Acceptable Daily Intake have such a large margin of safety that we don't have to worry about those? Maybe, maybe not. We already know that the assumptions used to determine cancer risk are highly uncertain and arbitrary. But there's an even larger gap, stemming from the fact that when an acceptable intake is determined for a pesticide, it is based solely on exposure to that pesticide alone. In reality, most of us are exposed to low levels of numerous pesticide ingredients. For instance, more than twenty suspected carcinogenic pesticides may be used on apples and tomatoes. The residues of numerous pesticides may be found in many processed and animal foods as well.

The National Research Council tells us, "The EPA sets acceptable levels for residues in food for each pesticide separately, although many combinations of pesticides are regularly used and detected on food crops."[12] The tests done on rats to determine cancer risk test only one pesticide at a time, but in reality we're exposed to many pesticides that can have similar effects on the body. The acceptable intake for a pesticide does not take into account the risk of taking in numerous pesticides that may all interact together. This means that even if your intake of a single pesticide is well below the Acceptable Daily Intake, you may be exposed to an illegally high level of similarly acting pesticides taken as a group.

The text *Pesticides and Human Health* explains, "An exposed individual may suffer adverse [long-term] health effects following exposure to numerous members of a class of pesticides . . . even though the exposure level for each pesticide was below the federally defined safe tolerance level."[13] In light of those facts, the studies that have shown the intake of a few pesticides throughout the population as being well below the Acceptable Daily Intake are essentially meaningless.

Perhaps the biggest gap of knowledge comes from trying to determine how all the tiny cumulative doses of pesticides interact in our body. Tolerance levels do not even attempt to take this into account. The National Research Council tells us, "Current regulations and standards do not assess or incorporate margins of safety reflecting the possibility of synergistic or additive effects."[14] Synergistic means that long-term tiny doses of a number of pesticides interacting together may do things to our body that one pesticide by itself could not do.

The lab tests upon which tolerance levels are based give no indication whatsoever of the carcinogenic or other risks of taking in numerous pesticides together, yet that is what is happening in the real world. This means that the true risks, instead of being below the upper risk estimates, are probably far above it, because we are ingesting numerous pesticides that act synergistically. Furthermore, some of those chemicals or their metabolites may accumulate in our bodies over the long term even though the dose in a given day is very tiny. Because of all this, the EPA's tolerance levels are of little value.

NO ONE REALLY KNOWS WHAT'S IN OUR FOOD

What's more, we don't even have a clear picture of how many residues are in our food. While the EPA establishes tolerances to cover all expected residues in food, it is the Food and Drug Administration that monitors food for compliance with those tolerances. The gaps in the FDA's enforcement of pesticide residue tolerances are so large that we really know very little about the extent of pesticides in the food supply. The FDA samples less than .002 percent of the food consumed.[15] In 91 percent of the samples tested by the FDA in recent years, only three pesticides were tested for, while hundreds of pesticide ingredients are on the market.[16]

The FDA simply does not have the capability to test for most of the pesticides that are on the market and in our food. What's worse, says the National Research Council, is that "the monitoring does not regularly check for many widely used pesticides, including a number of widely used compounds classified by the EPA as probable human carcinogens."[17] With regards to its own monitoring, the FDA says it is "impossible to monitor routinely for all possible chemical residues and to detect and remove each and every shipment of food and feed that might contain illegal residues."[18]

Even at legal levels, pesticides can be dangerous; but much of our food is likely to contain illegaly high levels of residues. There is no real safeguard to keep agribusiness farming from polluting our food with prohibited chemicals or illegal amounts of allowed chemicals. The potential for abuse is wide open. Many cases have, in fact, arisen where our own farmers have violated federal and state regulations in their pest control practices. And even when illegal residues are found, penalties are minor or nonexistent. For instance, in California in 1988, state inspectors recorded 9,287 violations of pesticide laws but issued only 600 fines.[19] And they were checking just a tiny fraction of all the food produced. Imagine how much illegal residue gets through that no one ever knows about!

Imported food from Mexico and other countries is even worse. Many countries don't even have tolerance levels, and their food can contain residues of pesticides that are outright banned in the United States because of their cancer risk. (Such pesticides include DDT, DDE, aldrin, dieldrin, stroban, mirex, chlordane, heptachlor, and others.) Imported food makes up a larger part of our food supply now than in the past.

As you can see, huge gaps exist in the monitoring of residues in our food supply. Despite the exposure studies that have been done, there is actually very little known about the quantity of pesticides we are getting through our food.

FDA Cover-Up

The FDA is clearly unable to monitor the food supply adequately for residues. Interestingly, the FDA has tried to skirt the whole issue of its inability to control pesticides by claiming that "natural carcinogens" that exist in food pose a greater cancer risk than spray residues and, therefore, it doesn't really matter anyway if they can't control pesticide residues. Don't you believe it.

Those spurious claims were based on the guesswork of FDA toxicologist Robert Scheuplein, who literally picked numbers out of his head to determine them. Naturally, he didn't take into account the additive and synergistic effects of numerous residues that greatly increase risk or the fact that many illegal residues are likely to get through FDA monitoring. But even ignoring this, and assuming the risk of cancer is as the EPA has estimated it to be, the FDA's claims don't hold water.

It's true that some natural chemicals have been identified by the International Agency for Research on Cancer as "possible" or "probable human carcinogens." These are found in bracken fern, ragwort, groundsel, rattlebox, and some wild mushrooms—none of which you're ever likely to eat. The fact is that the majority of natural chemicals found in everyday food are not even classified as "possibly carcinogenic," yet Scheuplein went ahead and considered them carcinogenic anyway.

He also assumed there are thousands of unknown natural carcinogens out there in food when there is, in fact, no evidence of that at all. The reason there is no evidence is because it is highly unlikely. The reason certain substances have been chosen for testing in the first place is because evidence has suggested they might be carcinogenic. Scheuplein's assumptions are pure speculation and bad science. But if that wasn't enough, he went on to make more outrageous assumptions.

He literally guessed at how much "natural carcinogens" we are likely to ingest, what their concentrations are, and what they will do in our body. Of course, most of what he considered natural carcinogens really are not. How does a figure 10,000 times more carcinogens from food than from pesticides sound? Sound good? Okay, that's what we'll use. That is what Robert Scheuplein did. Where did he get this from? He guessed! What about the potency of "natural carcinogens" compared with pesticides? It is known by science that true natural carcinogens as they are found in nature are far less potent than pesticides. Despite that fact, Scheuplein made sure all his estimates would show that food is more dangerous than pesticides. How did he do this? By essentially guessing.

As if that wasn't enough, the media misquoted him as saying that 98 percent of all cancer risk comes from natural carcinogens, but he didn't say that at all. He actually said he thought 98 percent of the risk of initiation of cancer might come from natural carcinogens. Risk of initiation is very different than total risk, because initiation is only half of what it takes to cause cancer. (The other half is a process known as promotion.)

What's really ridiculous about his claim is that many of the foods he says have "natural carcinogens," such as some vegetables, fruits, and grains, are the very foods that have proven to give us substantial protection against cancer. And Scheuplein himself admits we should eat more of those foods.

Some of Scheuplein's "natural carcinogens" are, indeed, potent carcinogens but are not natural at all. Meat that is grilled, charbroiled, cooked in smoke, or burnt anywhere creates cancer-causing polycyclic hydrocarbons—not exactly natural. Seafood that is smoked or grilled forms polyaromatic hydrocarbons. Meat with nitrites added to it, such as bacon, forms carcinogenic nitrosamines when cooked at high temperatures. None of those can be considered "natural" by any stretch of the imagination. Some of the other substances he bases his claim on are found in certain herbs and spices that are used sparingly anyway; cyto and myto-toxins, which result from spoiling food; and nitrates, which, while not carcinogens, can be turned into carcinogens—but there is little risk from this. Besides, nitrates are primarily found because of commercial agricultural practices anyway.

Any chemicals that are found naturally in foods normally consumed have been a part of the food chain for over a hundred million years and pose no risk. That is why animals on their natural diets never get cancer. Most pesticides, on the other hand, are concentrated and virulent poisons that have been created intentionally to kill animal and plant life. (For example, a dose of Albicarb one-fourth the size of an aspirin tablet will kill a grown man.) Instead of trying to cover up the danger of pesticides, the FDA should get on with its job.

WHAT PESTICIDES CAN DO TO US

Why are pesticides bad? What can they do to us? A prime risk is that DNA in the cells will mutate, which can eventually lead to cancer.[20]

Cancer is the end result of many factors. Cancer does not result from a single "hit" upon DNA; rather, multiple exposures must occur, leading to more than one mutation. This is known as initiation, but even this does not cause cancer. A DNA molecule that has been turned into a pre-cancerous cell will not turn into cancer on its own. The DNA can still be repaired. A pre-cancerous cell must continually be acted upon by promoters before a cancerous tumor finally develops. Promoters will not cause a tumor but promote its growth once a tumor exists. Two intensely studied promoters of cancer in the human body are high levels of animal fat and animal protein in the diet.

All those forces working together in the body cause cancer. The synergistic action of many tiny doses of pesticides may lead to many mutations, which can be a contributing factor to many types of cancer. However, if your exposure to pesticides is not excessive and your diet is otherwise healthy, DNA will be repaired without any tumor formation. No cancer has pesticides as its sole cause, but pesticides can be one of many factors in the total number of all cancers.

Pesticides also alter immune function (making us more vulnerable to disease), disrupt the nervous system, affect behavior, cause allergic reactions, and affect the body in other ways.[21]

Perhaps the greatest puzzle about pesticides is their potential to react with genetic material. Pesticides or pesticide intermediates (metabolites) acting in this way are called mutagens and have the potential of producing changes in our genetic makeup which may not be manifested for several generations. The text *Effects of Chronic Exposures to Pesticides on Animal Systems* tells us, "Pesticides could cause alterations in an individual's normal physiology, biochemistry, or behavior, or in the genetic material that an individual could pass on to future generations."[22]

The role of genetic illness is now becoming more apparent, with around 6 percent of all illness having a genetic factor.[23] And the more a disease is due to genetics, rather than environmental factors, the harder it is to prevent or cure. Present generations might now be seeing the effects of faulty genetic material that was first passed down forty years ago when pesticides came into heavy use.

A New Pesticide Menace

In 1989, the Mexican government rescinded long-term laws that had severely restricted foreigners from owning and operating agricultural land in Mexico. Now, Americans can buy, own, and operate farms in Mexico without restriction. Big investment money is reportedly going south of the border to buy up large fertile tracts of land for growing labor-intensive crops such as vegetables and fruits for which harvest is not mechanized.

There is a distinct competitive edge to farming operations in Mexico, which has cheap and plentiful labor but no social or environmental legislation with which to contend. On the United States side of the border, the minimum wage per hour may be eight to ten times higher than the rate at which the same labor can be had in Mexico.

These events promise to wipe out from the United States thousands of acres of farming that would require lots of hand labor. Over time, California will lose an estimated 50 percent of its market because of this. The inevitable result is that what is now grown in the United States will soon come from Mexico.

The ominous side effect is that there is no Environmental Protection Agency in Mexico. Growers there can use anything, anytime they want. Many chemicals, such as DDT and other organochlorine pesticides, are banned here but not banned there at all. This means that much of the produce you buy in the supermarket in the near future will likely be Mexican-grown and carry a nice thick layer of pesticide residues. Any meat from Mexico or other countries where organochlorine pesticides such as DDT are still in use will also contain residues in concentrations of ten times or more than what's in produce.[1]

With that in mind, it pays to grow as much of your own food as possible or to buy locally grown organic food whenever you can.

CONCLUSION

In summary, here is what we know about pesticides:

- Two-thirds of all pesticide ingredients on the market are not registered under current standards, and re-registration could take decades.
- Of the pesticide ingredients registered under current standards, a significant number are recognized as capable of causing tumors in laboratory animals.
- If the older pesticides were registered under current standards, many would be taken off the market or have their tolerances lowered because of carcinogenic risks.

- The assumptions used in setting legal tolerances are arbitrary and do not relfect actual cancer risk.
- The assumptions used in setting the Acceptable Daily Intakes do not take into account multiple exposures to other pesticides and synergistic actions between them although we are commonly exposed to many pesticide ingredients. This makes the EPA's tolerance levels of little value.
- The FDA checks only .002 percent of our food supply and most of the time just for three pesticides out of hundreds.
- Pesticides may interact synergistically and cause mutations leading to cancer or pass on defective genetic material to future generations.
- Moderate exposure to pesticides will probably not cause any permanent damage, because the body can repair damaged DNA and cleanse itself *if the diet is otherwise healthy.*

Even if the body can tolerate a certain exposure to pesticides, it's still wise to limit your exposure as much as possible, and the best

How to Get More Food Than You Can Grow

Would you like to have more fresh vegetables, fruits, and legumes grown with PowerCharged methods but don't have the time or space? Consider hiring someone to grow PowerCharged food for you. You can form a cooperative with some friends and hire a local farmer or someone with a large garden to grow some food for you using the methods in this book.

This is called consumer-supported agriculture, and it's becoming very popular. In 1990, NBC news reported on a big consumer co-op in Kimberton, Pennsylvania, involving forty families. Each family pays $375 a year to a small-scale local farmer and gets 500 pounds of fresh, spray-free fruits and vegetables as its share of the harvest. The farmer loves it because he's guaranteed a livelihood, and families living in a city enjoy getting to drive out to the country and pick organically grown food. Many city dwellers say this restores their sense of closeness to the land.

If you want to do this, make sure you find a grower who's willing to follow the methods in this book to grow a high level of minerals into the food and do it without sprays. Most farmers have not thought about growing food for maximum nutrition. They need to have an open mind and be eager to follow these scientifically proven methods.

way to do that is to grow as much of your own food as you can. You can also buy food labeled "organic" if you can afford it—it's often twice the cost—and if you know it is, in fact, organic. Some food sold as "organic" and said to be free of residues often is not.[24] Usually this is due to residue drift from adjacent farms and/or uptake from soils still containing pesticides even though applications have been stopped. As more states institute organic certification programs, a greater certainy may be brought to food sold as "organic."

Chlorinated hydrocarbons (organochlorines), known to be the worst type of pesticides, are still regularly found in meat in the United States despite large cutbacks in their use.[25] Also, animals are fed many crops that have been treated with fungicides for which there are no tolerances at all.[26] Of the total pounds of fungicides used, 90 percent are oncogenic, or tumor-forming.

Since a small amount of residues in plant tissue can become concentrated in animal tissues, consumption of animal tissue has been the chief source of pesticide contamination.[27] The main contaminant has been chlorinated hydrocarbons, which concentrate in animal tissues greatly. To this day, feed crops still pass chlorinated hydrocarbons on to animal tissue from residues that persist in the soil even when applications of chlorinated hydrocarbons have long since stopped.

In the United States, the one food you can buy that contains less residues than any other class of food is legumes.[28] Legumes, which include beans, peas, and lentils, are one of the healthiest foods on Earth, and we encourage you to grow and eat them. No single food is higher in protein, vitamins, minerals, fiber, and complex carbohydrates. Legumes are also low in fat and contain no cholesterol.

Now that you know how important growing your own spray-free, PowerCharged food is, let's start a new garden. . . .

5. *Site Selection and Layout*

WE'RE addressing this chapter to two kinds of gardeners: those who are already growing and those who would like to start. If you are already gardening, you might have already carried out most of the instructions here; if so, you can speed-read this chapter, catch only what interests you, and go on to the advanced gardening sections that follow.

If you just dabble in gardening but wish to get into it, this chapter is for you. Read all of it carefully. If you carry out the suggestions, you will be well along on the road to success in growing PowerCharged food.

Don't let the idea of an outdoor garden scare you off. You won't believe how much you can grow even in a tiny garden. Even a small flower bed is good. We like to have a square-shaped garden anywhere from 8 to 24 feet square, but some gardeners prefer larger gardens, from 32 to 64 feet square. And if that is not big enough, you can place two squares end-to-end to make a rectangle. We suggest you start with a square-shaped plot because it allows for the most efficient use of irrigation during long, hot, rainless summer months. You can also use flower beds that can be irrigated with drip irrigation lines.

PICK A SPOT

The first thing to do is find an area in the yard that's well away from trees and shrubs. Trees and shrubs are wonderful to have in a backyard but don't coexist well with a food garden. Trees and shrubs block out the sun, and their roots compete with your vegetables for water and nutrients. Shrubs and vines might also harbor insect pests and create a bird problem. If your yard is full of trees and shrubs and you really want to get into gardening, consider finding a house with a backyard not filled with trees. If no open area is available and moving is not practical, use scattered beds.

HARDPAN

Hidden under the soil surface sometimes is a layer of hard, cement-like material called hardpan or caliche. This stops subsurface drainage and interferes with root growth. To check a site for hardpan, sprinkle the soil thoroughly with water and use a posthole digger to see if you can dig a deep hole down to 36 inches without hitting hardpan. If hardpan is found, you will have to find another spot, move in heavy machinery to break it up, or use raised beds. (For details on raised beds, see "Raised Beds" inset beginning on page 54.)

LAYOUTS

You will need to choose a layout for your beds. The size, shape, and tilt of your land will help determine the best placement for your beds.

Beds Together Layout

If possible, put all your beds together side-by-side in a square or rectangle, for the sake of convenience and efficiency. (See Figure 5.1.) Some people believe there is magic in a circular garden; even if there is, we doubt there is enough difference to make it worth the inconvenience with which you would have to contend.

The minimum size you would want is about 10 by 10 (feet). A 20-by-20 square is an excellent choice if you have the space. It gives you room to plant a decent variety of food; and when you put it together with another square the same size, you get 800 square feet, which is a good size for a family. If you're just starting out or have limited space, consider a 20-by-10 or a 10-by-20 rectangle. Many beginners try to grow areas too big for them to handle. They then get discouraged, the weeds move in, and they give up. Don't let that happen to you. It is better to grow a single bed 2 by 8 or 4 by 8 and do it right than to have a larger plot with which you can't keep up.

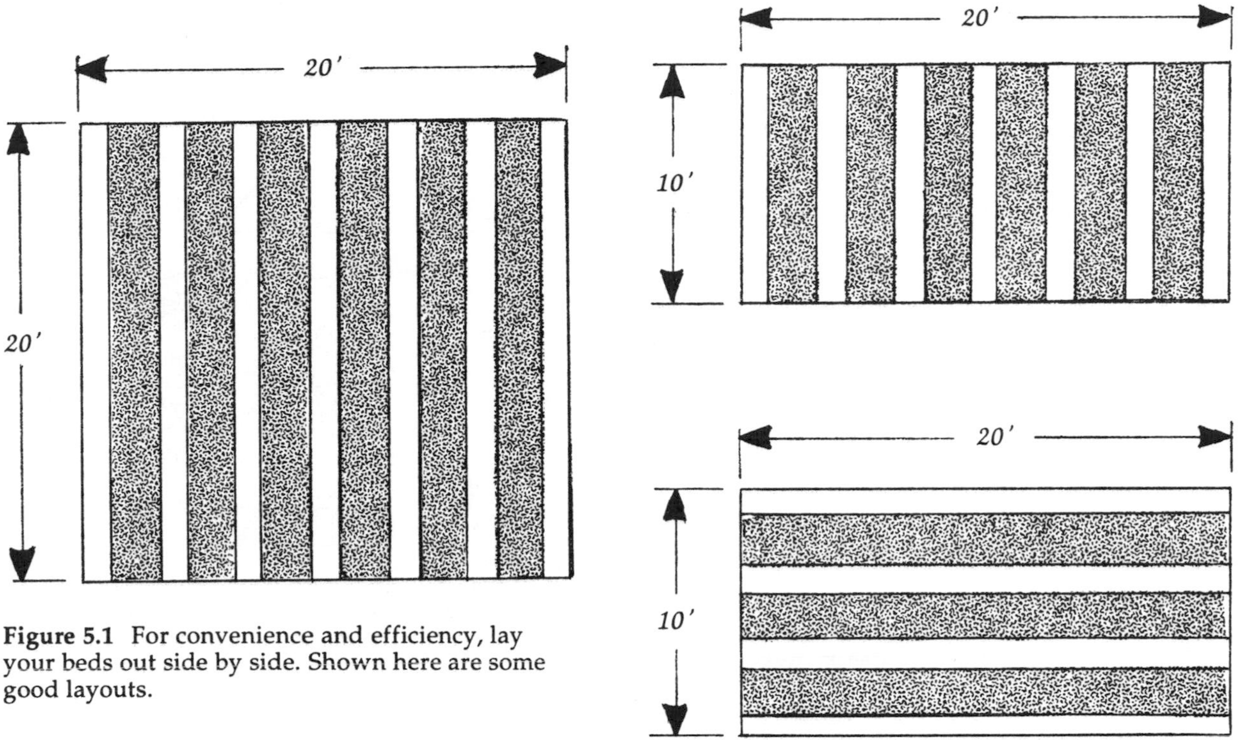

Figure 5.1 For convenience and efficiency, lay your beds out side by side. Shown here are some good layouts.

Scattered Beds Layout

Many backyards do not offer the open spaces that would allow for all the beds to be together side-by-side. Instead, there will be strips of open space here and there where you can make scattered beds. (See Figure 5.2.) Often, there are strips of good soil along the back and side fences or between shrubs. If you locate a bed near a tree or shrub, try to place it at least five or six feet from the drip line of the tree or shrub. (The drip line of a tree or shrub is a usually circular line on the soil surface beneath the tips of the branches all around the tree or shrub. For details on irrigation drip lines, which are quite different, see Chapter 12.)

Sloping Sites

If you have a hillside for a garden spot, make sure you run your beds across the slope, not down it, to prevent erosion. If the site is quite steep, you will need to use terrace gardening, whereby you build retaining walls of two-inch lumber or concrete blocks.

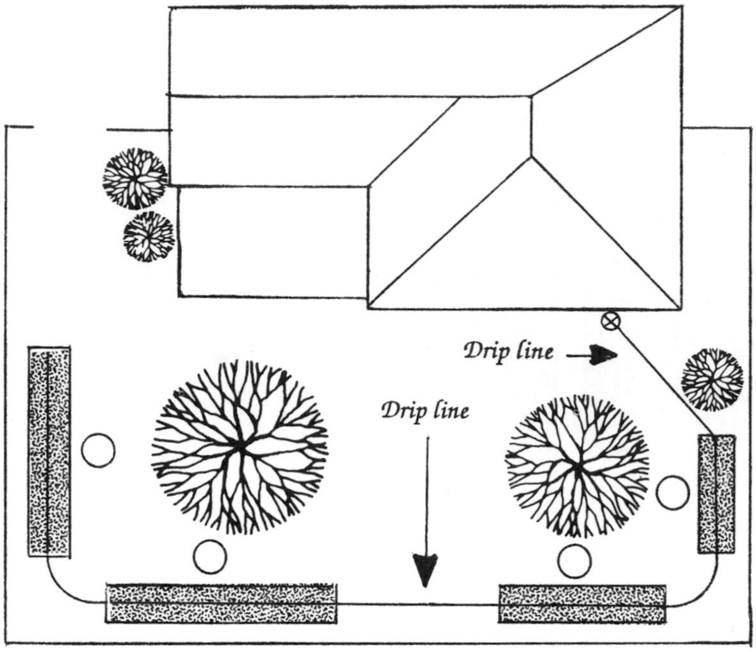

Figure 5.2 If you have no open area, use scattered beds. The scattered beds shown are under drip irrigation.

Permanent Beds

We always use permanent beds in our gardens and strongly recommend you do the same. Permanent beds are strips of soil that, once loosened and enriched, are never walked on again—except maybe once a year for working soil amendments or fertilizers into the soil. The walkways between the beds are never worked and provide permanent access.

BED WIDTH

You will see various bed widths advised, all the way from 16 to 60 inches. Since beds must alternate with walkways, you want a bed as wide as practical for more growing space. Suitable bed widths are based on the comfortable reach of the human arm. The typical reach is around 18 inches. That means if a bed can be reached from both sides, the maximum bed width should be 48 inches. But if the bed can be reached from only one side, the maximum width should be about 24 inches. If you go beyond those widths you will find it awkward to reach the center area of the bed and will have to lay boards on the surface of your nice loose beds to stand or squat on while you work the beds.

When deciding on bed width, one consideration is the use of a rototiller. We like a 36-inch-wide bed because our tiller tills 36 inches wide, but most standard tillers leave a tilled swath 24 inches wide. For that reason, you might want to use 24-inch-wide beds. In the following chapters, we will deal with 24-inch beds alternating with 16-

inch walkways for beds that are flat and neither raised nor sunken. (For more information on beds 36 inches wide, see Appendix E.) If beds are raised or sunken, walkways must be made wider for the curbs or for the sloping sides of the beds. (For more information on sunken beds, see the "Sunken Beds" inset on page 59.)

PERMANENT WALKWAYS

It is a good idea to loosen and fertilize all the soil inside your square growing area at the beginning, when you're first preparing it. But after that, permanent walkways need never be tilled again. Why till a walkway when all you will do is tramp it down again? You will see various walkway widths advised, some as narrow as 12 inches. The average person's foot with shoes on is not far from 12 inches long, and with 12-inch walkways your feet will inevitably get into the growing beds and pack them down. The best workable width for walkways is 16 to 20 inches.

SQUARE-FOOT GARDENING

This method calls for laying off small squares 4 feet per side, then marking off sixteen 12-inch squares inside the 4-foot squares. Then 12-inch walkways are placed around the outside of the 4-by-4 plot. This is the same as making a bed 48 inches wide, then breaking it into lengths 4 feet long. You can get a better effect by making beds 24 to 36 inches wide, then marking them off into segments 2 to 3 feet long with small skinny boards. (See Figure 5.3.)

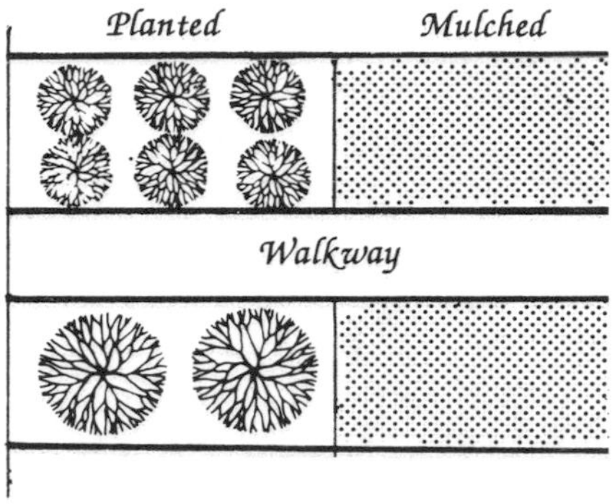

Figure 5.3 To get the same effect as a square-foot garden, you can mark off your beds in two- to three-foot sections. To keep out weeds, mulch any sections you're not using.

The square-foot method advocates using boards for the 12-inch walkways (which are really too narrow), but have you tried to buy or beg lumber lately? It certainly is too expensive to buy for boardwalks when the ground will do just as well. Besides, if the boards are nailed together, there will be a space that will harbor all kinds of insect pests.

The argument in favor of the square-foot system is that with standard beds, people get discouraged when they see a whole bed to be planted, so they plant part of it and let the rest grow up in weeds. But weeds do not come into a garden because of long beds, nor will they be kept out by square-foot gardening. Weeds are due to poor management.

Keep your garden small enough to handle. If you can afford the energy, time, and mulch for only one bed, by all means do your growing on just one bed. Keep the unplanted parts of beds mulched, and your seed problems will vanish like the morning dew. (To learn how to mulch, see Chapter 10.)

For small-plot growing interspersed and coordinated into an ornamental landscape plan, a few 4-foot squares can be useful for closely spaced plants such as lettuce, green onions, carrots, or herbs like

Raised Beds

We have gardened in all the major regions of the United States with great success while rarely ever using raised beds. We simply did "gardening on the flat," with our beds at the natural ground level. Most of you can do the same. Raised beds are hard to build and hard to maintain, so our advice is to try it on the flat first. But there are special situations where you need raised beds:

- Flat terrain with poor surface drainage, high rainfall, and slow runoff.
- Poor subsurface drainage due to a high water table or hardpan, so the soil stays soggy. (Dig a posthole 30 inches deep. If you strike water, you will need raised beds. If you don't strike water, then fill the hole with water; if it does not drain dry in 24 hours, you will need raised beds.)
- Lack of true soil—for instance, you have coarse sand or rocky or gravelly soil.
- Shallow soil. (Less than 18 inches deep.)
- You want to grow specialty crops such as herbs, which require small raised beds.
- Handicap situations or elderly persons with mobility limited so they need to sit on the edge of a concrete-block bed while they experience the joys of gardening.

BUILDING A RAISED BED

You can grow food in a bed that sits on a concrete slab if the bed is 16 inches deep and has drain holes at the bottom. But a more likely situtation is a rocky hillside where the soil is only a few inches deep. If that's the case, a good solution is to build a raised bed using redwood or concrete blocks. If using redwood, use lumber 2 inches thick by 10 feet long. (See Figure 1.)

If you use concrete blocks to make your bed, first lay a bed of sand 8 inches wide by 1 inch deep around the perimeter as a foundation for the blocks, and make this sand foundation perfectly level. Then sprinkle it down with water to make it firm. Use blocks 6 inches wide by 8 inches high and 16 inches long. If you lay the blocks two blocks high and make the ends three blocks wide and the sides sixteen blocks long, you end up with a bed with inside dimensions 16 inches deep by 36 inches wide by 21 feet, 3 inches long. For the second layer of blocks, be sure to stagger the joints. Fill the cells with something heavy, like dirt or sand, and you should not need mortar. Just stack them up. Though the depth of this bed is 16 inches, you get only 14 inches of net depth, because the bed is filled 2 inches down from the top. You can get by with the 14-inch net depth, but 18 is a lot better, so we hope you will have at least 4 inches of soil depth with which to begin.

The bed shown in Figure 1 when filled 14 inches deep requires about 100 cubic feet of soil mix and has about 64 square feet of growing surface. This bed takes some labor and expense to build and fill, but it will be the best investment can make if you have a situation calling for a raised bed. You'll be amazed at how much you can grow in this bed, which has the growing area of 128 ten-inch pots!

Curbs or No Curbs?

If you want to make a raised bed only 6 inches high without using curbs, you must make the bottom 36 inches wide to get a top bed width of 24 inches. (See Figure 2.) You can overcome this drawback by using wood curbs of 2-inch by 6-inch rot-proofed lumber. (See Figure 3.)

BASIC RAISED-BED SOIL MIX

What an opportunity for you to make the best soil you have ever made! You can tailor-make the ideal soil. It will be far superior to most garden soils. The first ingredient is good topsoil, the best topsoil you can find, hopefully a good loam. Next best is fine sandy loam, but you can even use plain sandy soil if it is not coarse sand.

The next ingredient is a soil amendment to keep your soil loose, mellow, and high in water-holding capacity. You can use vermiculite, peat moss, or finely ground bark. We prefer vermiculite because it stays in the soil without breaking down. If you use vermiculite, be sure it is horticultural grade, and buy it in the biggest bags or bales you can find. If you use bark, mix in 1 pound of

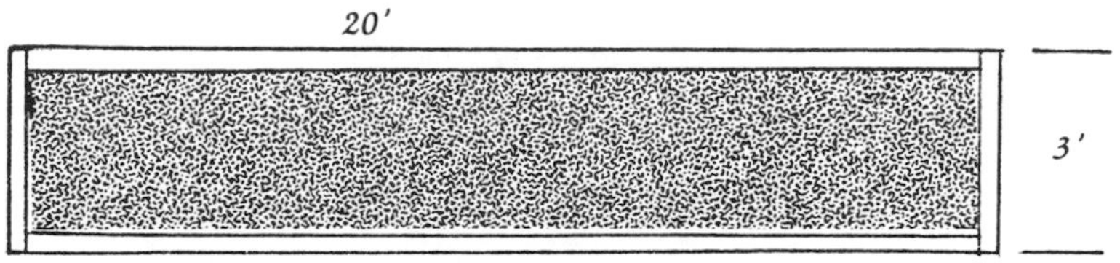

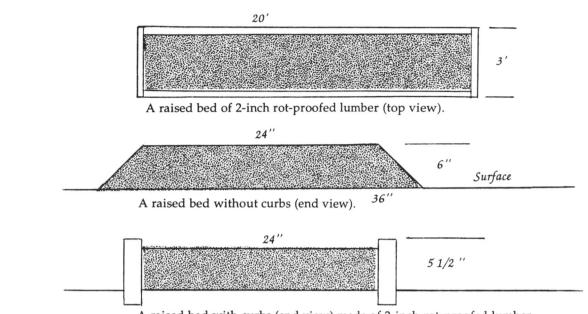

A raised bed of 2-inch rot-proofed lumber (top view).

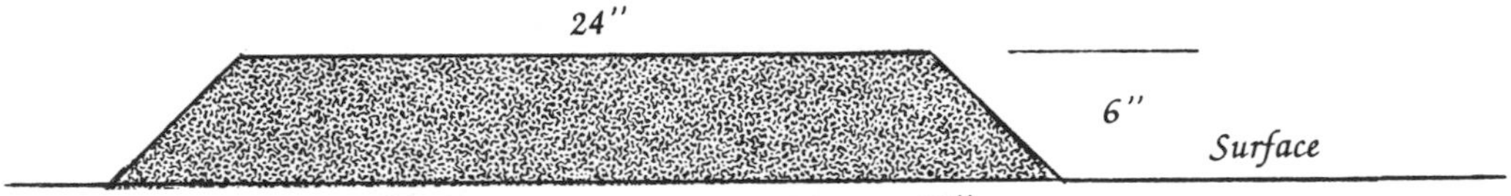

A raised bed without curbs (end view).

A raised bed with curbs (end view) made of 2-inch rot-proofed lumber.

actual nitrogen per 10 cubic feet to prevent nitrogen deficiency and supply phosphorus. A good fertilizer to use is one with an NPK analysis (explained in Chapter 6) such as 16-20-0. The composting organisms need both nitrogen and phosphorus to compost the bark.

When using ground bark, to get the 1 pound of actual nitrogen, spread the bark in a layer on a concrete slab, moisten it, and mix with a flat-point shovel. For each 10 cubic feet of bark, broadcast 6.25 pounds of 16-20-0 evenly on top of the layer of bark and mix again.

The bark and nitrogen-phosphorus mixture will need to incubate for at least three weeks at growing temperatures before planting. Incubation can be done in the soil, in a compost pile, or in a large plastic garbage can or pot with a drain hole at the bottom.

The basic mix to use for filling your raised bed is fifteen parts of topsoil to five parts of soil amendment. Parts can be gallons, shovel scoops, or any other measure of volume. We use a square-point shovel to shovel fifteen scoops of topsoil onto a concrete slab and rake it into a layer. Then we throw five scoops of vermiculite over the topsoil, spread it out, moisten it, then mix the two thoroughly. That makes 20 cubic feet, which goes into a wheelbarrow, then into the bed. Filling the bed takes a while, but take your time and know you are building a superior soil that will last for years. Fill your bed to within 2 inches of the top. Store any leftover mix in plastic bags and label them.

Topsoil Quality

Watch out for topsoil these days. For all you know, it may have come from a hazardous waste dump. Check it out before you have it delivered. It should be free of rocks, gravel, and debris. It might pay to send a soil sample to a good soils lab for a complete test. (See Appendix A for names of labs.) We know a man who bought a bunch of topsoil only to find it came from a former dump site and was terribly polluted.

CHARGE YOUR RAISED BEDS

You have just taken care of the structure of your soil by filling your bed with the basic mix. Now is the time to take care of the chemistry. In short, now is the time to PowerCharge your bed by injecting into it a good organic fertilizer (cottonseed meal), inoculating it with life (compost or dairy manure), and adding a small but potent dose of seaweed meal to provide over a a dozen trace elements essential for healthy, productive plant growth.

Table 5.1 shows the recipe for charging your basic raised-bed soil mix. The recipe for 100 cubic feet fills the bed shown in Figure 1 when filled 14 inches deep.

Table 5.1
Charging Raised-Bed Soil Mix

Ingredient	Amount to Use Per 100 Cubic Feet	Amount to Use Per 10 Cubic Feet
Cottonseed Meal	4 gallons	6.5 cups
Activator *	4 gallons	6.5 cups
Seaweed Meal	Quarter cup	1 teaspoon

* = Non-sterilized compost or dairy manure.

Mix the ingredients, moisten, spread evenly on the surface of the bed, and mix into the soil immediately 10 inches deep with a spading fork so the sun won't kill the soil life.

The Charging Ingredients

We like cottonseed meal as an organic fertilizer to supply the nitrogen, phosphorus, and potassium. Its analysis is 6.5–3–1.5. Garden centers sell this yellowish material in 5-pound bags, but we use so much of it we buy it in 50-pound bags from a feed store at much less cost. Feed stores are found even near big cities, in the outskirts. Where there are horses, there will be feed stores and free horse manure as well, if you can figure out a way to haul it.

The activator, though not essential, is very helpful to charge the bed with beneficial organisms. But it must not be heat-treated, since heat kills the beneficial organisms. Avoid bagged manure.

The seaweed meal supplies a dozen or more important trace elements not found in most soils or fertilizers. But it is very potent, so don't overdo it. Follow the recipe as shown and mix the small amount of seaweed meal thoroughly with the other ingredients before adding it to the bed.

BALANCING YOUR CHARGED SOIL

Plants grow best at a pH of 6 (slightly acid) to 7 (neutral). A soil pH of 6.5 is ideal and should be your target. Your soil pH may be all right, but if not, we suggest you adjust it to 6.5. This involves taking a soil sample for a simple test you can do yourself, or sending a sample off to a soils lab and getting a consultant to balance your soil. (See Chapter 6 for details.)

WATERING DOWN

When a raised bed is first filled, it is full of air and is so fluffy that it always settles down when watered. After you mix all the ingredients into your bed, water your bed down with a bubbler on the end of a hose. After all the water has soaked in, you'll be able to see the low places. Fill those with some of the basic soil mix and rake level so the surface is about 2 inches from the top of the bed. We like to make our bed surfaces perfectly level by using a wooden screed. Drag it along your bed, and it will leave an even, level surface a little bit down from the top of the bed. The empty space above the bed surface is a mulching and watering basin.

mint. For serious growing, though, your best bet is still on a bed or beds 24 to 36 inches wide by 8 to 24 feet long alternating with 16- to 20-inch walkways.

SITE PREPARATION

You have picked your growing spot or spots, and now you are ready to drive stakes to mark off the boundaries. To make this easy, get yourself a dozen 12-inch spikes from a hardware store, a hammer or hatchet, and some twine.

If all your beds are going to be together in a square or rectangular garden, lightly drive a spike at each corner. You can pace the distance between each corner to end up with an approximate square or rectangle. Then stretch twine around the four corner spikes. To make sure the plot is square, each diagonal should be the same length. (See Figure 5.4.) You can move the spikes around until the diagonals are of equal length. If you have to go for scattered beds, drive spikes at the four corners of each bed.

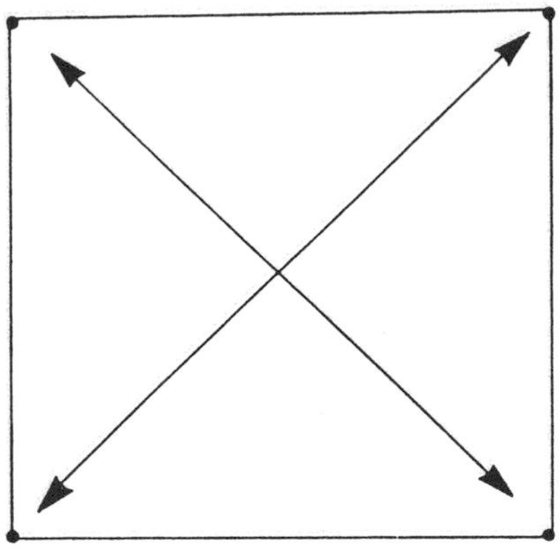

Figure 5.4 Lightly drive four stakes around your garden area. When the two diagonals in a plot are the same length, the plot is square. For example, in a 20-foot by 20-foot plot, both diagonals should be 28 feet, 3 inches.

PERENNIAL WEED REMOVAL

With most grasses and weeds, if you just rototill them under or cut the roots off with a hoe, you will never see them again. But in some areas, especially the South, sod is likely to be Bermuda grass and may also be infested with Johnson grass, bindweed, and nut sedge. All those weedy pest plants have something in common that makes them villians in your food plot: they all form fleshy, underground storage organs that generate new plants when you cut off the top of the plant. If you rototill an infested area and the tiller cuts an underground storage organ, such as a rhizome, into twenty parts, you get twenty new plants. It is important to kill those weeds before you go any further. If you're not sure you have them, the next growing season will show you.

If you have those weed pests, don't plant anything in the infested area. Instead, begin a weed removal program. You'll have to choose from two approaches: the mechanical way, which is hard work and time consuming; or the chemical way.

Mechanical Methods

There are three mechanical methods for removing perennial weeds.

One is mulching, where you lay large pieces of heavy black plastic sheeting over the infested area and cover the edges with two-by-fours to exclude all light. Mulch for the entire growing season until all the weeds are dead.

You can also cut your growing size way down, dig up the soil, and pick the rhizomes or other thickened underground parts out by hand or run the soil through a half-inch sieve. That is the way for you martyrs out there.

You can also go through your plot every week with a sharp hoe and continuously cut the weeds out until they're all dead. That might take an entire growing season.

The Chemical Way

By far, the quickest and easiest way to get rid of perennial weeds is to spray an herbicide called Roundup (glyphosate) on the leaves of the weeds when they are actively growing. Roundup is non-selective—it kills any green leaf it touches. It is systemic. That means the green leaves of the weed absorb the chemical, which circulates throughout all parts of the plant and kills the fleshy underground storage organs.

The good news for organic gardeners and environmentalists is that Roundup is applied within only a two-week period and is inactivated when it strikes the soil. It is *not* used over and over again, year after year; and, unlike many chemicals, it does not persist in the soil. You only use it once, when preparing your site. It will never have contact with any of your food plants.

To use Roundup effectively, wait until the weed you want to kill is growing vigorously, then spray the leaves thoroughly early in the morning when humidity is high and winds are down. Don't get impatient. Roundup works very slowly but very surely. You might see no change in the weed for a week, but within about ten days you'll see the green begin to disappear as the weed's leaves die. You will probably miss some spots, and those will show up as small islands of green; so mix up another small batch of spray and do those areas again.

Roundup kills any plant it touches, so be careful. If there are plants nearby that you want to protect, cover them with plastic. We recommend that you buy full-strength Roundup and mix it according to the label. It is the only herbicide we recommend, since it's a one-time thing, is non-persistent, and kills troublesome weeds, roots and all.

It is very important to use a stainless steel or plastic sprayer only. Use of a galvanized sprayer might generate explosive gases. Get a compression, pump-up type of sprayer. Do not use hose-end sprayers.

Follow-Up

For follow-up, use a hoe or deep mulch to prevent the survival of weed plants that arise from seed. Those seeds might already be in the soil or can blow in; if you let them grow, they will make seeds and regrow those bothersome underground storage organs. Weeds that arise from seeds are easy to control, since all you have to do is cut them off at the surface or throw some hay mulch on them and they die.

Sunken Beds

If you live in the arid West where the average annual rainfall is 20 inches a year or less and you want to use flood irrigation, you will find the sunken bed useful. This bed is sunk about 2 inches below the surface to catch and hold every drop of the scanty, precious natural rainfall and hold irrigation water until it soaks in.

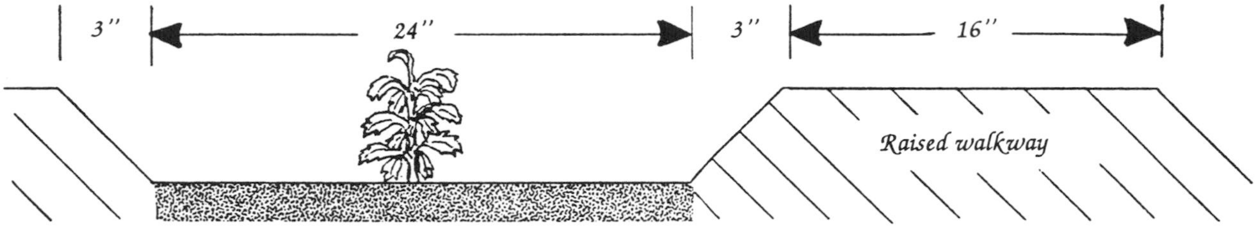

A 24-inch-wide sunken bed allows a 24-inch tomato cage to fit in the bed.

MINIMUM TILLAGE

We strongly recommend you grow plants with as little tillage as possible. Tillage means the mechanical loosening, stirring, or digging of the soil. The less you till your soil, the better; tillage disrupts soil structure by breaking up natural channels, and it discourages earthworms and their burrows.

We have used minimum tillage in our food gardens for years with excellent results and have used our rototiller only for bed preparation in the spring and sometimes in the fall for fall plantings. Cultivation to control weeds is best done by mulching. If you don't have mulch, a second choice is to shave off weeds at the surface with a sharp hoe.

LOOSENING THE SOIL

If no perennial weeds are present in the area you have staked off, all you need to do is rake it free of rocks and debris. Now is where a big powerful rear-tine rototiller takes over. If you had perennial weeds and have killed them with Roundup, the tiller can do the rest. If you have non-perennial grass or weeds, just rototill them under. For tough jobs, several passes might be necessary. Start by setting the depth control to shallow, and gradually increase it until you are loosening the soil the maximum depth, usually 6 to 7 inches. The deeper, the better.

Before arranging to rent a tiller and transport it to your yard, you might want to dig a hole about 18 inches deep to see what your soil

Figure 5.5

Loosening Your Soil With a Spading Fork

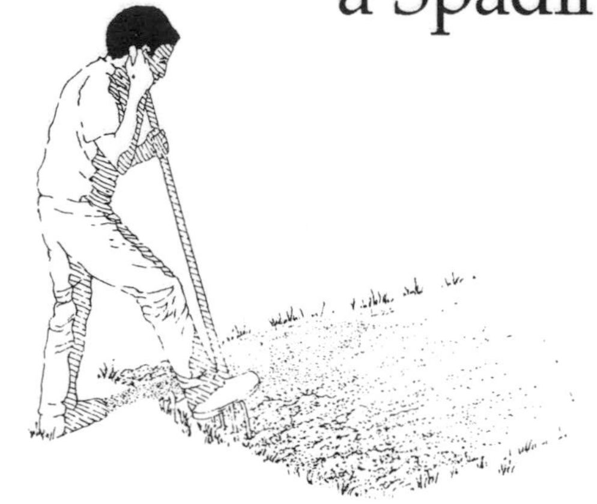

1. If you have only a small amount of bed space to loosen, you can use a spading fork. Push it down into the soil at one end of the bed.

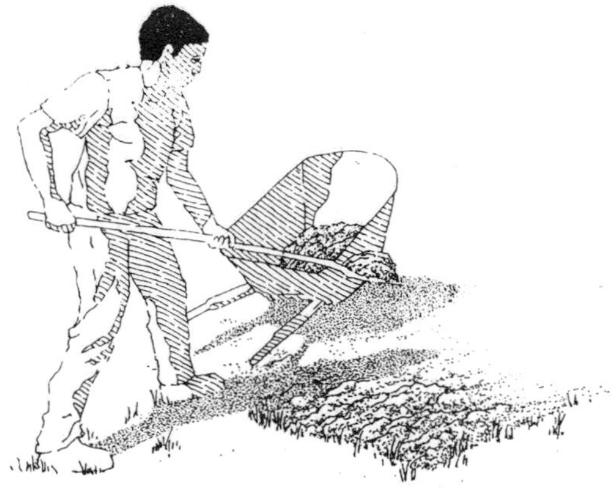

2. Pry up chunks of soil and throw them into a wheelbarrow.

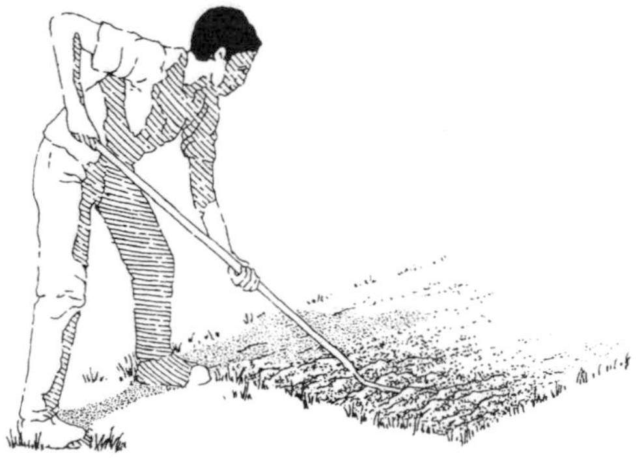

3. Spade the soil all the way across the bed.

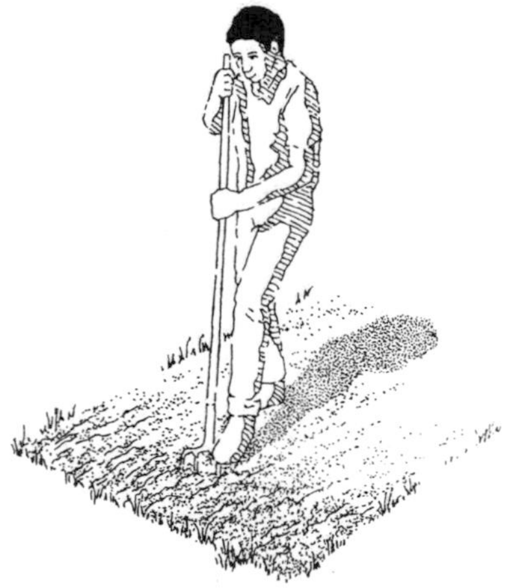

4. Reverse your position.

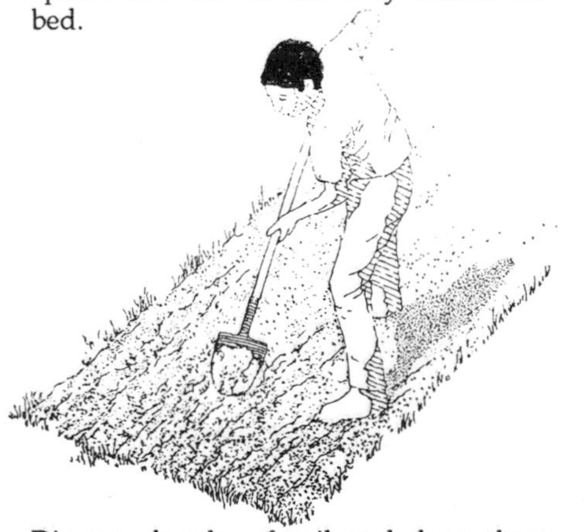

5. Dig up chunks of soil and drop them into the trench you just dug.

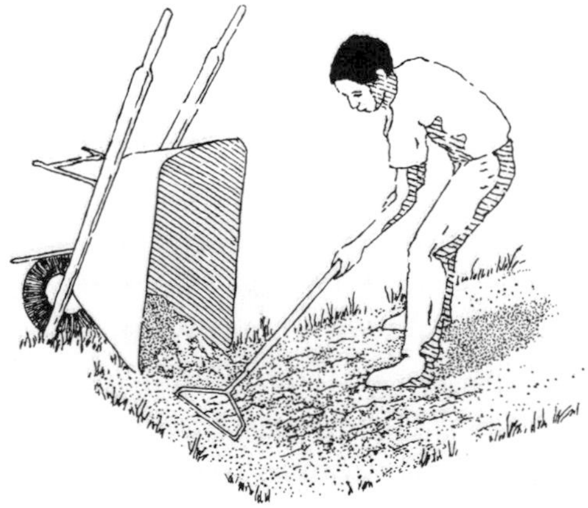

6. When the entire bed has been spaded, dump the soil from the wheelbarrow back into the bed, and rake it level.

is like. If it is gravelly or rocky, you might need to bring in tailor-made soil rather than loosen what you already have. If your test hole shows decent soil (see Chapter 6 for testing your soil) but has large rocks, you will need to rake out and remove the rocks as the rototiller unearths them.

For loosening the soil, a spading fork is suitable only if you're working a few small beds or reworking old beds that have been loosened within the past year or two. (See Figure 5.5.) But if your garden is going to be more than 50 to 100 square feet and loosened for the first time, then by all means use a powerful rear-tine tiller. After that, a short-handled spading fork will do a good job for you.

Double Digging

When you use a spading fork to spade garden soil, you usually go down about 10 inches. Some garden advisers suggest digging more than twice that deep, to about 24 inches. We don't know about you, but we're not about to dig that deep. Common sense and experience have proven to us that you don't need double digging to have a lush, productive garden. Yes, you do need good soil down to about 18 inches, but why do it mechanically with a great deal of back-breaking labor when nature will do it for you?

We have seen beautiful gardens created by rototilling permanent beds only 6 inches deep at the start of each season. The roots of plants, along with earthworms, do the rest. Unless there is hardpan, plant roots have no trouble penetrating the soil 24 inches or deeper.

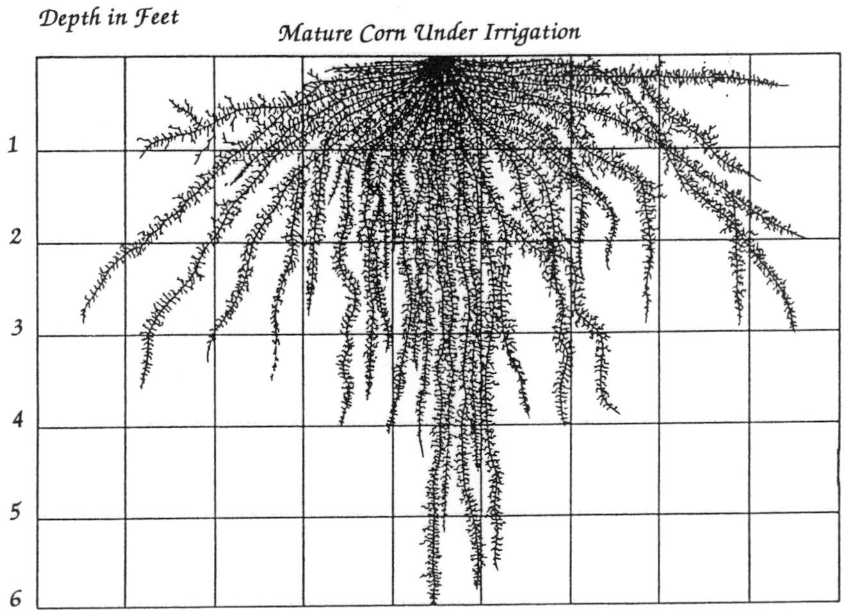

Figure 5.6 The roots of a mature corn plant will go down as much as 6 feet.

(Figure 5.6 shows that the roots of a mature corn plant will go down as much as 6 feet!) When roots die, they leave a small tunnel of organic matter. Earthworms in well-mulched garden soil will burrow down 24 to 36 inches along the root penetration. So why all this double digging? Biological gardening outlined in this book will do most of the digging you will ever need.

After your site is selected, the weeds removed, and the soil loosened, you're ready to get into the core of the PowerCharged method—charging your soil. . . .

6. *Charging Your Soil*

In this chapter you will learn a unique seven-step soil charging program that will enable you to grow food with the highest nutrition possible. The food produced by this new method is called PowerCharged food. PowerCharged food starts with the soil. Three things make a soil PowerCharged. First, PowerCharged soil contains the proper balance of all twenty-three nutrient elements needed for top plant and human health. Secondly, it contains the proper amount of organic matter. And finally, it is biologically active. These three factors interact in PowerCharged soil to produce food of superior nutritional quality.

HOW SOIL CHARGING RAISES NUTRITIONAL QUALITY

The soil is a storehouse of nutrients. It is like a kitchen with two pantries: one tiny, the other huge. The tiny pantry stores limited amounts of plant food and is called the soil solution; it is the watery solution between soil particles where plant roots feed. (See Figure 6.1.) The other pantry stores huge amounts of plant food and is composed of soil minerals and organic matter.

The key to growing food of superior nutrition is to stock the soil with nutrients through minerals and organic matter and then to unlock that storehouse of nutrients. Once this reservoir of nutrients is released into the soil solution, plant roots can easily absorb them.

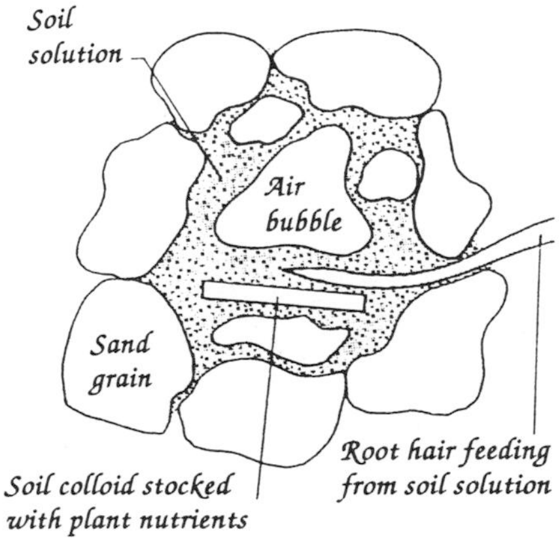

Figure 6.1 Plant root feeding from a soil solution containing colloid particles.

Unlocking this storehouse of nutrients requires soil microorganisms, or microbes. Microbes depend on organic matter to live. It's their source of food. As long as you have organic matter in your soil, you'll have microbes.

Microbes decompose organic matter and release nutrients into the soil solution in the form of electrically charged ions that were previously locked up in the organic matter. Microbial activity also breaks down the soil minerals into electrically charged ions that are released into the soil solution. Released nutrients are also stored on soil colloids, which are tiny soil particles that store nutrients readily available to plants. They're kind of like the plates on which food is served. The capacity of the soil to store nutrients on soil colloids is known as the soil's cation exchange capacity. The higher the cation exchange capacity, the more nutrients the soil can store.

Once the nutrients are in the soil solution or on soil colloids, they are easily absorbed by plants and converted into food that contains maximum levels of minerals, enzymes, vitamins, and protein. But without the help of microbes, most of the nutrients in the soil would stay locked up in the soil minerals and organic matter, making it hard for the plant roots to get them.

The first key to growing PowerCharged food, then, is to have soil high in organic matter that is biologically active with microorganisms. This is where the organic methods that rely heavily on organic matter make an important contribution to food quality. But organic matter is only half the story. Using lots of organic matter alone does not ensure food of high nutritional quality. There has to be an adequate amount and balance of nutrient elements in the soil to get food of high nutritional quality. Using locally produced organic matter or compost alone can just perpetuate existing soil deficiencies. How do you know if you have an adequate balance of nutrients in your soil? How do you know if essential trace minerals are present and available to your plants? Just putting organic matter in the soil alone is no guarantee. Organic matter can lack some essential nutrients.

In fact, you can get very unbalanced, inadequate soil by using organic matter without considering anything else. A great example of this is with nitrogen. Microorganisms in the soil that feed upon organic matter need about thirty parts of carbon to one part of nitrogen to do the best job of releasing nutrients into the soil solution. They use the carbon for energy as we would use carbohydrates, and they need the nitrogen for growth much as a youngster must have protein. Some organic matter has far too little nitrogen for the amount of carbon it contains. That forces the microorganisms to extract any existing nitrogen right out of your soil, causing a serious nitrogen deficiency. When that happens, microorganisms are said to have "robbed the soil of nitrogen." A proper amount and balance of

Test Results of PowerCharged Food

The nitrogen, phosphorus, and potassium supplied by chemical fertilizers today are being utilized poorly by plants in making nutritious food. They are overapplied and washed out of the soil quickly; there is a lack of organic matter and soil life to provide a steady stream of nutrients from the largest soil pantries; and depletion has often left the soil with inadequate amounts of many nutrients. As a result, our food is far less nutritious than it should be.

In our own research, we have regularly grown PowerCharged food that has nutrition two to twelve times higher than the levels shown in standard nutrition tables. The first table below shows the results of a test done in 1990 on tomatoes and romaine lettuce grown by Dr. Peavy, who prepared the beds according to the methods explained in this chapter. The samples were harvested, dried, and sent off to a lab along with some control samples. The lab determined the average values for five nutrients in the PowerCharged samples. (Lab analyses were done by A&L Labs, of Lubbock, Texas.)

The table compares those values with two other nutritional values given for the exact same foods: first, values shown in the 1975 edition of *Handbook of the Nutritional Contents of Foods* (Handbook 8) from the USDA; then, from the nutrition table appearing in the text *Understanding Nutrition* (Whitney and Hamilton, 1987), numbers based primarily on the newest 1985 and 1986 USDA nutrition tables.

The table shows two significant results. First, that by using the PowerCharged methods shown in this chapter you will be able to grow food 100 to 1,200 percent higher in mineral nutrition than shown in nutrition tables! Secondly, that for calcium, magnesium, and iron, there is a downward trend in mineral nutrition values going from the 1975 *Handbook 8* to the more recent values from 1985–1986 data. That indicates continuing soil depletion.

Interestingly, the PowerCharged samples also produced much higher values for protein. The second table below shows the percent of dry weight coming from protein in tomatoes and romaine lettuce. (Dry weight excludes weight coming from water.) The PowerCharged samples have about three times more protein than shown in *Handbook 8*. The gains in protein occur precisely because balanced plant nutrition interacts with organic matter and microorganisms to release a steady stream of nutrients to the plant.

Mineral Comparison (Milligrams per 100 grams of Fresh Weight)

	Potassium	Calcium	Magnesium	Iron	Zinc
Tomato					
PowerCharged	661	28.0	37.0	.91	.49
Handbook 8 (1975 data)	244	13.0	14.0	.50	—
Whitney (1985–1986 data)	207	7.3	11.4	.48	.11
Romaine Lettuce					
PowerCharged	1,117	290	72.0	1.6	.68
Handbook 8 (1975 data)	264	68	—	1.4	—
Whitney (1985–1986 data)	289	35.6	5.34	1.1	.32

Protein Comparison (Percent Protein in Dry Weight)

	Tomato	*Romaine Lettuce*
PowerCharged	17.6%	24.0%
Handbook 8	6.6%	7.8%

nutrients in the soil along with organic matter is vital in producing healthy plants and highly nutritious PowerCharged food.

DIFFERENCES BETWEEN COMMERCIAL AND POWERCHARGED METHODS

The PowerCharged method of providing optimal nutrition to plants contrasts sharply with conventional farming practices. Conventional farming uses very concentrated, synthetic forms of nitrogen, phosphorus, and potassium (NPK) fertilizer, usually as the sole source of nutrients to plants. Those fertilizers are commonly known as "chemical" fertilizers.

Chemical fertilizers, in and of themselves, are not necessarily bad if used properly. Unfortunately, they are generally not used properly. They are used in a way that bypasses or short-circuits the natural process of building the soil and supplying optimal nutrients through the plant's symbiotic relationship with microorganisms. (Symbiotic means the plants help the microbes and the microbes help the plants.)

Modern agriculture as it's now practiced and the misuse of chemical fertilizers have led to a number of problems that lower the quality of our food.

Chemical Fertilizers Saturate the Soil

Chemical fertilizers immediately saturate the soil solution and bind to the soil colloids but do nothing to enrich the soil permanently. The soil solution and colloids can store only a limited amount of nutrients that are immediately available for uptake by plants. This sudden availability of the three big nutrients gives the plants a surge in growth that produces big yields, but it is not a balanced, healthy growth. It's like receiving a dose of a stimulating drug. This saturation of the soil with chemical fertilizers blocks out the proper absorption of other nutrients.

Lack of Organic Matter and Microorganisms

High concentrations of chemical fertilizers hurt soil life. The high concentration of nitrogen thrust into the soil causes a rapid growth of soil microbes, which quickly devour any organic matter in the soil as a source of carbon. Since little organic matter is generally left in the soil from the previous harvest, what little remains is soon depleted. With nothing left to eat, the soil microorganisms die, leaving the soil biologically inactive. When someone says chemical fertilizers have "burned" the organic matter out of the soil, this is what they're talking about.

The use of chemical fertilizers without supplying the needed organic matter to support the soil microorganisms leaves the largest storehouse of nutrients—the soil minerals and organic matter—virtually untapped. Even if adequate nutrients are present in the soil, without soil microorganisms they'll remain largely locked up.

Soil Depletion and Leaching

To make matters worse, where chemical fertilizers have been used for years without the appropriate organic matter, soils are not only depleted of microorganisms but are often depleted of nutrients as well. Organic matter is essential both for sustaining the biological soil life to release nutrients and for holding those nutrients in the soil. Soils depleted of organic matter are highly susceptible to erosion. Organic matter increases the water- and nutrient-holding capacity of soil. It holds the soil together, preventing it from being washed or blown away. If strong rains or heavy irrigations are applied to soil depleted of organic matter, the excess water moves the rich soil solution out of the soil and into the drain water. The loss of plant food elements this way is known as leaching. Leaching is often accompanied by outright soil erosion, which not only removes the soil solution but carries away the soil colloids and minerals with it.

Not only is much of our cropland lacking in the soil life that would unlock nutrients from the huge pantries of the soil, but the pantries themselves are being emptied more every year. Year after year of chemical fertilizer use has left much of our soil in poor shape. Chemical fertilizers alone do absolutely nothing to replace all the depleted elements or rebuild the soil. They provide no organic matter, which would allow water to soak in slowly and feed microorganisms that aid in the release of nutrients. Instead, chemical fertilizers, as they're used today, promote soil compaction, erosion, and the leaching out of nutrients.

The lack of organic matter in the soil makes it easy for chemical fertilizers and pesticides to be leached out of the soil. When that happens, they pollute streams, lakes, and underground water supplies with nitrates and pesticides. Modern agriculture is now a major source of water pollution because of this.

Unbalanced Nutrition

Chemical fertilizers, often called "balanced" with only nitrogen, phosphorus, and potassium, are actually quite unbalanced. Plants need seventeen nutrient elements in adequate amounts; humans need those seventeen plus six more that plants don't need at all. When chemical fertilizers first came into use and soils were well stocked with nutrients, it was argued that enough beneficial "impu-

Balanced Plant Nutrition Produces High-Nutrient Food

Plants need seventeen elements as a part of their metabolism in producing food rich in minerals, trace-element-rich enzymes, vitamins, and even protein. A study done by the United States Marketing Service of Topeka, Kansas, illustrates this perfectly. The study shows that the protein content of Kansas wheat suffered a big decline from 1940 to 1951. That is exactly the period when concentrated chemical nitrogen fertilizers began being used heavily in place of more traditional practices such as using organic fertilizers and crop rotation. During that period, protein content (by weight) dropped from as high as 18.5 percent in 1940 to as low as 10.5 percent in 1951. The average over the entire state dropped from 17.2 percent protein down to 12.2 percent—a 30 percent drop in just eleven years.

Despite the increased use of concentrated forms of nitrogen, it wasn't getting turned into protein at the same rate as when the nitrogen was supplied in organic matter. That illustrates the importance of organic matter and microorganisms' releasing all the nutrients slowly over the growing season to produce food of maximum nutrition.

Kansas 1940

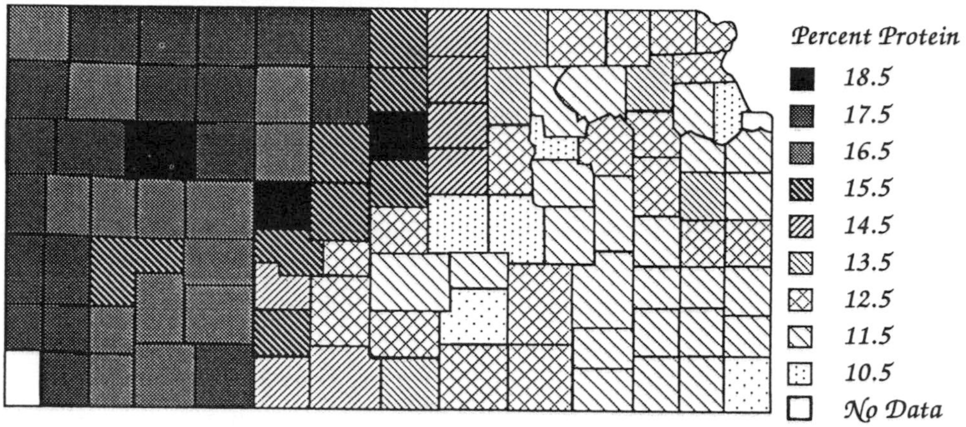

Kansas 1951

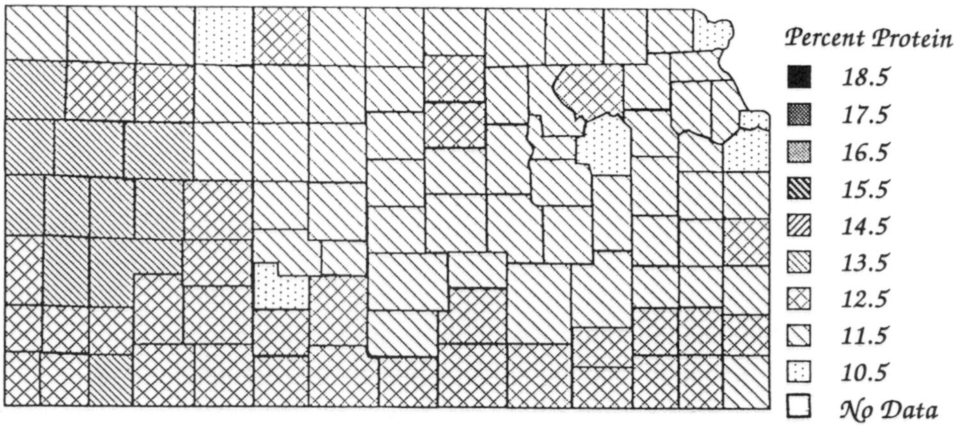

Decline in Protein Content of Kansas Wheat During the Rise of Modern Petrochemical Agriculture, County by County

rities" of trace elements were present in the fertilizer to replenish the soil; but today, with highly purified forms of chemical fertilizer, the only impurity is probably sulfur and not much else. Even if the fertilizer has some trace element impurities, it is not going to be balanced and would only fill the tiny pantry in the soil with inadequate amounts of trace minerals that are quickly depleted. Remember that nutrient elements bound up in soil mineral colloids and organic matter are the huge pantry of nutrients that must be tapped to get truly healthy plants and highly nutritious food.

Uneven Feeding

It's not only the presence of nutrients in the soil that is important in producing nutritious food, but the rate at which they're released. Every year, as soils are depleted, crops have more dependence on chemical fertilizers as their source of food. Plants grown with chemical fertilizers as their main source of nutrients take in too much nitrogen, phosphorus, and potassium (NPK) all at once and not a balanced mixture of nutrient elements over the growth cycle of the plant. Chemical fertilizers have little staying power in soils depleted of organic matter. To make up for that, they are often applied in rates far higher than the plants can use. That causes a rapid spurt of growth, but then the nutrients are gone quickly from the soil because of leaching and erosion.

Plants need all the nutrients released slowly as they grow. Charged soil that is high in nutrients, organic matter, and microorganisms supply just what plants need throughout the growing season. The warmer it gets and the faster plants grow, the higher the microbial activity in the soil, thus releasing more nutrients as the plants' needs increase. It's a perfect time-release system that produces food of optimal nutrition.

Vitamins

The concentration of vitamins depends mostly on food variety, maturity, and freshness but is also influenced somewhat by soil nutrients. For instance, copper is known to promote vitamin A formation. And there's evidence that adequate cobalt in the soil along with microorganisms produces vitamin B-12 in plants. Some plant foods—including many legumes, whole wheat, and nuts—have been found to provide a significant amount of vitamin B-12.[1]

GETTING STARTED

Once you have staked off, cleared, and loosened the soil in your food growing area, you are ready to charge the soil. If you already have a used garden spot, you can start right there. The best time to charge it is about eight weeks before the spring frost-free date in your local area. That means to charge in January or February down South and in March or April up North. Your local county extension office can give you the exact time. Don't worry if you miss the ideal time. The charging process can also be done other times. The rule is to finish the charging about three to four weeks before planting. Check the planting calendars for your area to see if you still have time to plant after charging.

In southern areas, you can charge your soil as late as June or July for August or September plantings. In northern areas, you can do the charging in the fall, before cold weather sets in, and let winter's cold put your charged soil on hold over the winter while you wait until spring for planting.

SEVEN-STEP SOIL CHARGING PROGRAM

The essential mineral elements in the soil are called mineral nutrients. The twenty-three nutrients needed to charge the soil are rarely already in correct balance, and some might not even be present at all. The first step in making sure all those elements are in the soil and in good balance and available to plants is to balance the major minerals and the pH of the soil. Here's how you do it:

1. Take soil samples.
2. Find soil pH.
3. Balance the soil.
   a) Basic soil balancing (the minimum program).
   b) Advanced soil balancing (a much better program).
4. Apply organic charging materials.
   a) Apply organic fertilizer.
   b) Apply organic matter.
   c) Apply trace elements.
5. Work charging materials into the soil.
6. Activate with water.
7. Wait before planting.

Step One: Take a Composite Soil Sample

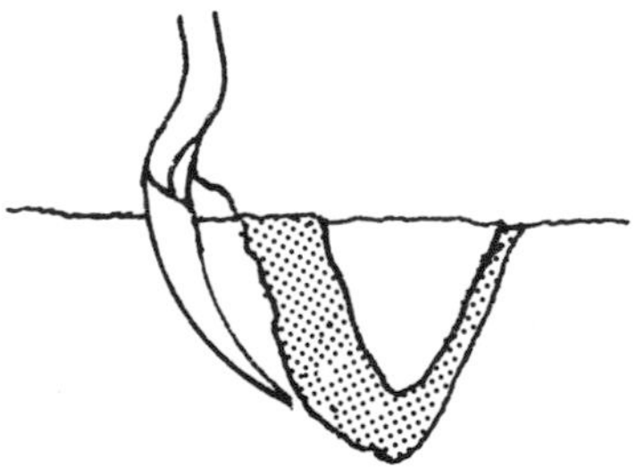

Figure 6.2 Getting a soil sample.

Take an inventory of your soil. The minimum inventory is a soil pH test, for which you need a soil sample. To sample the soil, use a trowel or a shovel to dig a small hole as deep as it will go. Scrape a layer of soil off the sides of the hole, and place the soil in a clean bucket. (See Figure 6.2.) Take several other samples scattered over your garden area, put them in the bucket, and mix thoroughly. (See Figure 6.3.) If the soil is moist, take out a cup and let it dry.

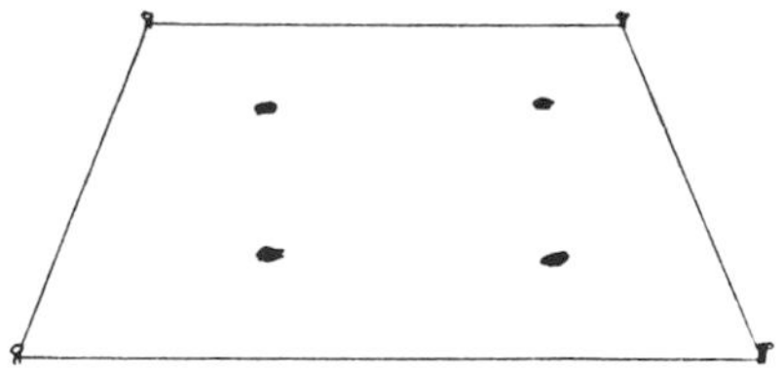

Figure 6.3 Take a soil sample from several spots in the garden plot.

Step Two: Find Your Soil pH

A soil pH test will find the acidity or alkalinity of your soil. The pH will tell you if you have a shortage or an excess of minerals. You can find soil pH yourself by testing the soil sample with a small soil pH kit. (See Figure 6.4.) The best one we know of is the Hellige-Truog soil pH kit from Nasco, which takes orders by phone at (800) 558–9595.

Step Three: Balance the Soil

You may choose between basic soil balancing and advanced soil balancing.

(A) Basic Soil Balancing

Plants grow best at a soil pH of 6 to 7. That range also provides for an optimal absorption of soil nutrients. If your soil falls within that range, leave it alone. If your soil pH is above 7, use the remedies given in the "High pH Western Soils" section later in this chapter. If it's below 6, you need to add some calcium-magnesium fertilizer to bring it up to about 6.5. Dolomite (dolomitic limestone), sold at garden centers, is the simplest thing to use and is readily available. It contains about 21 percent calcium and 13 percent magnesium.

Use Table 6.1 to determine how much dolomite to put in your soil. Let's say the pH is 5.5 and you have a sandy soil. First, locate 5.5 in the "Existing Soil pH" column. Move across the "5.5" row until you reach the "Sandy Texture" column. The number there is 3.0. So you would need to apply 3 pounds of dolomite per 100 square feet.

To identify your soil texture, you can get help from your county extension agent or you can approximate it yourself. (See "Determining Your Soil Texture" inset on page 74.)

That's all there is to balancing your soil in a quick, easy, and inexpensive manner. The result is a basic balancing job. But some readers might wish to go beyond that. Your soil can be balanced to a much greater precision with advanced soil balancing.

(B) Advanced Soil Balancing

Soil scientists have found that the highest quality food is grown from soil that has about 70 percent calcium, 12 percent magnesium, and 4 percent potassium. The most accurate way of finding out what's in your soil is to send your soil sample to a good soil testing lab. (See Appendix A.) A soil test report from a soil lab is an inventory of how

Figure 6.4

Using a Soil pH Test Kit

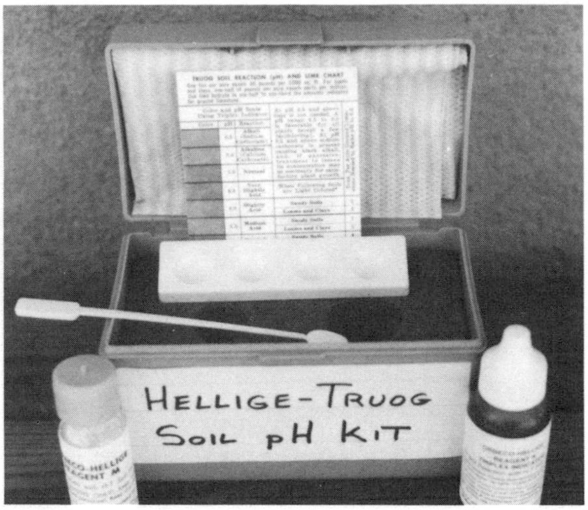

1 Start with a good soil pH test kit. We like the Hellige-Truog kit best. It is easy to use, durable, inexpensive, and accurate.

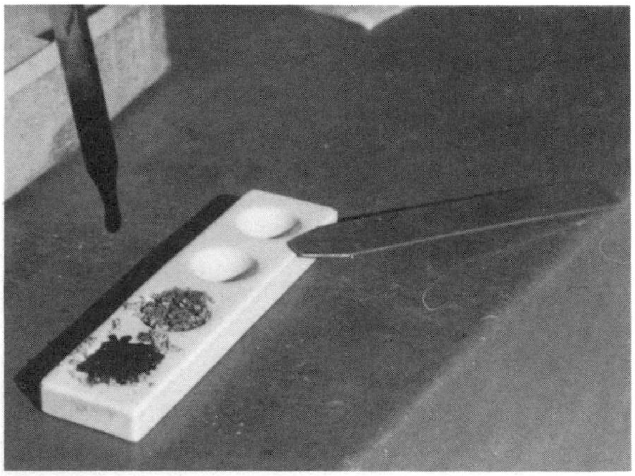

2 Take your soil sample, mix it well, dry it, and use the white plastic spatula to fill one of the cavities one-fourth full of soil to be tested. (Photo shows two tests being performed.)

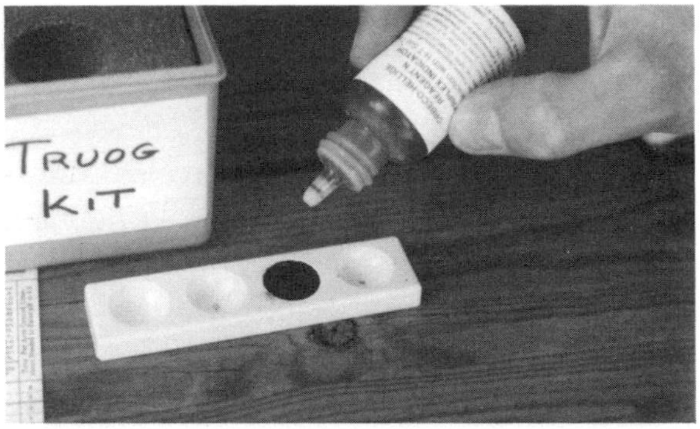

3 Squeeze drops of the liquid reagent onto the soil in the cavity until completely moistened. Mix with the spatula.

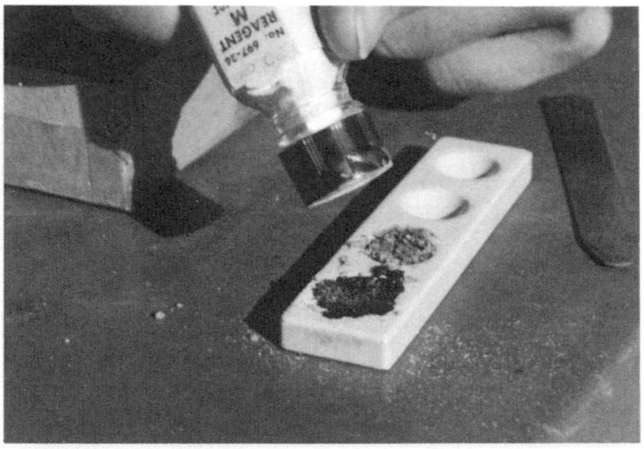

4 Remove the cover of the white reagent powder bottle and tap out enough of the white powder to cover the moistened soil surface.

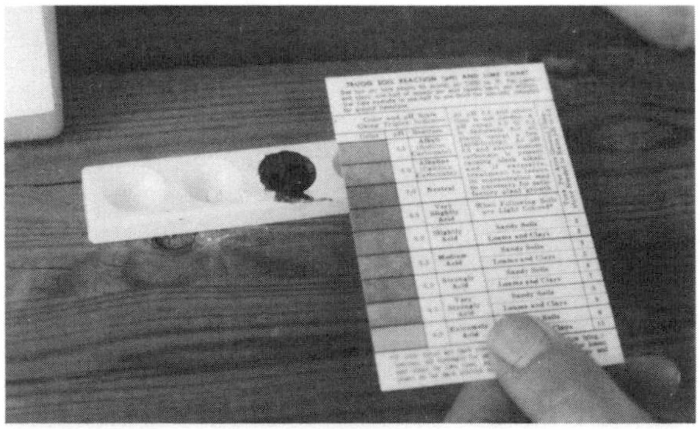

5 Wait 2 minutes, then place color chart on edge of test plate. Slide color chart along until you see a match. Look at the figure by the color. This is the pH of the soil sample. (The back of the color chart also tells you how to do the soil pH test.)

Table 6.1

Pounds of Dolomite to Raise pH in Top 6 Inches+ of Soil to 6.5

(Per 100 Square Feet)

Existing Soil pH	Sandy Texture	Loamy Texture	Clay-Loam Texture
5.0*	4.0	10.5	15.0
5.1	4.0	10.0	14.0
5.2	3.5	9.5	13.0
5.3	3.0	9.0	12.5
5.4	3.0	8.0	11.5
5.5	3.0	8.0	10.5
5.6	2.5	7.0	9.5
5.7	2.0	6.0	8.5
5.8	2.0	5.5	7.5
5.9	1.5	5.0	6.5
6.0	1.5	4.0	5.5
6.1	1.0	3.5	4.5
6.2	1.0	2.5	3.5
6.3	0.5	2.0	2.5
6.4	0.5	1.0	1.5

\+ Tables on soil fertility management assume a plow depth of 6 inches, which is the norm for most rototillers for the home garden. Standard round-point shovels and certain other hand instruments plow to a depth of 10 inches. If you're plowing that deeply, then use the table above but multiply the quantity of dolomote by 1.7.

* In the unlikely event your soil has a pH below 5, treat it just as you would soil with a pH of exactly 5.

much of those key three elements are present in your soil. The soil test will also show pH, soil texture (derived from the cation exchange capacity), organic matter, and the amount of phosphorus and other nutrients your soil contains.

A fertile, PowerCharged soil will contain about 60 parts per million of phosphorus. That is where a soil test comes in handy, since it shows how much phosphorus you have. If you already have enough, you do not want to add any more. The 60 parts per million of phosphorus is equal to 275 pounds of phosphorus oxide per acre, or 0.6 pound per 100 square feet.

The lab will send you this detailed information, but unless you're a soil scientist don't spend a lot of time trying to figure out what it

Determining Your Soil Texture

To balance your soil you must know its texture. Soil texture tells you how coarse or fine the soil particles are. Sand is made up of coarse particles, or grains; clay loam consists of very fine particles; and loam is a mixture of the two. To determine your soil's texture, put some soil in a saucer, pour in a little water to make a moist ball, then try to mold the ball into a cigar shape by rolling it between your thumb and forefinger. That is called "ribboning out" the soil. Another good test is to wet a pinch of the soil and rub it between your thumb and forefinger. That is called the "feel" of the soil. Now see if you can tell what kind of soil you have by using these guidelines:

- *Sand.* Made of coarse particles. Will not ribbon out. Feels gritty.
- *Clay Loam.* The opposite of sand. Made of very fine particles. Ribbons out easily to form a long ribbon. Feels slick when rubbed. Is plastic when wet.
- *Loam.* The ideal soil. A combination of sand, silt, and clay particles. Ribbons out fairly easily depending on how much clay it contains. Feels smooth wet or dry. May feel floury when dry. Loams usually have about 50 percent sand, 15 percent clay, and 35 percent silt particles.

means. The soil test report will tell you what you have but will not tell you what to do to bring your soil into proper balance.

A professional consultant can look at this inventory, see what needs to be added to bring your soil into balance, and tell you what materials to add and how much of each. Here is a three-step advanced soil balancing program:

1. Take a soil sample as already described under the regular soil charging program.
2. Send the sample to a good soil test lab for a standard soil test. Brookside Labs and A&L Labs are good. (Labs are listed in Appendix A. A sample cover letter is in Appendix C.)
3. When your soil test report comes back, send a copy of it to a good consultant to do soil-balancing computations and to instruct you what to do. If you can't find a consulting soil scientist in your area, write to us. (See address in book's Conclusion.)

Step Four: Apply Organic Charging Materials

There are three things you need in this step of the soil charging process: organic fertilizer, organic matter, and trace elements.

Organic Fertilizer

Organic fertilizers provide a steady release of nitrogen and other nutrients throughout the growing season without getting leached out and are much better than salt-type, chemical fertilizers in almost all cases. For the small growing area, cottonseed meal is the best choice. It's the main source of the three big nutrients—nitrogen, phosphorus, and potassium—and has an NPK analysis of 6-3-1.5.[2]

Cottonseed meal is an oilseed meal made by squeezing the oil out of cottonseeds. The result is a yellowish powder that is high in nitrogen, odorless, and weed-free. Since the seed from which the meal is derived is buried deep inside the plant, it's protected first by the outer boll, then the lint, then the seedcoat; so you don't have to worry about pesticide residues. You can buy cottonseed meal in 5-pound bags at garden centers or at wholesale prices in 50-pound bags at feed stores. Check your Yellow Pages for the nearest feed store.

How much cottonseed meal should you use? Your plants will need about half a pound of actual nitrogen per 100 square feet, but at first you'll need to apply twice that much because only about half the nitrogen in organic fertilizer becomes available the first year. To apply the needed nitrogen the first year, apply about 20 pounds (4 gallons) of cottonseed meal per 100 square feet. Each year thereafter, apply about 10 pounds (2 gallons) per 100 square feet. When calculating the square footage of your garden, count beds and walkways.

NPK ANALYSIS

N, P, and K are the respective chemical symbols for the elements nitrogen, phosphorus, and potassium. Good fertilizer companies, whether dealing with organic or chemical products, will place on their bags of fertilizer three numbers known as the fertilizer's NPK analysis. For instance, if the numbers are listed as 2-1-1, that means the fertilizer contains 2 percent nitrogen (N), 1 percent phosphate (P_2O_5), and 1 percent potash (K_2O).

Organic Matter

Organic matter is necessary for soil life. It increases the water- and nutrient-holding capacity of the soil and provides some nutrients to the soil solution. How much organic matter do you need? Let nature be your guide. Soils that have not been tampered with by people average about 1.5 percent organic matter by weight in the southern coastal plains of the United States, while virgin soils in the northern prairies average about 5.5 percent. Those percentages by weight might seem low but actually represent a very high content by volume. Set a goal for your soil based on those figures. How do you tell how much organic matter to add? If your soil is soft, spongy, and easy to work, you probably already have an adequate amount of organic matter. If it's a new plot and the soil is fairly hard, apply at

Using Bark for Organic Matter

With bark, mix 1 pound of actual nitrogen per 10 cubic feet of bark, and let it incubate three weeks at growing-season temperatures before planting.

If, for example, you want to spread a layer of ground bark 3 inches deep over a plot of land 10 feet long by 10 feet wide, what should you do?

First, find the volume of bark you'll need. Bark is sold in cubic feet. You compute the cubic feet by multiplying the length of the coverage (10 feet) by the width (10 feet) by the depth (3 inches, or .25 foot). In this case, that means you will need 25 cubic feet of bark (10 x 10 x .25).

Next, compute the pounds of nitrogen you'll need. Tests have shown that about 1 pound of actual nitrogen is required to balance every 10 cubic feet of bark. Since you've already calculated you'll need 25 cubic feet of bark, you divide the 25 by 10, resulting in 2.5. That's how many pounds of nitrogen you'll need.

But since the nitrogen is only one component of the fertilizer, how do you know how much fertilizer to apply to provide those 2.5 pounds of nitrogen? You use this formula:

$$\text{Pounds of Fertilizer to Apply} = \frac{\text{Lbs. of Nitrogen Wanted} \times 100}{\text{\% of Nitrogen in Fertilizer}}$$

Suppose your fertilizer is ammonium phosphate, which has an NPK analysis of 16-20-0. That's 16 percent nitrogen. You want 2.5 pounds of nitrogen. Multiplying by 100 gives you 250. Dividing by the percent of nitrogen in the fertilizer (16 percent) gives you the final answer of how much fertilizer to apply: about 15 pounds.

least a 3-inch layer of organic matter and then rototill it in, 6 to 8 inches deep.

The best sources of organic matter are peat moss, compost, and leaf mold. If you want to use ground bark, you have to take an extra step to bring the carbon-to-nitrogen ratio into balance. (See "Using Bark for Organic Matter" inset above.)

Trace Elements

The best source of trace elements at the present time is seaweed meal. Dried seaweed meal is most valuable for the seventeen trace elements it contains that are essential in plant and human nutrition. Dried seaweed is very concentrated, so a little bit goes a long way. Apply half a cup per 100 square feet by mixing it in thoroughly with the cottonseed meal. If you're tempted to use more on the feeling that "if a little bit is good a lot must be better," don't. While half a cup sounds like a small amount, it is very concentrated, and research indicates it is plenty. It is possible to get too much into your soil and do more harm than good.

Another way of applying seaweed is by using a water-soluble seaweed extract that can be sprayed on the leaves as a foliar spray. We recommend the spray method be used in addition to placement in the soil, especially if you live in an area where the soil pH tends to be high, just to ensure your plants get enough trace elements. In high pH soils, some of the trace elements can become tied up and poorly available, especially iron, manganese, zinc, and copper. (See Figure 6.5.) Foliar feeding with seaweed extract completely overcomes that problem. (See the "Foliar Feeding With Seaweed" section in Chapter 12 for details on using seaweed spray.) If your garden center does not have either kind of seaweed and can't order it for you, you can order it yourself. (See Appendix A.)

Step Five: Work Charging Materials Into the Soil

You have already loosened your soil with a rototiller or lots of spading. Now you are ready to mix your charging materials into the soil. Spread the dolomite, if needed, and the cottonseed meal mixed with seaweed evenly over the surface of the beds. On top of that, spread the layer of organic matter, which you might want to sprinkle down lightly so it doesn't blow around. Then mix all the ingredients into the soil thoroughly. If you have a new garden, spread the materials over the entire plot and work it all in. You can work the materials in with a spading fork, but a tiller is much better, especially if you have a new garden space, where the soil tends to be harder. In that case, apply all the materials over the whole plot and rototill the whole thing. If you don't have a rototiller, you can probably rent a lightweight front-tine tiller that will fit in the trunk of a car.

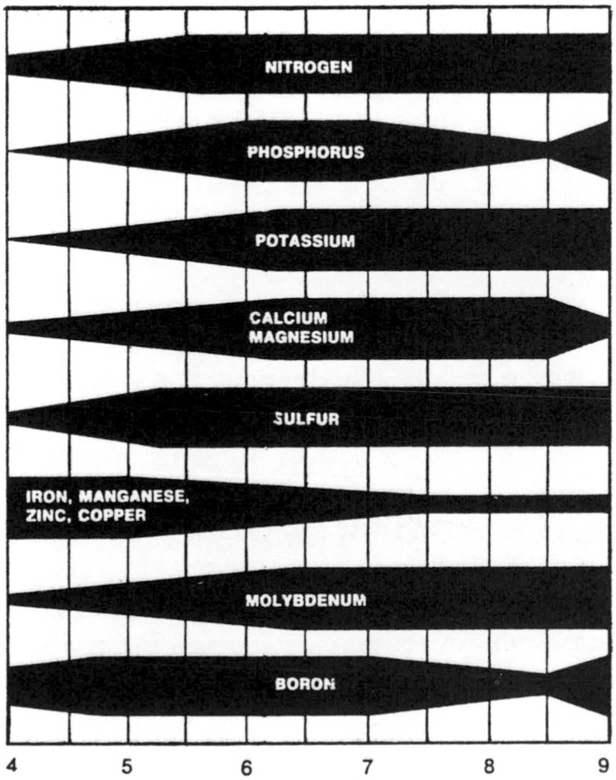

Figure 6.5 The wider the band for each nutrient, the more available that nutrient is for uptake by most plants. When the band narrows, uptake is suppressed. A pH of 6.3 to 6.5 is ideal, for that's where most of the bands are widest, showing greatest availability of the nutrients identified within the bands.

Step Six: Activate With Water

You now have all the charging materials in place except one: water. Unless rain falls within a week, turn on your sprinkler to apply half an inch of water. You can stand empty tin cans across the garden plot to determine when you've watered half an inch.

Step Seven: Wait Before Planting

It is best to wait three to four weeks to allow the soil life to work on the charging materials you have worked in. If you have a new plot, you can go ahead and mark off your beds immediately after charging the soil.

RECHARGING YOUR BEDS

After the initial soil charging treatment, work only with the beds and leave the walkways alone. Your beds will need recharging each year. Generally, there is no reason to apply any fertilizers more than once a year if you use the PowerCharged method. You recharge your beds by basically repeating the seven-step soil charging program.

The soil pH should be checked once a year and, if needed, balanced with dolomite. Apply the same amount of seaweed meal, but cut the amount of cottonseed meal in half. Work the charging materials in with a spading fork or a rototiller. We advocate a permanent bed system, so just work with the beds and leave the walkways alone. As far as organic matter is concerned, that can actually be provided by surface mulch, which will work its way down into the soil as the soil life breaks it down. More on surface mulch later.

HIGH PH WESTERN SOILS

If you live where the average annual rainfall is less than 25 inches, you will probably have high pH soils, which present special challenges. A pH of 7 is about neutral. A soil with a pH over 7 is alkaline. The ideal soil pH is 6.5. When the soil pH is too high, plants have a hard time getting certain nutrients, especially important trace elements such as iron, zinc, and copper. (Figure 6.5 shows you what high soil pH and low soil pH do to the availability of plant nutrient uptake.)

High soil pH is due to excessive amounts of calcium, magnesium, potassium, or sodium. If your soil pH is above 7, you should leach once a year. You leach by running lots of water through a soil to wash excess minerals out—like washing dirty clothes. (See "Leaching" inset on page 79 for the mechanics of leaching.) Water alone will do the job unless you have too much sodium. If you have too much sodium, then special steps have to be taken. If you get a soil test, you'll know whether your high pH is caused by excessive sodium or by other minerals. Without a soil test, you can guess by looking at the pH. If the soil pH is 8.5 or higher, it's likely due to sodium.

Sodium Injury

With too much sodium in the soil, plants are stunted and grow slowly. Some plants are more sensitive than others to sodium. Lettuce, for example, is much more sensitive than tomatoes. So, growing in the same sodium-excessive soil, tomatoes might do fine and bear well while lettuce fares poorly.

When sodium gets into the soil, it locks onto the soil colloids with an electrical charge and is difficult to dislodge. If you have too much sodium, you first have to apply gypsum or sulfur to the soil and then do the leaching before you even begin the soil charging program. The sulfur or gypsum you add is known as soil amendment. (Table 6.2 shows how much sulfur or gypsum should be used.) Work the

Leaching

If your soil pH is over 7, you need to leach the soil. If a soil test shows the high pH is due to excess sodium, or if you don't have a soil test but your pH is 8.5 or higher, you need to work sulfur or gypsum into the soil several weeks before leaching. To do the leaching, use sprinkler irrigation and deliberately overirrigate to wash the salts down and out of your soil. The idea is to apply excessive amounts of water.

What amounts are excessive? The answer, as Table 12.2 (in Chapter 12) tells us, is that it depends on your soil. Let's assume you have sandy soil and want to wash the salts out of the top two feet of it. The table tells us that one inch of irrigation water will fill the sandy soil, so do that first. You can use the "can test" (also explained in Chapter 12) to determine how long you will need to run the sprinklers to produce one inch of water. (Chapter 12 tells you how to apply the water evenly.) After that first inch of water has been applied, the leaching can begin.

Continue to run your sprinklers to apply three extra inches of water. You can use a continuous run of the sprinkler, so long as the water soaks into the ground and does not run off. If water starts to run off, stop the sprinklers and let the soil dry out a little, then apply three more inches of water the next day. Then take a soil sample down to twelve inches deep, let it dry, and test its pH. If the pH is below 7, the leaching has worked. If the pH is above 7, keep applying water in three-inch amounts until the pH falls to between 6 and 7.

Table 6.2

Amount of Soil Amendment to Lower Soil pH to 6.5

(Pounds per 100 Square Feet)

Soil pH	Sandy Soil		Loam or Clay Loam Soil	
	If Using Sulfur	If Using Gypsum	If Using Sulfur	If Using Gypsum
7.5	1.5	8.1	2.0	10.8
8.0	3.0	16.2	4.5	24.3
8.5	4.5	24.3	6.0	32.4
9.0	6.0	32.4	8.0	43.2

amendment into the soil. After several weeks, apply excessive amounts of water (leaching) to move the salts down and out. Make sure you do that before applying any of the soil charging materials. Once that is done, and your soil pH is around 6.5, you can begin the soil charging program.

7. *The Planting Plan*

MOST gardeners find that they end up with too much harvest coming off all at once and later have nothing to harvest at all. That is due to a lack of planning but is easy to correct by making a planting plan. This plan is your road map to success. It will enable you to grow a continuous supply of just the right amount of fresh PowerCharged food throughout the growing season for your family's needs.

If you make a good planting plan, everything else becomes so much easier. Your plan will show you what to plant, how much to plant, when to plant, and where. Things go a lot better when you plant by a plan. It is much better to make your mistakes on paper than to make them in the garden. A stroke of your eraser will correct mistakes in your plan on paper; but once you get several beds planted, you can't unplant them. With a good plan, you will always have plenty without waste.

WHAT TO PLANT

From a health standpoint, every gardener should have at least one cruciferous vegetable growing in the garden. These vegetables of the brassica family include cabbage, broccoli, cauliflower, Brussels sprouts, rutabagas, turnips, kohlrabi, and certain dark green leafy vegetables such as kale, mustard, collard greens, and turnip greens.

Cruciferous vegetables have proven to be powerful protectors against cancer and should be eaten often.

Another consideration in deciding what to plant should be the nutritional value of various foods. Some foods grown in properly mineralized soil are so rich in vitamins and minerals that eating them is like taking a supplement except it's better, because you're assured of getting the highest biological value possible in addition to great taste. Fortunately, many of the cruciferous vegetables are also very high in vitamins and minerals, so there will be some overlap. To see which foods have the highest content of specific minerals and vitamins, look at Table 7.1. Foods are listed in descending order, starting with the richest source of the nutrient.

Another yardstick for the selection of what to plant is based on a combination of what gets the maximum yield in the smallest space, the dollar value of the harvest, and how long it takes to get a harvest. (See Table 7.2.)

HOW MUCH TO PLANT

It is much better to plan a small food-growing area of 400 square feet (20 feet by 20 feet) and do it right than to have a larger space and become overwhelmed by weeds or too much work. But if you have the space, time, and interest, you can plan 400 square feet of space for each adult you wish to feed. (Table 7.3 shows the amount to plant per person. Figure 7.1 shows the number of rows and the spacing between plants that should be planned.)

THE PLANTING PLAN WORKSHEET

Table 7.3 shows you how much to plant per person.

Take lettuce, for example. Let's say your family has four people who like to eat lettuce. Looking at Table 7.3, you see that the allotment per person for lettuce is 7 to 10 total feet, or an average of about 8 total feet per person. Enter "8" in the planting plan worksheet (Table 7.4) in the "Total Feet to Plant per Person" category. Then, since four people are eating, you need 32 total feet of lettuce for the family. Enter this.

Now look at Figure 7.1. Find lettuce. (It is one of the four-row plants.) Four rows are planted along the bed. Enter "4" on the worksheet under "Rows per Bed." This means that each foot of bed you plant equals 4 total feet of lettuce. Since you need 32 total feet, you will need to plant 8 feet of bed. One foot of bed equals one bed foot. Enter "8" on the planting plan worksheet in the column headed "Bed Feet Needed."

Now take green onions as an example. Figure 7.1 tells you that onions are a seven-row plant. This means you can plant seven rows along the bed with the rows spaced only 3 inches apart. This means

Table 7.1

The Best Garden Sources of Specific Minerals and Vitamins

Calcium

Bok Choy Cabbage
Turnip, Collard, and Mustard Greens
Broccoli
Looseleaf and Romaine Lettuce
Kale
Okra
Regular Cabbage
Summer Squash
Green Beans

Magnesium

Spinach
Beets, Greens, and Roots
Broccoli
Summer Squash
Turnip and Mustard Greens
Bok Choy Cabbage
Asparagus
Cucumber
Green Beans

Iron

Spinach
Swiss Chard
Bok Choy Cabbage
Mustard and Beet Greens
Looseleaf Lettuce
Green Peas
Jerusalem Artichoke
Kale
Broccoli

Zinc

Collard Greens
Spinach
Bok Choy Cabbage
Looseleaf Lettuce
Summer Squash
Asparagus
Beet Greens
Black-Eyed Peas
Mustard Greens

Copper

Tomato
Lima and Green Beans
Asparagus
Cabbage
Broccoli
Spinach
Potato
Beets
Sunflower Seeds

Vitamin C

Sweet Pepper (especially red)
Cauliflower (normal cooking considered)
Bok Choy Cabbage (cooking considered)
Regular Cabbage
Broccoli (normal cooking considered)
Strawberries
Kohlrabi
Mustard Greens (normal cooking considered)
Brussels Sprouts (normal cooking considered)
Looseleaf Lettuce

Vitamin A

Carrot
Spinach
Turnip and Mustard Greens
Sweet Pepper (especially red)
Bok Choy Cabbage
Sweet Potato
Green Onions
Winter Squash
Looseleaf Lettuce

Vitamin B-6

Bok Choy Cabbage
Spinach
Turnip Greens
Cauliflower
Broccoli
Sweet Pepper
Asparagus
Summer Squash
Regular Cabbage

Folacin

Spinach
Looseleaf Lettuce
Turnip and Collard Greens
Asparagus
Regular and Bok Choy Cabbage
Broccoli
Cauliflower
Beets
Summer Squash

Table 7.2

Most Valuable Foods to Plant Based on Yield, Dollar Value of the Harvest, and Time to Harvest

(Using a Standard Scale of 1 to 10)

Rank	Kind of Food	Value Rating	Rank	Kind of Food	Value Rating
1*	Tomato	9.0	18	Spinach	6.2
2*	Onion (green bunching)	8.2	19	Lima Beans (pole)	6.1
3	Lettuce (leaf)	7.4	20	Radish	6.1
4	Turnip (greens and roots)	7.4	21	Cabbage	6.0
5*	Summer Squash	7.2	22	Leeks	5.9
6	Peas (edible pod)	6.9	23	Collard Greens	5.8
7	Onions (bulb)	6.9	24	Okra	5.7
8*	Snap Beans (pole)	6.8	25	Kale	5.6
9	Beets	6.6	26	Cauliflower	5.3
10	Snap Beans (bush)	6.5	27	Eggplant	5.3
11	Carrot	6.5	28	Green Peas	5.2
12*	Cucumber	6.5	29	Brussels Sprouts	4.3
13*	Sweet Pepper	6.4	30	Celery	4.3
14	Broccoli	6.3	31	Black-Eyed Peas	4.3
15	Kohlrabi	6.3	32	Sweet Corn	4.1
16	Swiss Chard	6.3	33	Winter Squash	3.8
17	Mustard Greens	6.2	34	Melons	3.8

SOURCE: National Garden Bureau, 1980. Based on a survey of thirty-six home garden experts across the United States. Value rating was based on total yield per square foot, dollar value per pound, and time from seeding to harvest.

* = The most popular food plants, based on a separate survey of home food growers.

that if you plant only 1 foot of bed, you will have planted seven rows of onions, each row 1 foot long. This gives you a total of 7 feet of green onions.

The allotment for green onions from Table 7.3 is 3 to 5 feet, or an average of 4 total feet per person. With four people eating, you would need 16 total feet. One bed foot of onions will give you 7 total feet. Two bed feet of onions will give you 14 total feet, and that is close enough. You can plant 14 total feet of green onions by planting only 2 bed feet.

Table 7.3

How Much to Plant

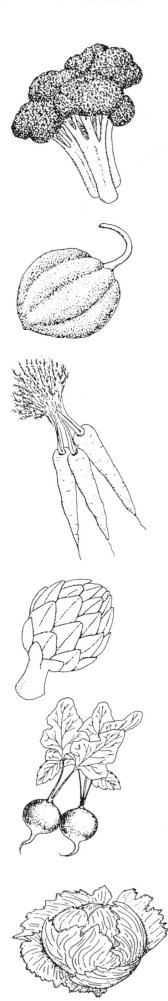

Crop	Total Feet to Plant per Person
EARLY PLANTING	
Asparagus	15
Beet	5–10
Broccoli*	4.5–9
Brussels Sprouts*	2–4
Cabbage*	3–5
Carrot	5–10
Cauliflower*	5–10
Celery*	6
Chard	1–2
Collard	5–10
Kale	5–10
Kohlrabi	3–5
Lettuce	7–10
Mustard	5–10
Onion (green)	3–5
Onion (bulb)	30–50
Pea (green)	15–20
Potato	50–100
Radish	3–5
Spinach	5–10
Strawberries*	4–8
Sunchoke (Jerusalem Artichoke)	2
Turnip	5–10
MEDIUM PLANTING	
Beans, general	15
Green Snap Bean (bush)	15
Green Snap Bean (pole)	5
Lima Bean (bush)	15
Lima Bean (pole)	5
Soybean	10–15
Sweet Corn	10–15
Tomato*	6–15
LATE PLANTING	
Black-Eyed Pea	10–15
Cantaloupe/Honeydew	6–12
Cucumber	2–6
Eggplant*	3
Okra	4–6
Peanut	6
Summer Squash	6
Sweet Pepper*	4–8
Sweet Potato	10–20
Watermelon	12–24
Winter Squash	6

* = Use transplants from a garden center to start these plants for the small garden.

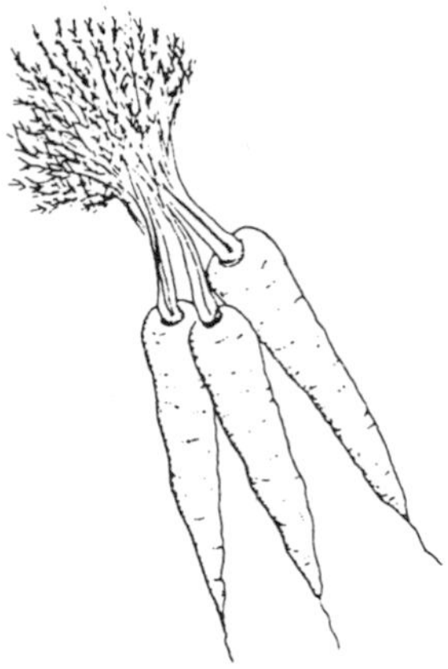

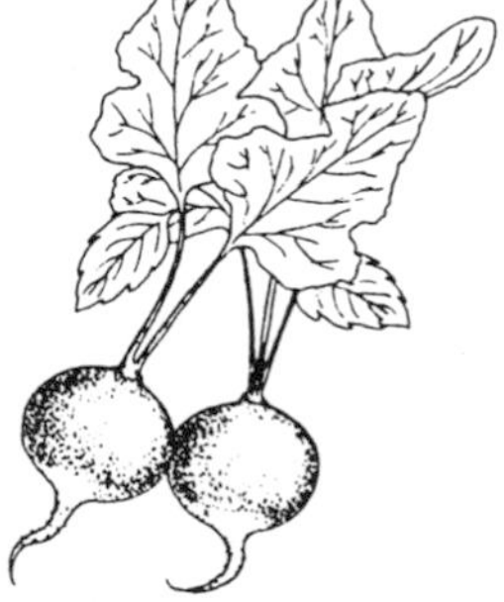

Figure 7.1

Plant Spacing

(Number of rows and spacing between plants in 24-inch-wide beds)

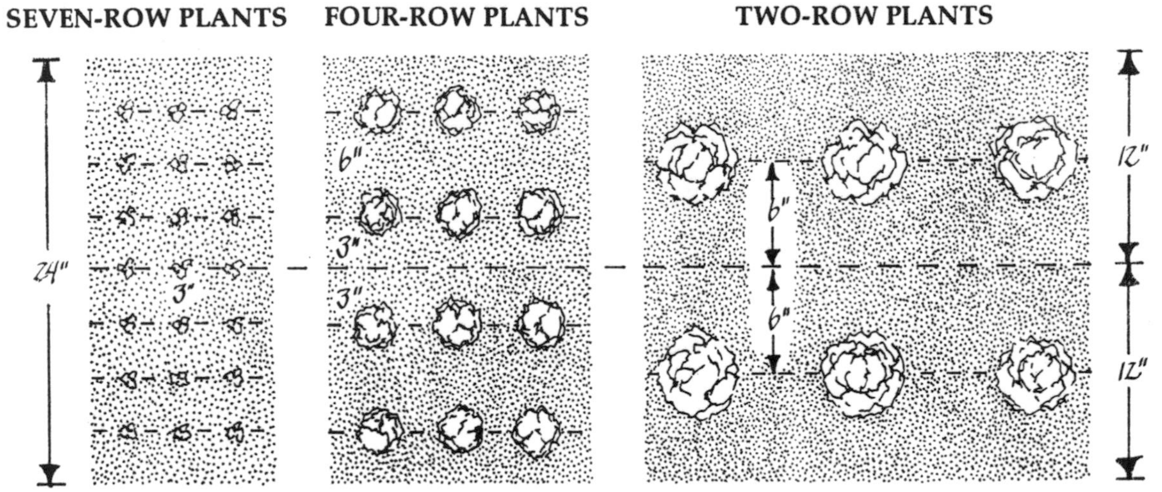

PLANTING INSTRUCTIONS FOR A SEVEN-ROW BED

❑ Leave 3 inches between rows.
❑ Plant the first row on the centerline.
❑ The distance between plants going along the bed is as follows:

Onion: 3 inches
Radish: 1 inch

PLANTING INSTRUCTIONS FOR A FOUR-ROW BED

❑ Leave 6 inches between rows.
❑ Plant center rows 3 inches off the centerline, and plant the other rows 6 inches apart.
❑ The distance between plants going along the bed is as follows:

Lettuce: 6 inches
Strawberries: 6 inches

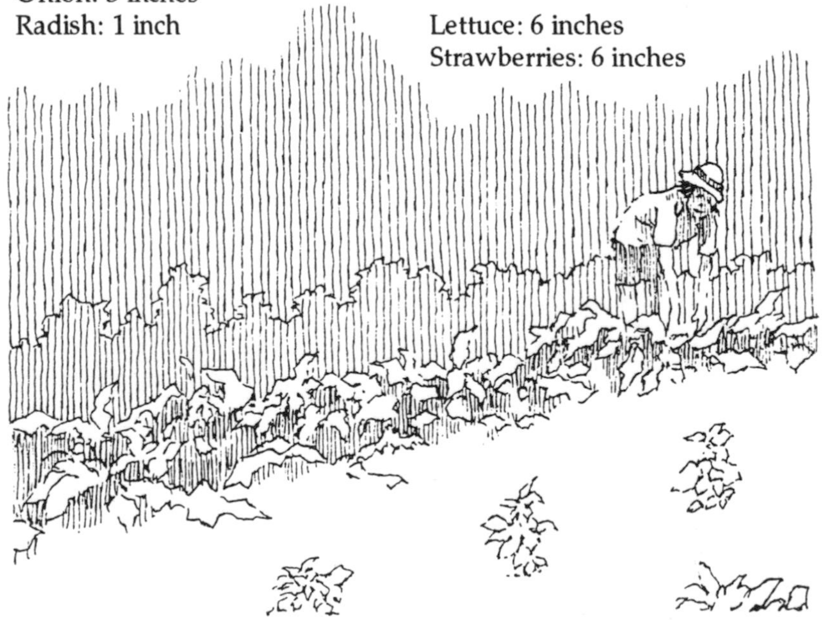

PLANTING INSTRUCTIONS FOR A TWO-ROW BED

❑ Leave 12 inches between rows.
❑ Plant the rows 6 inches off the centerline.
❑ The distance between plants going along the bed is as follows:

Beans, general: 5 inches
Snap Bean, bush: 5 inches
Beet: 3 inches
Brussels Sprouts: 12 inches
Cabbage: 12 inches
Carrot: 2 inches
Celery: 6 inches
Chard: 6 inches
Collard: 12 inches
Corn: 10 inches
Garlic: 3 inches
Kohlrabi: 12 inches
Lettuce, Romaine: 12 inches
Mustard: 6 inches
Pea, Green: 2 inches
Pea, Southern: 6 inches
Peanuts: 8 inches
Spinach: 5 inches
Turnip: 3 inches

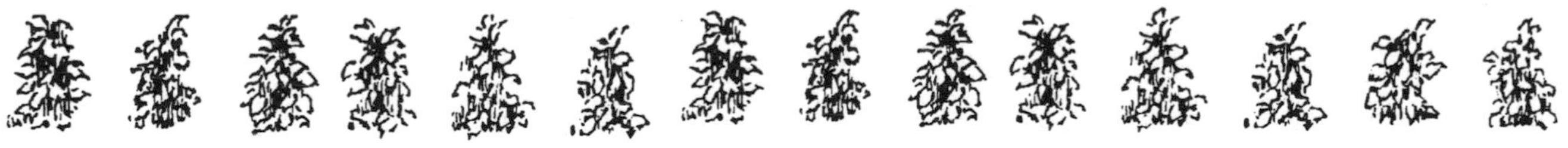

ONE-ROW PLANTS

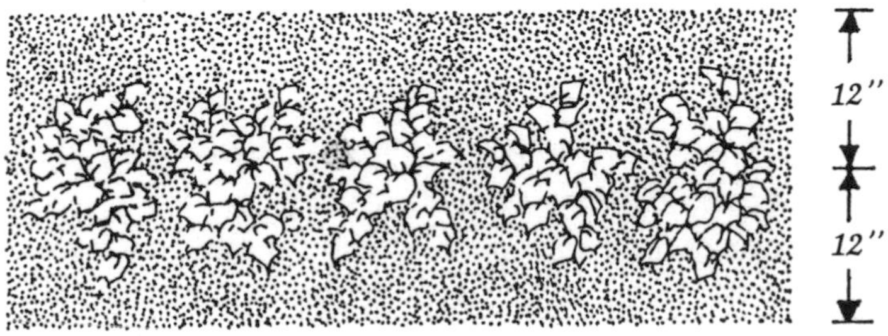

SKIP-BED PLANTING

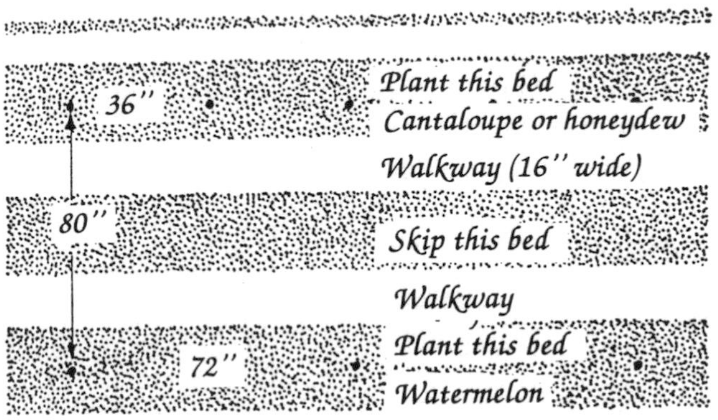

PLANTING INSTRUCTIONS FOR A ONE-ROW BED

❑ Plant one row along the centerline.
❑ The distance between plants running along the bed is as follows:

Asparagus: 18 inches
Black-Eyed Pea: 3 inches
Broccoli: 18 inches
Cauliflower: 18 inches
Corn: 6 inches
Cucumber: 12 inches
Eggplant: 18 inches
Kale: 12 inches
Okra: 18 inches
Pepper: 12 inches
Potato: 10 inches
Snap Bean, pole: 6 inches
Soybean: 3 inches
Squash: 36 inches
Sweet Potato: 12 inches
Sunchoke: 12 inches
Sunseeds: 12 inches
Tomato: 36 inches (use trellis)

PLANTING INSTRUCTIONS FOR SKIP-BED PLANTS

❑ Plant a bed, skip a bed.
❑ The distance between plants running along the bed is as follows:

Cantaloupe: 36 inches
Honeydew Melon: 36 inches
Watermelon: 72 inches

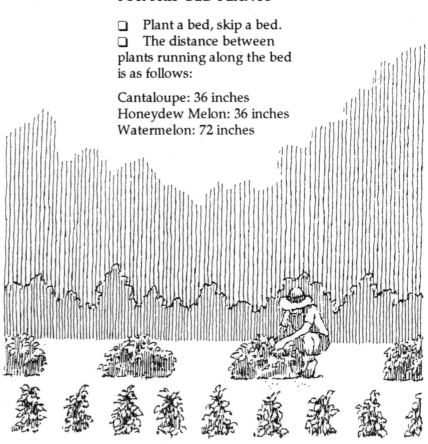

Here's how your planting plan worksheet would be filled in for those two vegetables:

KIND OF PLANT	NUMBER EATING	TOTAL FEET TO PLANT PER		ROWS PER BED	BED FEET NEEDED	WHEN TO PLANT	BED NO.
		PERSON	FAMILY				
Lettuce	4	8	32	4	8		
Green Onion	4	4	16	7	2		

Note the easy math that enables you easily to work out how many feet of bed to plan for each kind of plant. (See "Easiest Way to Fill Out the Planting Plan Worksheet" inset below.)

WHEN TO PLANT

All planting dates are based on the average spring freeze-free date and the average fall freeze date in your local area. To learn what those dates are, call your county officials and ask for the county extension agent. Enter these dates at the top of the "When to Plant

Easiest Way to Fill Out the Planting Plan Worksheet

The planting plan worksheet (Table 7.4) is meant to be an aid to successful gardening. Have fun with it! Here's an easy way to work with it:

Write down every food you want to eat, then fill in all the columns through "Bed Feet Needed." At first, don't worry too much about how much space you have; just fill in what you want to eat.

Add up all the numbers in the "Bed Feet Needed" column and write the total at the bottom of the worksheet.

Figure out how much bed feet you have available. A garden of 20 by 20 feet would have 6 beds, each 20 feet long, giving you 120 bed feet. Record the total bed feet available at the bottom of the worksheet.

If you totaled more bed feet needed than you have available, figure out how many bed feet need to be cut. Then go back through your list, cut out or reduce some of the foods, and fill out the worksheet again until the bed feet needed equals the bed feet available. Make copies of the worksheet and fill it in as many times as needed.

If you have more bed feet available than you need, you can do one of two things: add more foods or leave a part of a bed unplanted.

Worksheet" (Table 7.5). Then use a calendar to determine the planting dates for your area. Once you do that, you can fill in the "When to Plant" column in your Planting Plan Worksheet (Table 7.4), and you're done. You might also want to note on a large wall calendar the dates for planting each food.

It will be helpful to keep in mind that there is an overlap of planting periods, that nature is quite forgiving, and that the precision of launching a rocket is not required. Planting periods are guidelines, and it is not necessary to follow them with strict exactness. For instance, strawberries and lettuce could be planted at the same time with no problem, even though their planting dates are not identical.

PLANTING MAP

You'll find it helpful to sketch a bird's-eye view of your food-growing area, showing what you're going to plant and for how many feet. It's also helpful to show the number of rows for each food and the dates you've chosen for their planting. For this sketch, you can show the beds only. Figure 7.2 shows a sample planting map for a 20- by 20-foot garden containing six beds, each 20 feet long. This planting map could be used as a model garden for two adults. It is based on the top-ranked vegetables from Table 7.2. The spring freeze-free date is assumed to be May 15.

VARIETIES

The best varieties for a food in one area may or may not be the best for another area. What you need is good localized information showing varieties that have been tested in your area and proven to be good producers. One source of information is your local county extension agent. Another source is the experience of good local gardeners.

Tomatoes are the nation's number-one vegetable crop. If you grow tomatoes and wish to compute your total yield, you have to pick the ripe fruits every two to three days, weigh them, record the weights, and at the end of the season add up the figures, This is usually repeated for about two years. A big test in which Dr. Peavy was involved called for studying the yield of forty tomato varieties planted in the high desert of El Paso, Texas. (Partial results are given in Table 7.6.)

If we had to pick the top two tomato varieties, they would be Early Girl and Fantastic. One source for both varieties is Porter & Sons Seeds. (See Appendix B.) Early Girl, as the name implies, is very early. If you want a giant tomato fruit, you might want to try Beefsteak. Under the test conditions in the Southwest it did not bear any fruit, but it might do better in your area. Better Boy bore large 11-ounce fruits, but the yield was only half that of the top two.

Table 7.4

Planting Plan Worksheet

KIND OF PLANT	NUMBER EATING	TOTAL FEET TO PLANT PER		ROWS PER BED	BED FEET NEEDED	WHEN TO PLANT	BED NUMBER
		PERSON	FAMILY				
EARLY							
MEDIUM							
LATE							

TOTAL BED FEET NEEDED

BED FEET AVAILABLE IN GARDEN

BED FEET TO BE CUT OR ADDED

Table 7.5

When to Plant Worksheet

Spring Freeze-Free Date ____________ **Fall Freeze Date** ____________

	FOR SUMMER GARDEN		FOR FALL GARDEN	
KIND OF FOOD TO PLANT	WEEKS FROM SPRING FREEZE-FREE DATE	WHEN TO PLANT	WEEKS FROM FALL FREEZE DATE	WHEN TO PLANT
EARLY				
Asparagus	4–6 before		8–10 before	
Beet	4–6 before		10–16 before	
Broccoli	4–6 before		10–16 before	
Brussels Sprouts	4–6 before		10–16 before	
Cabbage	4–6 before		10–16 before	
Carrot	4–6 before		12–14 before	
Cauliflower	4–6 before		10–16 before	
Celery	2 before–2 after		—	
Chard	2–6 before		12–16 before	
Collard	2–6 before		8–12 before	
Kohlrabi	2–6 before		12–16 before	
Lettuce	6 before–2 after		10–14 before	
Mustard	Freeze-free date–6 after		10–16 before	
Onion	4–6 before		8–10 before	
Peas, Green	2–8 before		8–12 before	
Potato	4–6 before		14–16 before	
Radish	6 before–4 after		8 before–freeze date	
Spinach	4–6 before		8–10 before	
Strawberries	4 before–4 after		8–10 before	
Sunchoke	4 before–4 after		freeze date–4 after	
Turnip	2–6 before		8–10 before	
MEDIUM				
Beans, general	2–8 after		8–10 before	
Bean, Lima	Freeze-free date–4 after		8–10 before	
Bean, Snap	Freeze-free date–4 after		8–10 before	
Corn	Freeze-free date–6 after		12–14 before	
Tomato	Freeze-free date–8 after		12–14 before	
LATE				
Black-Eyed Pea	2–10 after		10–12 before	
Cantaloupe	Freeze-free date–6 after		14–16 before	
Cucumber	Freeze-free date–6 after		10–12 before	
Eggplant	2–6 after		12–14 before	
Garlic	—		4–6 before	
Okra	2–6 after		12–16 before	
Peanut	Freeze-free date–2 after		—	
Pepper	1–8 after		12–16 before	
Squash	1–4 after		12–15 before	
Sweet Potato	2–8 after		—	
Watermelon	Freeze-free date–6 after		14–16 before	

Table 7.6

The Six Top-Yielding Tomato Varieties

Variety	Average Yield per Plant (Pounds)
Early Girl	18
Super Fantastic	16
Quik Pik	14
Earliana	13
Big Set	12
Floramerica	11

Note: Celebrity and Ace are also good varieties.

For cucumbers, be sure to try the Lemon variety (also available from Porter & Sons). It looks something like a lemon but definitely tastes like the most delicious cucumber you ever ate. For lettuce, Romaine (Cos), Buttercrunch, and Bibb—all leaf lettuces—are the highest in nutrition and taste. By all means, try black-eyed peas (Southern Pea or Cowpea). Good pea varieties are California Black-Eye and Purple Hull. For sweet pepper, try Paprika and California Wonder. (We do not recommend hot peppers, for health reasons.) For snap beans, Kentucky Wonder is a good pole variety and Blue Lake a good bush variety.

For sweet corn, most varieties are hybrids, which give much higher yields than non-hybrids. But there's a price to be paid for those high yields, and it is quality. Food grown from hybrids is inferior in nutritional quality. Some good non-hybrid sweet corn varieties are Country Gentleman and Golden Bantam. High-yielding hybrids include Golden Cross Bantam and Merit.

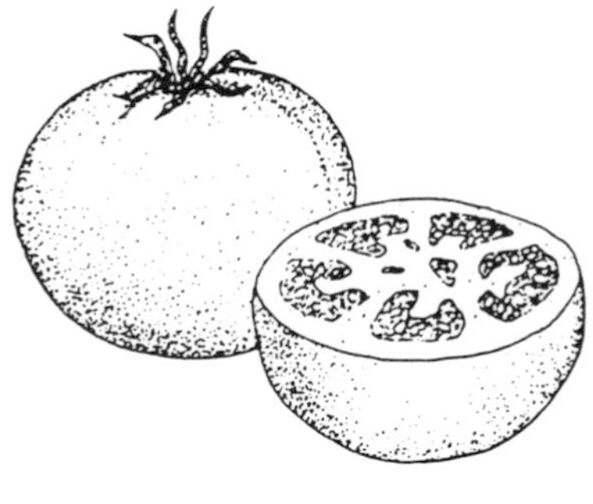

There is a pressing need for research into creating open-pollinated (non-hybrid) varieties that combine superior nutritional quality with good yields. Two good sources of non-hybrid seeds are Bountiful Gardens and Seed Savers Exchange. (Both are listed in Appendix B.)

Using your planting plan worksheet, list one vegetable at a time on the seed order worksheet, which you can make by copying onto a sheet of blank paper the format given in Table 7.7. From your county extension agent, local gardeners, this book, and seed catalogs, select one or more varieties and enter in the table. To figure out how much seed you wish to order, it's helpful to know how many seeds

Figure 7.2

Planting Map

Top View of a 20-Foot by 20-Foot Food Garden With 24-Inch-Wide Beds
(Walkways Not Shown)

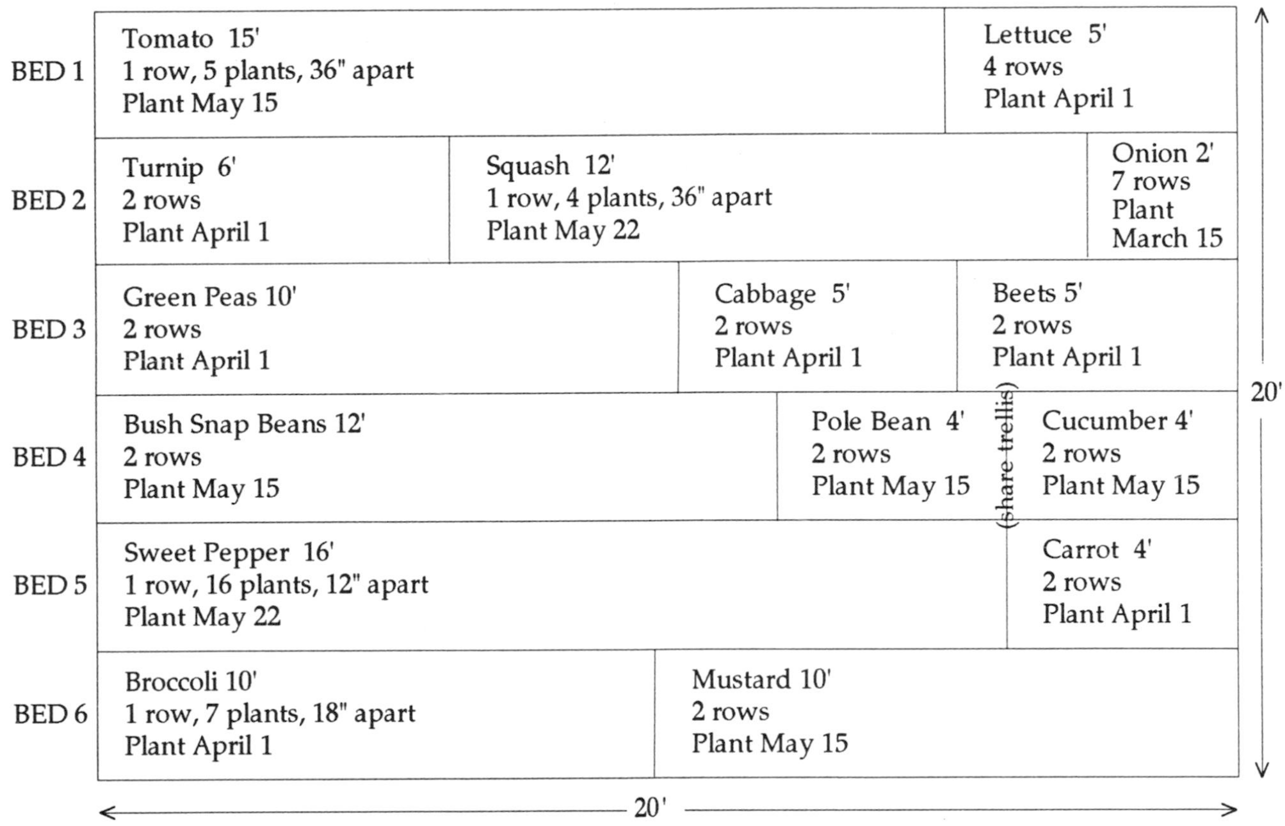

are in an ounce. For small seeds, the answer can be found in Table 8.1 (in Chapter 8). For large seeds:

Vegetable	**Number of Seeds per Ounce**
Lima Beans	25–75
Snap Beans	100–125
Southern Peas	about 225
Sweet Corn	120–180

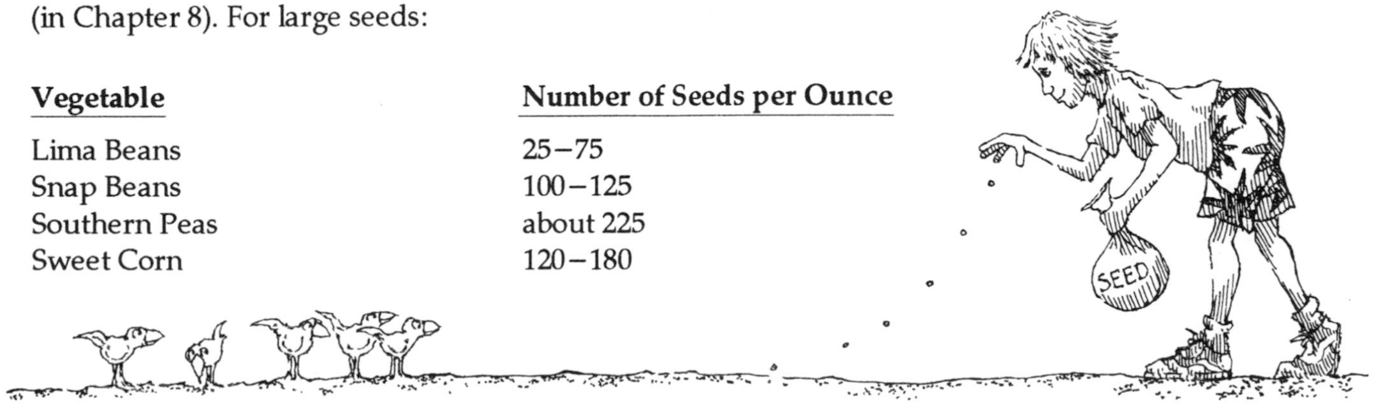

Table 7.7

Format for Seed and Transplant Order Worksheet

Food Plant	Variety	Amount of Seed Needed	On Hand	To Order	Source	Catalog Page
Tomato	Celebrity	—	—	—	Local garden center (plants)	
	Roma	—	—	—	Same	
Snap Bean (Bush)	Blue Lake	.5 lb.	0	.5 lb.	Porter	11
Cucumber	Lemon	3 packets	2 packets	1 packet	Porter	15

8. *Planting With Ease*

BEFORE you plant anything, you'll need to stake off the centerlines of your beds so you'll know where to plant. As described in Chapter 5, we suggest you use beds 24 to 36 inches wide, alternating with walkways 16 to 18 inches wide. Most of the time, a 24-inch bed is best since most good rear-tine tillers till a swath that wide. That gives you 40 inches from bed center to bed center if your walkways are 16 inches wide. If you have an extra-wide tiller that tills 36 inches, then make your beds 36 inches wide and your walkways 18 inches wide. That would give you 54 inches from bed center to bed center.

STAKING OFF BEDS

A practical way to mark your bed centers is to use 12-inch steel spikes from the hardware store. Use a hammer or hatchet to drive a row of them into the ground 40 inches apart (54 inches apart if you use an extra-wide tiller) in a straight line along both ends of your food plot. (Figure 8.1 shows the beds and centerstakes for a 20- by 20-foot garden using 24-inch beds and 16-inch walkways.) Move out into firmer, non-loosened soil to drive the spikes so they will stay firmly in the ground. Now you have your centerstakes.

Besides marking off centerlines, you might want to stake off your beds so nobody will walk on them. To do this, use another set of 12-inch spikes to stake off bed corners. With the bed center spikes in place, drive four more spikes into the ground to mark off the four corners of the first bed. Stretch a strong twine taut between the corner spikes. Now take a hoe and mark the bed outline by digging a shallow trench along the lines you have stretched. The four corner spikes and the twine are no longer needed at the first bed, so they can be pulled up and used to mark off another bed. Remember that bed outlines will alternate, with 16- to 18-inch walkways in between.

Wood Stakes

Even better than steel spikes are wood stakes, 1 by 2 by 16 inches, driven in to mark the centerline of each bed. We like the wood stakes, especially along one end of the beds, because we can use a black felt pen or some stencils and spray paint to mark the stakes with consecutive numbers for each bed. That helps us to do a better

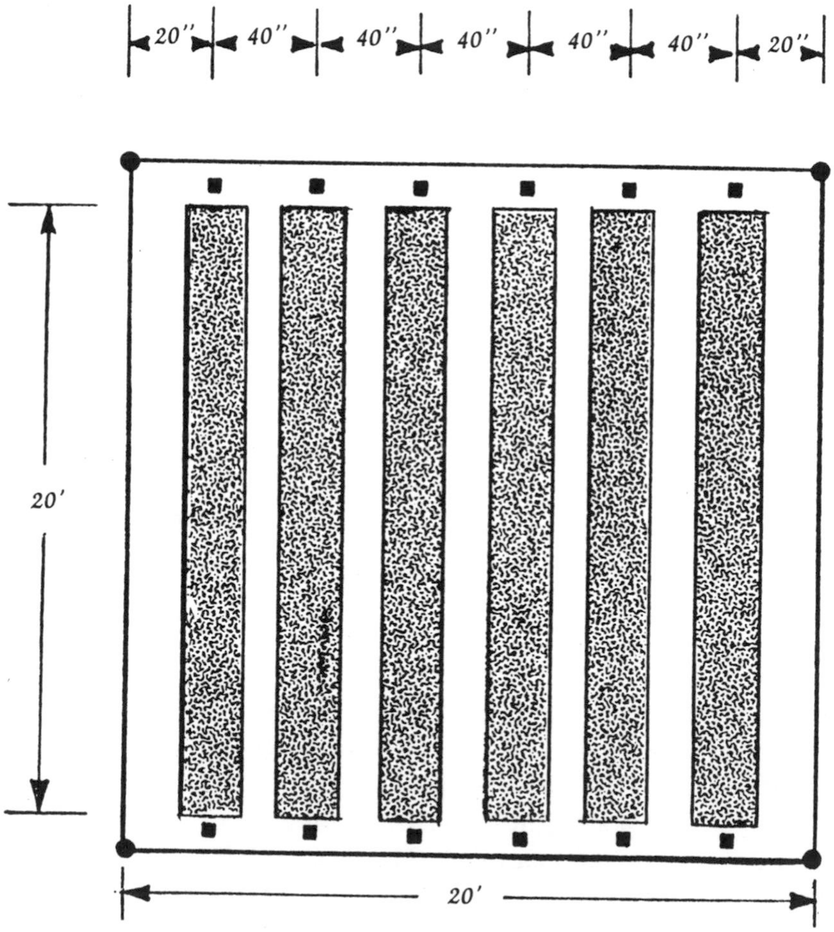

Figure 8.1 Beds and center stakes for a 20-foot by 20-foot food garden with 24-inch beds and 16-inch walkways.

job of planning and to keep up with what was planted where and when—vital information when it's time for crop rotation.

Soak the bottom 10 inches of each stake in rot-proofing solution, then dry thoroughly, and only then drive them into the ground. It is a good idea to paint the top of the stakes with white latex paint, which preserves them against the weather and makes them easy to see. Otherwise, some people might stumble over them. When putting in stakes, make sure the sharp end goes into the ground and that either edge of the protruding end is on the centerline.

If you choose *not* to have steel spikes or wood stakes at each end of each bed, then be sure you have a reference stake or some other reference point near your growing area so you can always locate a corner of Bed 1 by measuring from the reference. After a season or two, your permanent beds will be fairly easy to see, since they are loose and tend to be slightly raised above the walkways.

PLANTING BEDDING PLANTS

To get nutrition from the PowerCharged soil you have built, you have to populate it with green plants. To populate your food plot, you will need to plant seeds or set out bedding plants (transplants). For the smaller food garden (20 by 20 feet or smaller), it is usually best to buy bedding plants from a nursery; if some plants are unavailable, then get them going by planting seeds.

If organic fertilizer (except compost) has been applied, it is best to wait three to four weeks before transplanting or planting. Tomatoes are usually established by transplanting small plants into holes in the ground. Other plants also good to transplant include pepper, cabbage, broccoli, and cauliflower.

Transplants have a top that is 2 to 6 inches tall and a rootball 2 to 3 inches in diameter by 2 to 4 inches long. Valuable time is saved by transplants. You get a jump on the season. Suitable outdoor growing temperatures for tomatoes are not reached until the average spring freeze-free date, but indoors you can start six weeks earlier and have nice big plants a month sooner.

A bulb planter is very helpful for taking a chunk of soil out of the ground to create a hole just the right size for the rootball of a bedding plant. If a bulb planter is not available, use a trowel to dig the holes.

Conditioning Transplants

Do not take plants directly out of a greenhouse, your windowsill, or the garden center and then transplant them to the garden. They will be too tender to withstand the sudden change from a safe, sheltered environment indoors to the harsher conditions outdoors. Plants need to be conditioned, or "hardened off," before being transplanted outdoors. To harden them off, gradually expose the plants to the outdoors and reduce their water. About a week before you wish to transplant them outdoors, put them out in a sheltered place in bright light for an hour or two, then bring them back in. The next day, put them out in the same spot but expose them for two to four hours. The third day, put them in full sun for perhaps six hours—and so on until you can leave them out all day. After four to seven days, they are ready to be transplanted outdoors.

When to Transplant

The best time to set plants outdoors is late afternoon. This gives the young plants about twelve hours of darkness for the roots to grow into the soil of their new home. It reduces transplant shock by cutting down on transpiration (loss of water from the breathing pores of the leaves) while the roots are getting into position to absorb water from the soil. This way, your plants will be all set the next day to absorb the water the leaves will need when the sun comes up.

How to Transplant

Most of the plants you will transplant are quite widely spaced, so you will need a garden line (such as twine) and a rule to show you where to make planting holes. You can use a yardstick laid along the garden line. When transplants are to be spaced twelve inches apart or less, a planting template will save you lots of time. A good template is a piece of board (such as a one-by-two) eight feet long with a mark showing where each plant goes.

When you're ready to set plants out, take your transplants (which are sitting in small cups of potting soil), a bulb planter or trowel, and a bucket of water with a small can for dipping water. Here is a good transplanting procedure (illustrated in Figure 8.2):

1. Water all plants thoroughly until a little water drains out at the bottom.
2. Stretch a line between the center stakes and use a yardstick or template to mark planting spots. Then take your bulb planter or trowel and dig planting holes so the plants will end up at the same level as they were in the cup. (Tomato plants need to be set much deeper, because their stems will sprout roots and will need protection from the wind.)
3. Your transplants must be removed properly from their potting soil. Hold out one hand, palm facing up. Turn the cup upside down onto that hand, with the stem between your fingers. With your free hand, tap the bottom of the cup. That should loosen the rootball enough so you can lift the cup off. Handle the transplant by the rootball only, not the stem.

Figure 8.2

A Good Transplanting Procedure

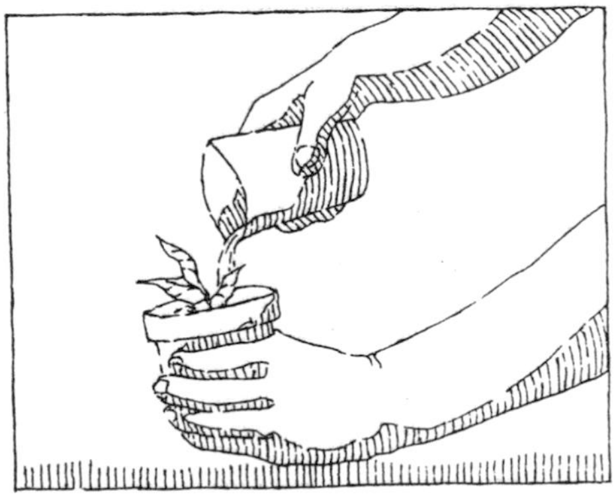

1. Water the plant thoroughly.

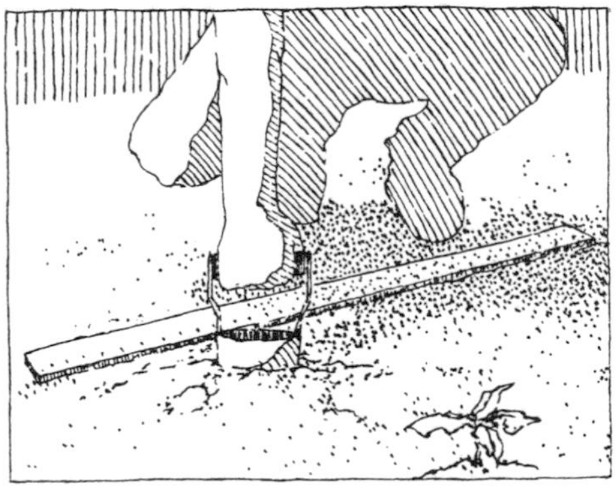

2. Mark off and dig your planting holes.

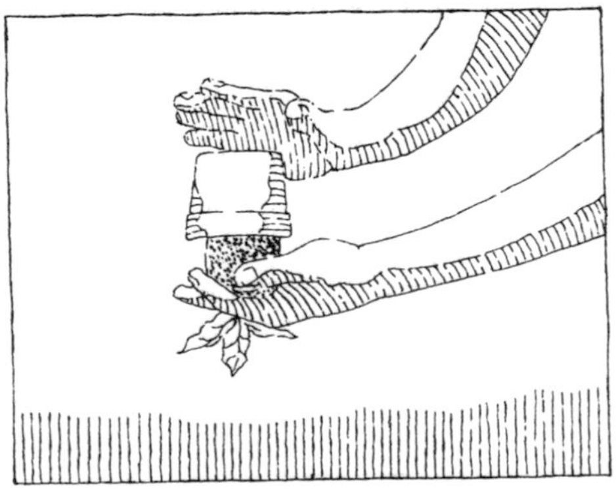

3. Lift the cup off the transplants.

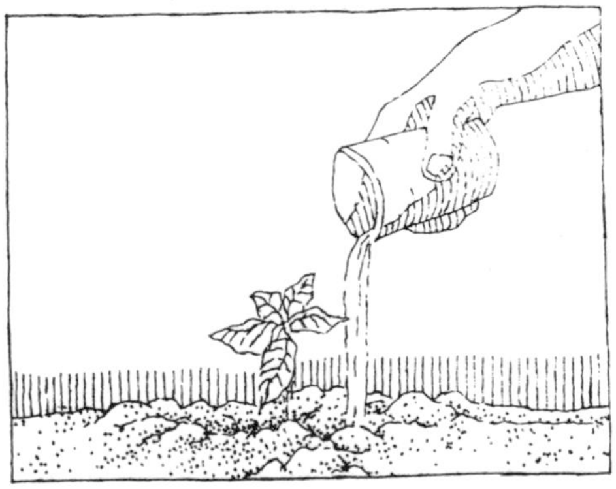

4. Place the rootball of the plant in the hole; water thoroughly.

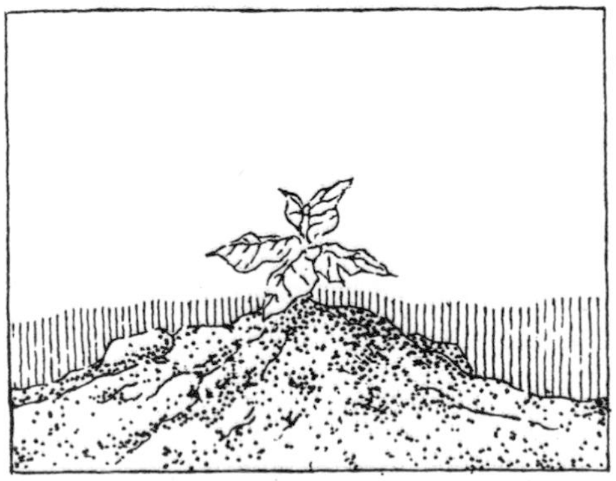

5. Firm the soil around the plant, and mound up earth to protect it from wind.

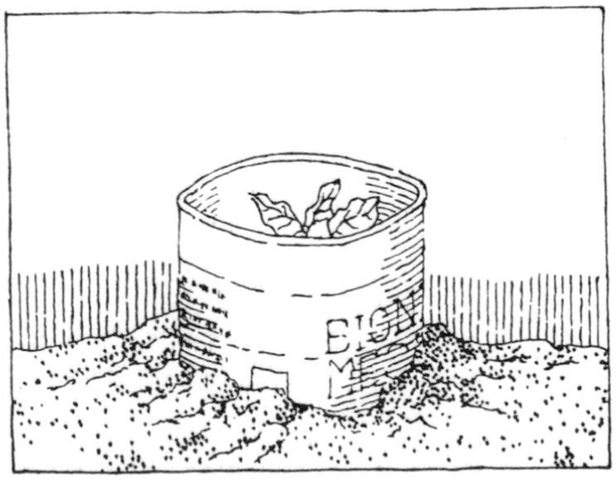

6. Install wind protection, such as a coffee can with its top and bottom removed.

4. Carefully place the rootball of the plant in the hole. If tomato, bury the stem up to the first set of true leaves. All of the buried stem will grow roots. With other transplants, set the plant at the same depth it had grown in the cup.
5. Pour water around the sides of the rootball sitting in the hole, and fill in the spaces with loose soil.
6. After the water has dried, place more soil around the rootball of the plant, and press down firmly on all sides of the stem. This is to collapse all big air pockets and to be sure the rootball is in good contact with the soil. Mound up the earth around the stem of the plant a little to lessen its getting whipped around in the wind.
7. Install wind protection. Most areas have damaging winds in the spring. Be prepared with protection such as:

   - An empty can, such as a three-quart coffee can with the bottom cut out. Place this cylinder of thin metal around the plant and push it down into the soil an inch or two to anchor it. If you have the plastic top that came with the can, snap it in place at the top and leave it until the plant reaches the top. If you don't have the plastic top, then cover the top with a board when the sun is not shining, but at all other times leave it uncovered so sunlight can strike the plant.

   - An empty milk carton or a large paper bag. Cut the bottom out of the paper bag, leaving a flap. Place around the plant, bottom side first, and put soil on the flap to anchor the sack. If an empty milk carton, cut off the top and the bottom, except on the bottom leave a flap on which to pile soil as an anchor. With either cover, mound soil up around the base an inch or two to hold the cover in place.

Starter Solution for Bedding Plants

You may be advised to use a starter solution when setting out bedding plants. This means that instead of just pouring plain water into the hole around the rootball, you first mix the water with a special compound, usually a high-phosphorus fertilizer. Phosphorus is often advised since it is said to stimulate rooting, and that is true—but only if the roots are forming on a germinating seed. Phosphorus has no effect on roots of bedding plants unless the soil already has a phosphorus deficiency.

Root Stimulator

You may see bottles or jugs of "root stimulator" offered for sale. This is the same as "starter solution," and most of what you are buying is water. Since you have water already, you can make up your own starter solution or root stimulator by mixing any high-phosphorus fertilizer with water. For instance, mix 1 teaspoonful of BR-61 (a fertilizer that has a 0-60-0 NPK analysis) per gallon of water, or mix 3 teaspoonfuls of plain superphosphate (0-20-0 NPK) per gallon of water. These are likely to be more effective in soils low in phosphorus.

Cold Protection

If you're planting early in the season, you'll need some protection from the cold. Here are several methods.

Hotkaps and Row Covers

Hotkaps are miniature tents made of wax-like paper placed over early planted transplants. (See Figure 8.3.) They not only protect from light frosts but raise the early season temperatures around early set, heat-loving plants such as tomato and peppers and give you an earlier harvest. For a few plants, you can turn buckets upside down over them in the late evening to protect against cold injury, but hotkaps are better.

A new type of hotkap is the row cover. The floating row cover is especially useful because it takes no framework to hold it up. You just lay it over newly seeded beds or over a row of newly set transplants; it is so light, the plants will just lift it up as they grow. (See Appendix A for sources.) Row covers often come 60 inches wide. If your beds are narrower, then cut the cover into strips.

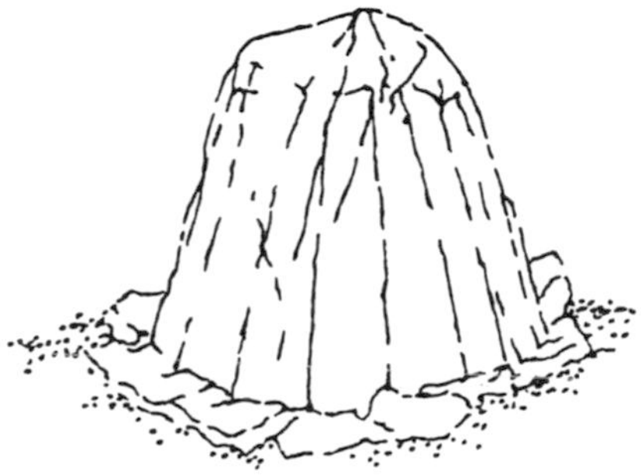

Figure 8.3 Place a hotkap over your transplant to protect it from the cold.

Water Walls

You can also protect plants from cold by using a water wall. It does about the same thing as a hotkap or a row cover but has a number of plastic sleeves attached to form a circle about 12 inches in diameter and 18 inches high. You fill the sleeves with water and set it down over plants just as with hotkaps. Daytime sunlight heats up the water, which is released at night as temperatures drop below freezing.

We are testing water walls and are not sure yet if they are that much better than hotkaps. It appears that hotkaps are about as effective as water walls but cost much less. (When hotkaps were selling for 30 cents each, water walls were selling for $2.50 each. However, water walls can be re-used up to six times.)

PLANTING SEEDS

Be sure your seeds are viable. Viable seeds are those with living germs that will germinate and emerge through the soil surface to give you a good, healthy row of plants. Keep seeds dry and cold by storing them in your refrigerator. For long-term storage, you can even use the freezer.

If you are unsure about some of your seeds, give them a germination test. It's easy. Fold a paper napkin in half, unfold it, place either half on a saucer, moisten that half to hold it down, then count out ten seeds and place them on the moistened napkin about an inch apart. (See Figure 8.4.) Cover the seeds with the other half of the napkin, moisten again, and slide the saucer into a plastic bag. Fold the bag under to seal it off, and place the saucer on top of your hot water heater or some other warm spot. Tape a note to the door of the hot water heater closet to remind yourself to check the seeds for germination on the third day and every day thereafter for several more days. If your seeds are good, nine out of ten will germinate, giving you 90 percent germination. If germination is less than 90 percent, you should compensate by planting extra seeds—the lower the germination rate, the more the extra seeds. How many more seeds? Divide 100 by the germination percentage. The result tells you how many seeds to plant for each seed that is figured into the standard seeding rate. For instance, if you get 50 percent germination, meaning only half the seeds germinate, you should plant twice as thick to compensate for those that won't come up.

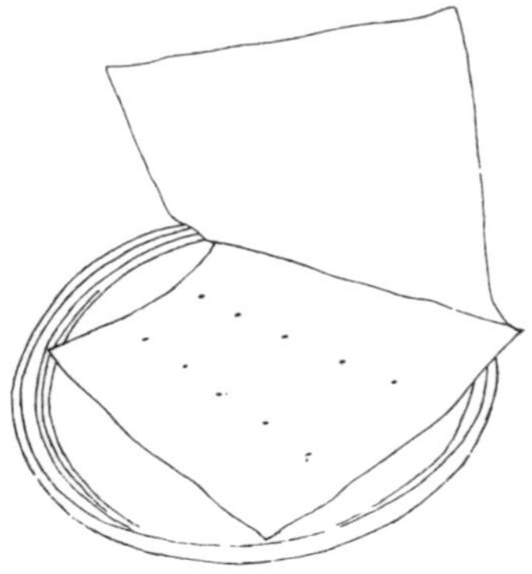

Figure 8.4 A germination test lets you know the viability of your seeds.

To align your rows, stretch twine between the centerline stakes of the bed.

Planting Large Seeds

Plant large seeds, such as corn and beans, about 1 to 1.5 inches deep. Use the corner of a narrow, long-bladed hoe—or, better, a V-bladed hoe—to open a deep planting trench. Look back at Figure 7.1 to find the proper spacing for the seeds along the bed. For insurance, you can plant your seeds double thick, then thin out the extra plants if they all come up. That means if the proper spacing is 5 inches, plant a seed every 2.5 inches if you want insurance. In addition, if your germination rate is around 50 percent, plant two seeds every 2.5 inches.

Don't worry if it seems like you're planting too many seeds. It's better to be safe than sorry. You can easily thin later. If you plant one seed according to the spacings in Figure 7.1 and every seed comes up, you are in good shape and will not have to thin. But if the bugs or the worms or the birds get some of the seeds, you can end up with a poor stand.

Hold a few seeds in the palm of one hand while dropping one or two at a time into the trench with the other hand. Then backfill the trench until the seeds are covered to the proper depth. Firm the soil over the seeds to eliminate air pockets by lightly tamping with the back of the hoe blade or rake.

Planting Small Seeds

Small seeds, such as onion and lettuce, require a different planting method. Because they are so small in size (Table 8.1 indicates just how small), they must be planted very shallow, about three-eighths to half an inch deep. Special care is needed to keep the seedbed moist until emergence.

Just before planting, take a rake and rake off the top crust of the bed. If the soil in the bed is not loose for half an inch deep, then use the rake to loosen it. That is the depth at which you will need to make a seedbed in the form of a planting trench. A good way to make planting trenches for small seeds is to use a heavy-duty yardstick. With your garden line stretched between the centerline stakes of the bed, place the long thin edge of the yardstick on the soil surface and press down about half an inch. Then wiggle it a little, side-to-side, to keep the sides of the trench from falling when you lift the yardstick out. (See Figure 8.5.)

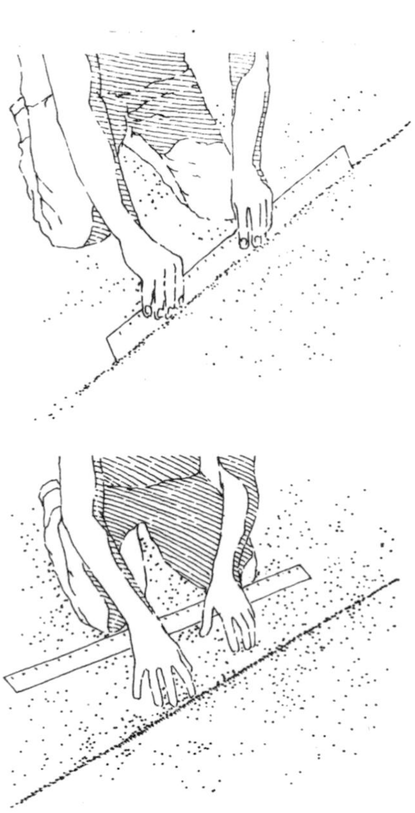

Figure 8.5 Make a planting trench for small seeds by using a yardstick.

Planting Onions

You can sow onion seeds directly out of the seed packet. Snip off about the top quarter-inch from the packet, then fold the packet in half, creating a vertical crease. Hold the packet an inch or two directly above the planting trench, and shake the packet to let seed fall

Table 8.1

How Small Are Small Seeds?

Vegetable	Seeds per Ounce
Very Small	
Celery	72,000
Lettuce	25,000
Carrot	23,000
Turnip	15,000
Mustard	15,000
Small	
Broccoli	9,000
Brussels Sprouts	9,000
Cabbage	9,000
Cauliflower	9,000
Collard	9,000
Kale	9,000
Kohlrabi	9,000
Onion	8,500

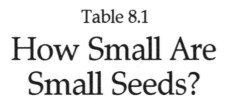

slowly out as you move along the trench. You might need to practice. One seed every quarter-inch is a good rate of seeding. This is about forty-eight seeds per linear foot. This will give you a nice thick stand, which you can thin early—and you can even eat the thinnings. Don't worry too much initially about the spacing. That will be taken care of later on by thinning.

We suggest you cover small seeds in the planting trench with a seed covering mix. Good mixes are compost; a mixture of half screened soil and half compost; half soil and half vermiculite; and sphagnum peat moss. Moisten the mix and use it to cover the seeds and to fill the trench. Then firm the covering mix above the seed by tamping gently with the back of a hoe or rake.

Planting Lettuce

Lettuce is spaced much more widely than onions. To make planting easy, make planting trenches as with onions, then lay a planting template along those trenches for "hill-dropping" lettuce seed. Hill-dropping means you grasp one to three seeds and drop them in the planting trench every 3 to 6 inches. You can drop seeds every 2 to 3 inches just for insurance, since thinning is easy with this much space between seed drops. Cover and tamp the same as with onions. Instead of hill-dropping, you can sow more thickly directly out of the seed packet after creasing it like you would with onions.

Keep the Seedbed Moist

Small seeds are planted only about half an inch deep or shallower, and the soil surrounding the seed must be kept moist until the seedlings emerge. First of all, be sure you plant in soil that is moist from the surface to at least 6 inches deep. Then keep the soil around the seeds moist until plants emerge and become about 1 inch tall.

The first few days after planting are critical because the top half-inch of soil can dry out quickly. You can keep the top inch of soil moist by mulching the seedbed to stop surface drying. Then, starting the third day, lift up a few inches of the mulch to see when emergence begins. When the first sprouts are seen, rake all the mulch off to one side. Organic mulch can be used, but so can wooden boards or strips of burlap. We like burlap because you can buy it in rolls and cut narrow or wide strips to fit any situation. The only time you wouldn't want to use mulching is in the early spring, when you would want the sun to warm the soil.

Another way to keep the seedbed moist is to lay a soaker hose up against the line of planted seeds on the soil surface, and turn on the water every day just long enough to wet a band of soil about an inch wide.

Still another way is to sprinkle the seedbed lightly with a sprinkler can held close to the soil (to prevent splash erosion). Or mist with a misting nozzle on the end of your hose every day until emergence. Some seeds will come up in two to three days. Others require five to eight days. (See Table 8.2.) Soil temperature and planting depth determine how long it takes for seeds to emerge as plants.

The preceding methods enable you to keep moist only the beds that are planted. Still another way, if you have a solid-set sprinkler system, is to turn on the four sprinklers at each corner of your garden every day just long enough to apply about a quarter-inch of water. When all is said and done, that might be the easiest way.

THINNING

A common mistake is failure to thin a row of direct-seeded food plants. But it is fatal not to do so. You cannot feel sorry for the plants. Where there are too many, none can grow properly. There is a final spacing that is best for all plants. (See Figure 7.1.) It is a good idea to reach the final spacing gradually. Use two or more thinnings for insurance against the possibility that natural forces will help you thin and leave you with skips.

Thinning Lettuce

We have found the following procedure to be the best for thinning lettuce. It requires that you get down on your hands and knees or be able to squat. You might want to get yourself a pair of kneepads to make kneeling easier. Here is the procedure:

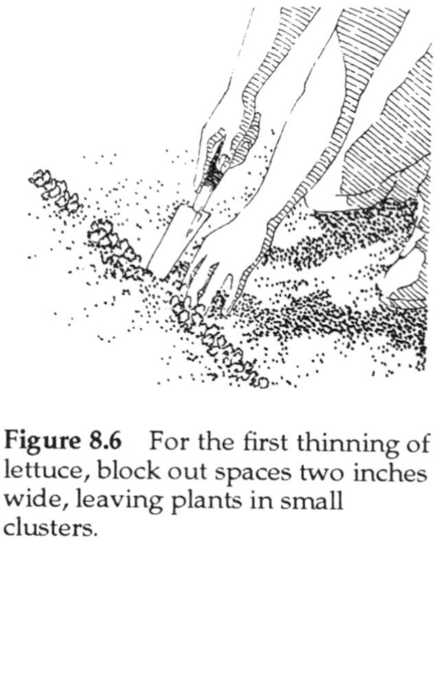

Figure 8.6 For the first thinning of lettuce, block out spaces two inches wide, leaving plants in small clusters.

1. *First Thinning.* This step applies to a thick stand of lettuce seedlings where the seeds have been sown rather than hill-dropped. (If hill-dropped, go to the next step.) Slide a sharp putty knife or mason's trowel on the surface across the line of plants with a swift movement to cut off the stems of the plants in its path. Leave blocks of space about two inches wide. (See Figure 8.6.) Try to leave one to three plants in a cluster.

   Go over the area again and thin back to one plant every two inches. Select the largest, healthiest-looking plant in each cluster to save, and use a sharp knife or your fingers to thin the rest. You will now have a nice row of lettuce plants, with a single plant every two inches.

   When should you do the thinning? When plants first emerge, you will see two tiny leaves. These are seed leaves, not true leaves. Soon you will see a third leaf start to form. That is the first true leaf. Try to do the first thinning after the first true leaf starts to grow but before the second true leaf emerges. (See Figure 8.7.)

Table 8.2

Days to Emergence

(For Seeds Planted Half an Inch Deep)

	Soil Temperature				
	86°F	77°F	68°F	59°F	50°F
Bean, Lima	7	7	18	—	—
Bean, Snap	6	8	11	16	—
Beet	5	5	6	10	17
Cabbage	4	5	6	9	15
Carrot	6	6	7	10	17
Cauliflower	5	5	6	10	20
Celery	—	—	7	12	16
Corn	4	4	7	12	22
Cucumber	5	4	6	13	—
Eggplant	5	8	13	—	—
Lettuce	3	2	3	4	7
Okra	7	13	17	—	—
Onion	4	4	5	7	13
Parsley	12	13	14	17	—
Parsnip	32	15	14	19	—
Pea, Green	6	6	8	9	14
Pepper	8	8	13	25	—
Radish	3	4	4	6	11
Spinach	6	5	6	7	12
Tomato	6	6	8	14	—
Turnip	1	1	2	5	5
Watermelon	4	5	12	—	—

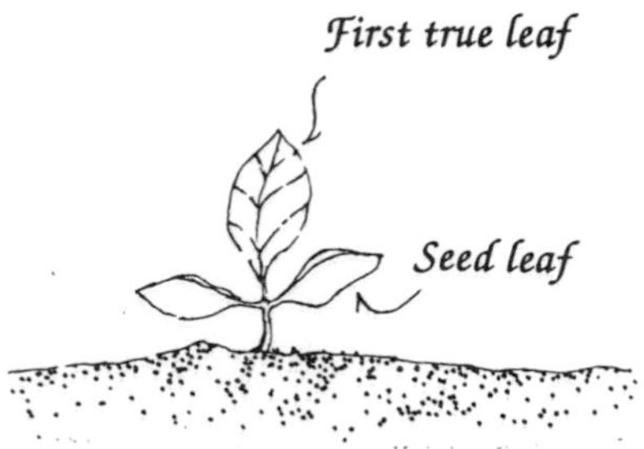

Figure 8.7 Try to do the first thinning after the first true leaf starts to grow but before the second true leaf emerges.

2. *Second Thinning.* After a short time, there will be no vacant spaces in the lettuce row. All the two-inch blocks you had cut out will now be filled with plant growth. Take out every other plant so that the remaining plants are now spaced four to six inches apart. The plants you just took out will be large enough to eat. You are now almost at final spacing.
3. *Harvest Thinning.* The second thinning left spaces four to six inches wide. Soon, all that space will be filled in and you will have mature lettuce plants ready for harvest. As before, harvest by taking out every other plant. This gives eight inches between the plants that are left for a little extra growth. For romaine (cos) lettuce, each maturing plant needs ten to twelve inches of space, so you might need to do one additional thinning.

Table 8.3

Life Cycle of Food Plants

Crop	Days to Harvest From Seed	Length of Harvest (Days)
EARLY PLANTING		
Asparagus	730	60
Beet	50–60	30
Broccoli	60–80	40
Brussels Sprouts	90–100	21
Cabbage	60–90	40
Carrot	70–80	21
Cauliflower	70–90	14
Celery	100	30
Chard	45–55	40
Collard	60	60
Kale	70–90	60
Kohlrabi	55–75	14
Lettuce	45–90	21
Mustard	30	30
Onion (green)	90–120	40
Onion (bulb)	120–150	One Time
Pea (green)	55–90	7
Potato	75–100	One Time
Radish	25–40	7
Spinach	40–60	40
Strawberry	90	Until Frost
Sunchoke	120	Over Winter
Turnip	30–60	30
MEDIUM PLANTING		
Beans, general	90	One Time
Green Snap Bean (bush)	45–60	14
Green Snap Bean (pole)	60–70	30
Lima Bean (bush)	65–80	14
Lima Bean (pole)	75–85	40
Soybeans	120	One Time
Sweet Corn	70–90	10
Tomato	70–90	40
LATE PLANTING		
Black-Eyed Pea	60–70	30
Cantaloupe/Honeydew	85–100	30
Cucumber	50–70	30
Eggplant	80–90	90
Okra	80–120	Until Frost
Peanut	120–150	One Time
Summer Squash	55–60	40
Sweet Pepper	60–90	90
Sweet Potato	100–120	One Time
Watermelon	80–100	30
Winter Squash	85–100	One Time

Thinning Onions

As soon as onions are large enough to grasp with your fingers, water the bed to loosen the soil and then thin the plants to about a quarter-inch apart. (Half an inch apart is okay, too.) When you thin, you will leave small blocks of empty space. Soon, the plants you leave will fill in this space, and at the second thinning the green onions will be large enough for you to eat the thinnings. Remember that the green top is exceedingly rich in vitamin A. Continue to thin and to eat the thinnings as green onions until the space between plants is two to three inches wide. At this point you have two choices: continue to harvest and eat the onions as green bunching onions; or let them grow and form mature bulbs two to three inches in diameter.

Thinning Large Plants

For crops grown from large seeds, such as corn and beans, use thinning procedures somewhat similar to the process for lettuce and onions, except you can't eat the thinnings. The idea is that when the plants are still small, you should have more of them than when they reach their final spacing. The temporary excess provides: insurance against loss of plants to weather, birds, or insects; shade for the soil surface; and a supply of organic matter from thinnings. One difference with these large plants is that you simply pull the surplus plants up out of the ground with your fingers or cut off the stems with scissors.

REPLANTING VACANT BEDS

Radish is the quickest food plant to mature (thirty-five days) and garlic the slowest (thirty-two weeks). Table 8.3 shows the time from seed to harvest and the number of days of harvesting you'll get from various food plants. When harvest nears, look at the When to Plant Worksheet (from Chapter 7) to see if there is still time to plant some other crop in the space about to be vacated.

9. *Weed Control*

WEEDS probably drive more gardeners away from gardening than any other single cause. They also are a great problem to commercial growers, leading to frequent and heavy dosings of the soil with chemical weed killers year after year. These weed killers, called herbicides, can be picked up by the plants and passed on to you when you eat food grown from this soil. That is another good reason for you to grow some of your own food in soil free from herbicides.

GOOD WEEDS AND BAD WEEDS

Weeds are plants that appear in your food plot as growths that you didn't plant and don't want. They steal nutrients, light, and water from your food plants. This will result in reduced harvest or no harvest at all, so you must control weeds or they will control you.

Some weeds are worse than others. The "good" weeds are the annuals, which are easily killed by cutting the weed off at the surface of the soil. The "bad" weeds are the perennials, which form storage organs underground such as swollen roots. You can cut perennial weeds off at the surface, but that does not kill them. Instead, the underground storage organ just sends up another shoot, and this is repeated time after time. The biggest offenders in this group are Bermuda grass, Johnson grass, bindweed, and nut sedge. (See Figure 9.1.)

THE BEST WEED CONTROL

Figure 9.1
The pesty perennial weeds.

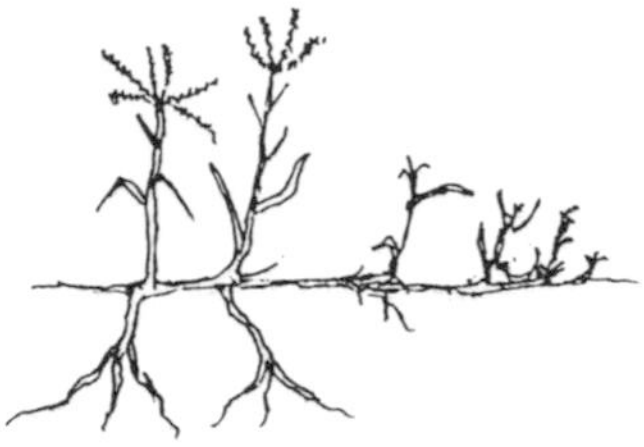

Bermuda grass

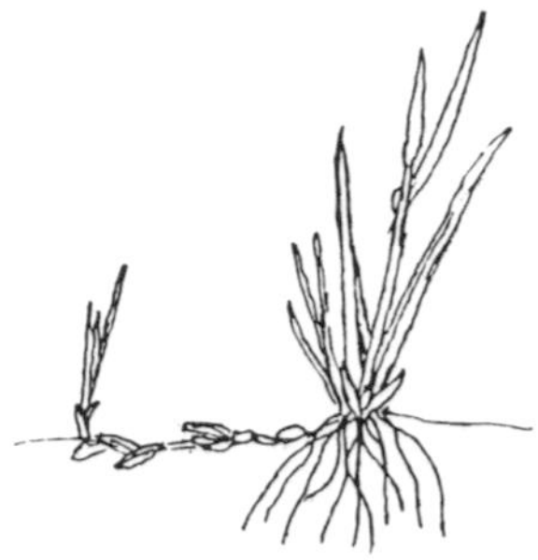

Johnson grass

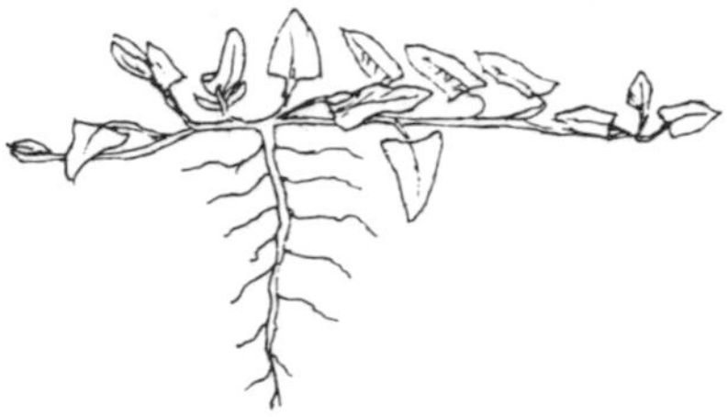

Bindweed

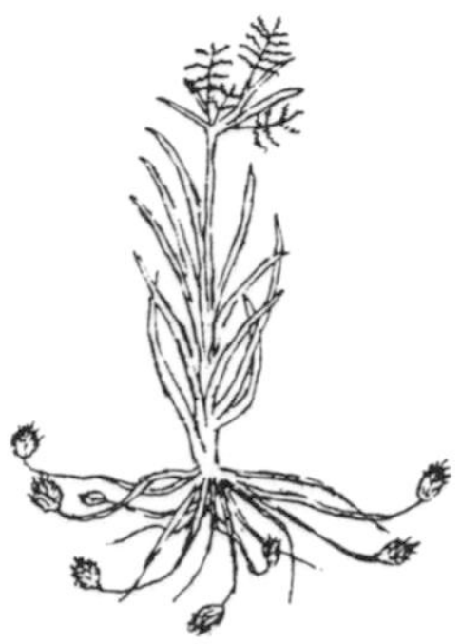

Nut sedge

The best way to control weeds is by prevention: don't let them come up and start growing. Do this by depriving weed seedlings of light and by avoiding cultivation of the soil. To cut their light off, keep the soil surface covered with mulch. (For details on this, see Chapter 10.)

Cultivation, or tillage, means mechanically loosening the soil, and the less this is done the better. Nature never tills. She mulches by maintaining a bed of decaying leaves, grasses, and other plants on the ground at all times. You should cultivate only when you prepare beds for planting or work with soil-improving materials. Most soil contains at various depths thousands of weed seeds that last for years and stay dormant if you leave them be. But cultivation brings them up to or near the surface, where conditions are ideal for germination. Avoid tillage, and you avoid activating weed seeds.

PESTY PERENNIALS

These are the weeds that come up and regenerate from underground storage organs. If you pick a food-growing plot that is free of these weed pests, you are lucky. Just go into a mulching program, never let a weed grow up and go to seed, and you're home free.

Alas, this is often not the case. You may have a Bermuda grass lawn you want to convert to food growing. Or you may have bindweed or some other perennial weed pest. Here is where we make an exception to the rule of "no herbicides in the home garden" and advise use of a special systemic weed killer called glyphosate, sold under the trade name of Roundup. We make this exception because Roundup is used once or twice within a two-week period and then no more; it is inactivated when it strikes the soil; it is absorbed by the leaves of the weed, then circulates throughout all parts of the plant, killing even the troublesome underground storage organ; and it is quick, thorough, and permanent. (For details on using Roundup, see the "Perennial Weed Removal" section of Chapter 5.)

We strongly advise you to get rid of perennial weeds before planting your food plot. Once you get rid of perennial weeds, you will easily be able to keep any weeds under control with mulching and mechanical methods such as hoeing.

WEED CONTROL BY HOE

If you choose not to use mulch for weed control or have to wait for some reason to go the mulching route, try the nursery hoe. (See Figure 9.2.) This hoe is an excellent tool to get the weeds. It has a long narrow blade about three inches tall and seven inches long. No gardener should be without one. If you cannot find one locally, you can order one from Nasco. (See "Weed Control" listing in Appendix A.)

How to Sharpen a Hoe

A hoe, to be used effectively, must have a sharp knife-like blade. It is actually a knife blade mounted on a long handle for use while you are standing upright. The blade of the hoe is moved into or along the soil surface. But there are often small rocks in the soil, so the hoe's cutting edge suffers nicks and becomes dull, causing it to cut poorly. At this point, the cutting edge needs to be sharpened.

A file (from a hardware store) is the most common tool used to sharpen the nursery hoe and other sharp-bladed tools. To sharpen any tool, hold it firmly and slide the surface of the file over the surface of the cutting edge. A small vise mounted on a sturdy table is the best way to hold the hoe firmly in place. If you don't have the vise or the table, place two bricks on edge parallel to each other and about 3 inches apart on a concrete slab. Place the hoe in the slot between the bricks, with the cutting edge up. (See illustration below.) Hold the hoe firmly by placing one knee on it as you kneel down over the blade to sharpen it.

HOE-SHARPENING TECHNIQUE

The top end of the file is a thin piece of steel designed as a handle. If you're right-handed, grasp the top end (the handle end) of the file with your right hand and the opposite end of the file with your left hand. Move the file downward against the blade of the hoe at an angle of about 45°. Move the file firmly to remove or grind off all the nicks and blunt edges and restore the sharp cutting edge. After each stroke, lift the file up, return it to the original position, and repeat the stroke. Move across the blade of the hoe to the other edge. Repeat until the cutting edge is sharp. Several passes may be needed.

Be careful. The sharp blade will cut your hands if you push against it. Don't let your right hand get down too close to the blade of the hoe.

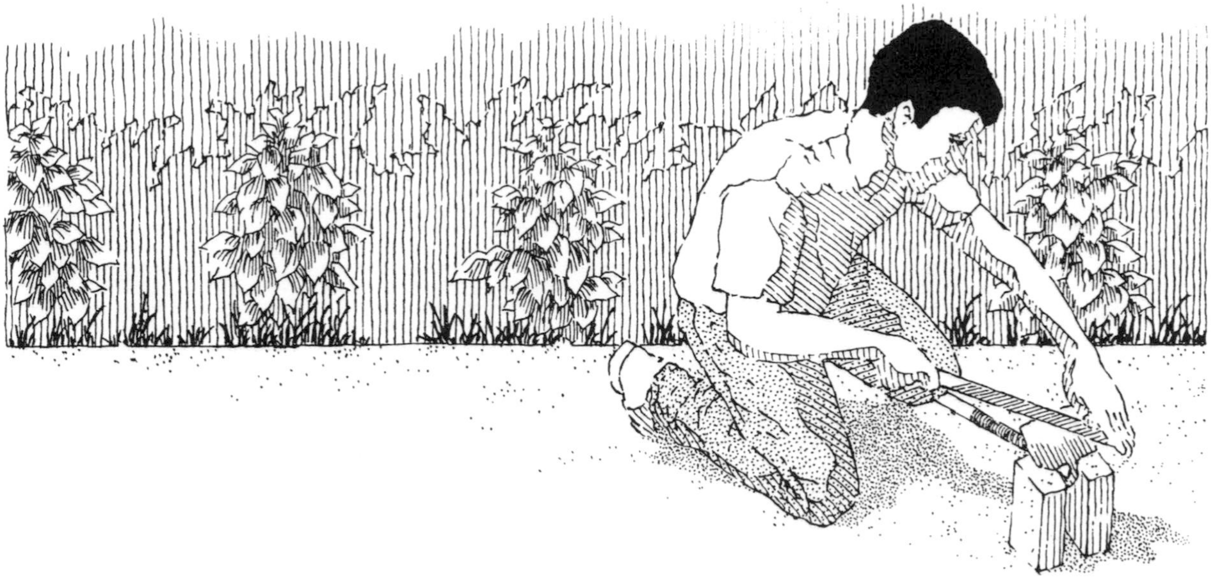

Another good hoe is the sliding hoe. (See Figure 9.3.) It is D-shaped with a thin sharp blade. It is also known as a "swing head hoe." You don't chop with this hoe; instead, you slide it back and forth along the soil surface. It actually shaves the weeds off at the surface of the soil just like you shave whiskers off your face or hair off your legs. You don't have to lift it for each stroke as you would

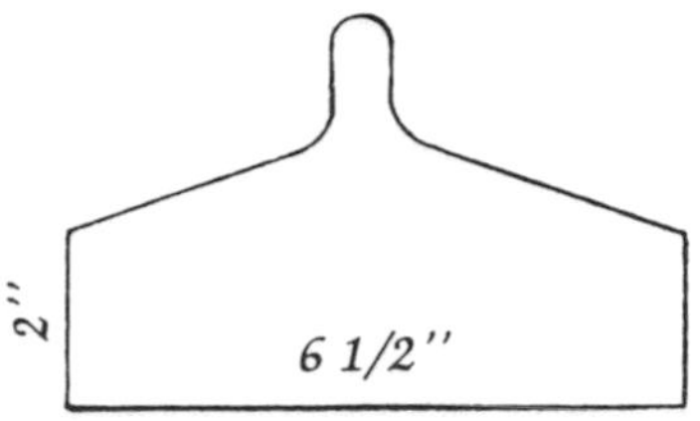

Figure 9.2 Blade of a nursery hoe.

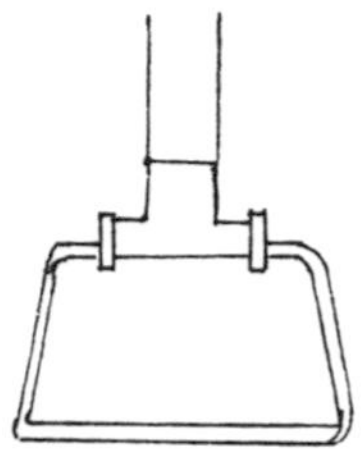

Figure 9.3 Blade of a sliding hoe.

with other hoes. It is the easiest way to shave weeds off the surface we have ever seen.

Be sure to keep the hoe blade sharp. (See "How to Sharpen a Hoe" inset on page 111.) Go to your local hardware store for a hoe-sharpening tool called a file, and ask them to show you how to use it if you don't already know. A sharp hoe blade is like a razor on the face. This leaves the soil undisturbed. Go through your garden at least once a week and cover every square foot. Go up one row and down the next. After shaving the weeds off at the surface, leave them as a mulch.

In areas where spring comes late and you need to leave the soil uncovered so it will warm up, this hoe is especially useful. It handles small weeds best, so you can easily catch them before they get too big.

10. *Mulch, Magic, and Compost*

MULCH is a covering you place over bare soil. Examples include spoiled hay, straw, stable cleanings, lawn clippings, shredded leaves, ground bark, and similar materials. Those are all organic mulches, which admit air and water but exclude light and furnish organic matter for the soil and for feeding earthworms.

Straw is very convenient to use because it comes in bales. It is sold at some garden centers and at feed stores.

But before using leaves, they should be shredded with a grinder or a lawn mower or placed in a leaf pen several feet deep to age for six to twelve months. Otherwise, they lie like shingles on a roof, impeding rainfall and sprinkler irrigation from entering the soil.

Organic mulches should cover the soil constantly to protect it from direct exposure to sun, wind, and rain, with certain exceptions. One exception is in areas with a late, wet spring, when you want the soil to be moist and bare to absorb solar energy to collect warmth. Another exception is at planting, when mulch is raked aside.

Organic mulch is our favorite because it is readily available, inexpensive, can be grown yourself, and breaks down into humus. It is also bulky and takes some work to gather, to bring into your backyard, and to spread. But it's worth all the trouble.

THE MAGIC OF MULCH

Don't like the hard work of spading or the trouble and expense of renting a rototiller? Then let mulch do its magic for you. Let it biologically soften up that stubborn soil you might have. We once had a weed-infested area for a garden space and little time to cut the weeds or spade the soil. Was this a problem? Not at all. We hauled in spoiled hay and laid down an 8-inch organic mulch over the whole area. After sprinkling, we noticed the mulch had settled into a layer about 4 to 6 inches deep and, eventually, only 2 to 3 inches deep as it turned into humus on the underside.

After a month or two, we dug a patch of mulch away and, lo and behold, no more seeds nor hard crusty soil. Instead, we found a thin layer of dark, rich-smelling humus at the underside of the mulch layer and on top of the soil surface. The soil had become so soft and mellow that we could dig a trench with our fingers. A little later, we staked off bed centers, raked the mulch into the walkways, made planting trenches, and planted seeds. All this had been done without digging or spading or rototilling or fertilizing. Several weeks later, when the plants were up several inches in the rows, we just raked the mulch back onto the bed and in between the plants to cover all bare soil.

What made this magic possible? Simple. We just copied nature. We enlisted natural, biological forces instead of the usual high-tech, power method of killing weeds and loosening the soil. If we follow nature's lead, the rule of thumb is to keep the soil covered. Nature abhors bare soil and in productive areas never permits the soil to be bare for long. Nature keeps the soil covered with leaf mold in forests and with living or decaying grass on the prairies.

Does this mean that when you start a new garden you can avoid the loosening that was talked about in Chapter 5? Only if you have a huge amount of mulch, have a lot of time to wait for it to do its thing, and if the soil is fairly decent to begin with. When we used mulch instead of loosening by a rototiller or spading, we had access to a huge amount of a farmer's surplus hay and could wait many months for it to work its way into the soil. For most of us, this is not practical. But mulch is critically important in keeping your soil in good shape and weed-free after it has been charged.

When you cover the soil with organic mulch, you protect its surface from baking in the sun, drying out from wind erosion, and suffering splash erosion from raindrops. By excluding light, you are stopping weed growth in its tracks while allowing air and water to flow slowly through the mulch and into the soil without causing erosion. You provide a home for millions of beneficial soil organisms that feed on the mulch layer and loosen the soil by burrowing into it like millions of tiny spading forks. You have invited earthworms in to loosen the soil with their tunnels.

OTHER MULCHES

Though organic mulch is our choice, you can use other kinds of mulch. Burlap bags make an excellent temporary mulch for covering newly planted seeds. You can buy burlap bags from feed stores or rolls of burlap from supply houses such as Mellingers. (See Appendix A.) Strips of old carpet may be used. Boards from a half-inch to one-inch thick may also be used. But only organic mulches break down into humus.

Sawdust and Shredded Limb Prunings

Use these with great care. They are unbelievably high in carbon but low in nitrogen. They will play havoc if they get into your soil, suck-

Horse Manure for Compost or Mulch

Horse manure is excellent mulching or composting material. Horse manure has a lot going for it. Unlike dairy manure, it has very little odor. Horse manure comes in the form of light fluffy pills that are difficult to work into the soil and awkward to use as mulch. To be effective as a mulch, it needs to be run through either a compost shredder or a compost heap to make particles small enough to pass through a half-inch mesh screen.

COMPOSTING HORSE MANURE

If horse manure is mixed with stable cleanings, you might be able to use it as is and cover your bare soil with a layer about 4 inches deep or more.

A better way is to let the compost heap break down the large chunks of horse manure into small chunks. Because this manure is so light and fluffy, you might need several big bins. Circular wire bins holding about 1 cubic yard each may be used, or you can build square bins of wood 4 feet wide by 4 feet long by 4 feet tall with removable boards at the front for easy loading. For aeration, leave a quarter-inch crack between boards or use concrete block with no mortar between the joints.

A good plan when making horse manure compost is to spread a layer of the manure or stable cleanings about 6 inches thick, then sprinkle on a thin layer of fertile soil or compost as an activator, then gently hose down the material with a gentle spray to moisten it. Repeat this process until full height is reached. Unless natural rainfall occurs, sprinkle your compost heap about once a week until a little water runs out the bottom.

ing up all available nitrogen and thereby starving and stunting your plants. Sawdust and similar products should really be composted before being used as mulch. To do this, mix equal parts (by volume) of dairy manure and sawdust; or mix 1.25 pounds of 16-20-0 salt fertilizer per 10 gallons (1.33 cubic feet) of sawdust. The salt fertilizer supplies about a fifth of a pound of actual nitrogen. You could also mix the 10 gallons of sawdust with other fertilizers, such as one pound of ammonium sulfate (which has an NPK analysis of 21-0-0) or half a pound of urea. We much prefer mixing sawdust or other wood-type products with manure.

Black Plastic Mulch

This mulch sheeting works fairly well if you prepare your beds and install drip irrigation (explained in Chapter 12) on the surface, then cover the beds, the drip line, and the walkways with the plastic sheeting. This kind of mulch works best with widely spaced crops like tomato; you just cut holes in the plastic wherever a plant is to be set. But with closely spaced crops like beans, you might have plants two inches apart; in that case, the black plastic mulch does not work quite so well. Closely spaced crops are usually started by planting seeds, so you would have to cut a slit where your rows are to be placed and then plant the seeds through the slit.

MULCH ELIMINATES WEEDING

Weeds. You chop them down, and they grow right back. You cultivate the soil, and the weeds still come back. How discouraging, especially to beginning gardeners. But put on a good thick layer of mulch, maintain it, and your weed problems are gone. Mulch gradually turns to humus and disappears, so you have to renew it from time to time. Always try to keep your layer of mulch two to three inches deep.

Sometimes a few weeds escape and come up through the mulch, but they are spindly and can easily be pulled up and added to the mulch layer. Or you can use the Ruth Stout method for handling weeds that come up through mulch. This grand lady of mulch gardening simply forked up some hay with her pitchfork and deftly threw it on top of the weed. So simple! Mulch blocks light from the soil surface; weeds cannot grow without light; so mulch blocks weeds, too.

MULCH ENCOURAGES EARTHWORMS

The earthworm is the gardener's best friend. They studied soil chemistry and soil science long before any professor at an agricultural college did. They are not only master biochemists but master soil aerators as well, and you can judge the quality of your garden soil by its worm count.

Earthworms increase nutrient availability and aerate the soil with miles of tunnels as they burrow down into the soil. They must maintain a moist skin at all times, and they need protection from light and birds. Mulch, irrigation, and rainfall provide the needed moisture; and mulch alone provides earthworms with protection as well as the organic matter that is their food. Earthworms are discouraged by ammonium sulfate, a salt fertilizer, so use it with care, if at all.

Earthworms and Mulching

To "Super PowerCharge" your soil, introduce earthworms into it and protect them with a mulch of straw, grass clippings, ground bark, or other organic material. The earthworms will burrow all the way to the bottom of your bed and mix in the charging materials you have dug into the top six inches. Bait shops sell these worms. If you keep your bed covered with organic mulch to feed soil life, no more earthworms should be needed. (To find out if your soil already has enough earthworms, see the "Earthworm Count" inset directly below.)

Earthworm Count

A good test of biological gardening is to find out if a soil has earthworms and, if so, how many. To find out, make an earthworm count. Earthworm count is based on how many worms are present in the soil under each square foot. Note that we need to count the worms in the soil under the square foot, not on the surface. (You won't find these useful creatures on the surface.) Soil scientists have found a favorable earthworm count is six to twenty-three worms per square foot.

One way to make an earthworm count is to push a round-point shovel into the soil to the hilt, pry up a chunk of soil, spread it out on a flat surface, and count the worms present. The chunk of soil you pried up will leave a hole with a surface area about one-third of a square foot, so a suitable count would be two to seven worms per shovelful.

Another way is to use a posthole digger to dig a hole about 8 inches deep and 6 inches in diameter—about a fifth of a square foot. One to four worms per hole would be a favorable count.

Don't be surprised if you find no worms in bare soil. Earthworms usually appear in the garden only after the soil has been mulched for several months.

MANAGING MULCH

If you live where spring comes late and the soil warms up slowly, rake your beds bare about two weeks before you plant and leave them bare (and moist) until the weather warms up. Mulch will block the sun's rays from striking the soil, thus insulating it from solar heating. After your plants are several inches tall, apply mulch over all the surface.

Another way is to let your mulch get thin before planting, then rake the thin layer of mulch off your beds and into the walkways. After you have planted the beds and the plants are up several inches, rake the mulch back onto the beds and between the plants. At this time, you will probably need to add more mulch.

We prefer to keep our food plot covered with a deep organic mulch all during the growing season and to let it peter out toward the end—but always keeping a thin layer over all the surface to protect against splash erosion from falling raindrops. About January or February, we add organic fertilizer and other PowerCharging materials if needed, rototill or spade, and rake the beds level, then lightly mulch the beds to keep the soil surface covered. (See Figure 10.1.) At planting time, we just rake the mulch to leave a band of bare soil about six inches wide, for our planting trench, and leave this strip bare temporarily until plants emerge and grow several inches tall. (See Figure 10.2.) Then the beds get heavily mulched to cover the soil between the plants in the rows and all other bare areas. (See Figure 10.3.) That is the minimum-tillage method of soil management.

THE NON-TILLAGE SYSTEM

After your initial soil preparation when you first put your food plot in, you might want to try a non-tillage system. This is the next step up from minimum tillage. Instead of rototilling or spading your beds early in the spring, you just use a rake to move mulch around or do a little cosmetic leveling. To recharge beds, just rake the mulch off and spread a thin layer of organic fertilizer (and minerals, if needed) on the surface. (For details on recharging, refer back to Chapter 6.) Then just rake the mulch back on the beds. Let the earthworms move these materials down into the soil.

We have not yet tried the non-tillage method, but Japanese author and farmer Masanoba Fukuoka has. His book *One Straw Revolution* describes how he treats his whole mini-farm this way. (For sources, see Appendix A.)

SOW BUGS AND MULCH

There is a cute little insect-like creature that lives in compost bins and under mulch called the sow bug. Touch it and it curls up into a

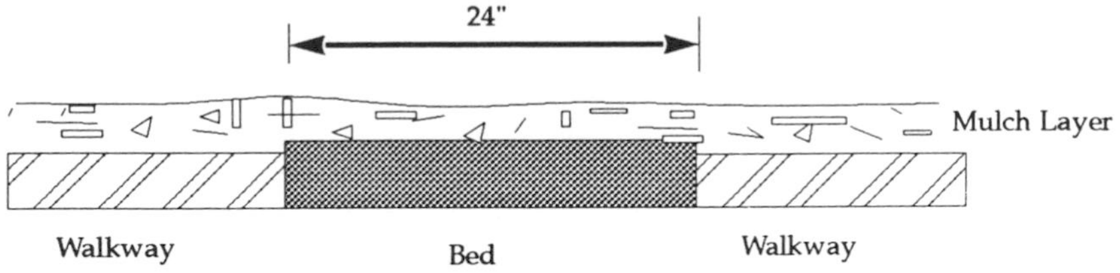

Figure 10.1 Before planting, the food plot is covered by a mulch layer 2 inches deep.

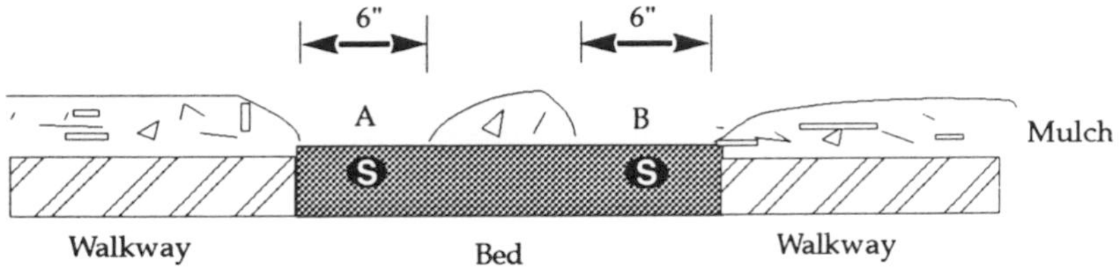

Figure 10.2 At planting time, the mulch is raked to one side, creating a bare band of soil along rows A and B. Seeds (S) are planted in the rows.

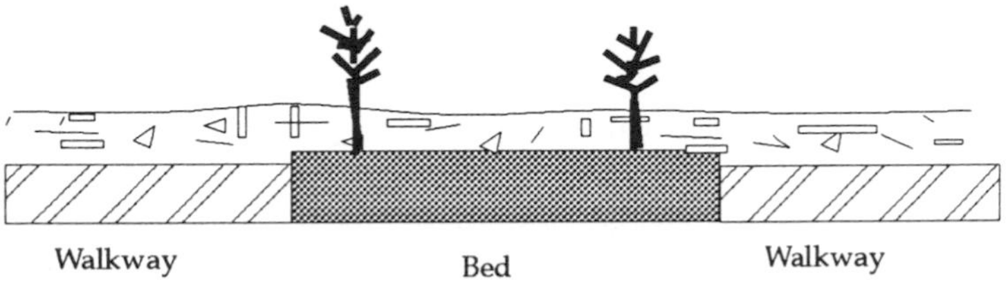

Figure 10.3 After the plants grow 2 to 3 inches tall, the mulch is raked back to cover the bare soil.

ball, hence its other name, pill bug. Soil science books will tell you that dead organic matter is all they eat, but we have found that that's not all they eat. They will also nip off the tips of emerging seedlings and kill the plants or even gnaw through the stem of a big tomato transplant much like a beaver cuts down small trees.

The sow bug can be a useful creature, but you can't put up with its bad habits. You can control it chemically or biologically. (See Chapter 11.)

WHEN NOT TO MULCH

At times, it is better not to mulch. You should not mulch newly seeded beds, squash, or (in cold soil) early spring plantings.

Newly Seeded Beds

Sow bugs hide under the mulch; then, when seedlings are beginning to emerge, they come out and nip them off. Keep the mulch raked three to four inches away from each row until seedlings are an inch or two tall.

Squash

Squash bugs, like sow bugs, hide under mulch, so keep the soil under the plants raked clear of all leaves and all mulch the entire season.

Early Spring Plantings When Soil Is Cold

Mulch blocks solar energy from heating the soil. To warm up beds for early spring planting, rake away the mulch and keep your beds moist for six inches deep. This allows solar energy to heat the soil and the stored water.

MULCH AND COMPOST

All organic mulch materials are also good for making compost. In its simplest form, compost is made by spreading a two- to three-inch layer of mulching materials over the soil surface for the soil organisms to break down. This is called sheet composting and is virtually the same as mulching. The numerous advantages of mulching or sheet composting include weed control, helping earthworms, slowing surface evaporation of water, and protecting the soil surface against wind and water erosion.

You can actually make compost by working composting materials right into your soil and letting the compost organisms get busy making compost. If you use this method, wait eight to twelve weeks before planting, because plants don't grow well or at all in a heap of raw compost that is breaking down. This differs from sheet composting, which has a thin layer of materials breaking down on top of the soil instead of in the soil. With finished compost, you can work it into the soil and plant immediately with great results.

Nature makes compost slowly by sheet composting. She does not make compost in a heap. But nature has lots more time than you or we do, so you will probably also want to have a regular compost heap or a compost bin. Another disadvantage of sheet composting is that some kinds of organic matter won't compost well that way—for instance, vines and long tough stalks such as okra or corn. You must somehow reduce these to small pieces before using them as mulch. The only easy (but high-tech) way to do this is by using a compost shredder. A slow, labor-intensive way is by using a hatchet and a chopping block. You can compromise by putting big, long, tough stalks and vines in your compost bin but placing other materials that are already in small pieces directly on the soil as a mulch.

WAYS OF COMPOSTING

We think the main reason for composting in heaps is to balance the carbon and nitrogen in the raw composting material. It also enables you to compost stalks and vines and to recycle kitchen trimmings easily. The simplest way to compost is just to build a heap of composting materials. This can, however, look messy, and it cuts down on the efficiency of the composting process. For tidy, efficient composting, use a compost bin.

Some people might tell you that a big benefit of a compost heap is that it heats up and kills weed seeds. It is true that a well-made heap will heat up to about 170°F, quite hot, but that is only in the interior of the heap. The parts of the heap along the outer edges, even in a bin, do not get nearly that hot. We have tried but have never found a practical, effective way to turn the cool outside parts of a compost heap into the inside. Turning the heap when there are heavy stalks and vines present is a difficult if not impossible task. We don't turn the compost heap inside our bin, but it makes perfect compost anyway—it just takes longer.

Pit Composting

Most composting materials become available in October or November, when in most of the country cold weather sets in. But the coldness slows or virtually stops the composting process. One way to help protect against the freezing temperatures that stop the biological activity necessary for composting is to go underground. Dig a pit about 18 inches deep by 36 inches wide by 48 inches long or longer.

Pit composting won't work in water-logged soil, because of an absence of air, so build your pit on high ground, preferably in sandy soil. When the pit is filled, cover the top with a 12-inch layer of straw or a similar organic mulch.

The Circular Wire Bin

The minimum critical size for a compost pile in a bin is one cubic meter (about one cubic yard, or 27 cubic feet). The simplest, easiest bin is made of welded wire, sold in hardware stores. Your bin should be 24 inches tall and have a diameter of 54 inches.

The welded wire is available in the needed height, usually with meshes of 1 inch by 2 inches. For the diameter, you can ask the hardware store to cut off a piece of wire 14 feet long. Bend this into a circle, fasten the ends together, and you have a durable circular wire compost bin that is easy to fill. If your compost material is shredded and falls out between the meshes in the wire, line the inside of the bin with several thicknesses of old newspaper.

WHEN TO COMPOST

Even though cold comes along with the composting materials in the fall, you can go ahead and fill your compost bin anyway. Next spring, when the weather gets warm enough to allow it, the composting process will proceed. You will want to tidy up your yard in the meantime, so why not store the materials in the compost bin? If you filled your compost bin in the fall, you should have finished compost next summer. If you begin composting in the spring, unturned compost will take about three or four months to complete composting, possibly delaying your compost harvest time until late summer, which is too late for current season crops. But this is no problem. Just harvest the compost and store it for use next spring.

BUILDING THE COMPOST PILE

Compost organisms work best when the ratio of carbon to nitrogen is 30:1. After the organisms finish their work, the ratio of the final compost is about 20:1. You can achieve these ratios with a mixture of compost materials that average out to about 1.7 percent nitrogen content. Most crop residues, including leaves, stems, roots, and straw, have a much lower nitrogen content, so to balance the pile we add a high-nitrogen material such as animal manure or cottonseed meal or even salt fertilizer. On the flip side, pure cattle manure has a carbon-to-nitrogen ratio of about 14:1, which is too rich in nitrogen unless you add some high-carbon material to it.

The practical way to build a compost pile, whether in or outside a bin or in a pit, is in layers. Make the bottom layer 6 inches of coarse plant residues, then spread on a 2-inch layer of cattle, horse, or rabbit manure or lawn clippings (for high nitrogen), then add a sprinkling of fertile soil. Repeat the process until the pile reaches the top of the bin or pit. (See Figure 10.4.) Moisten the materials as you add the layers. For the high-nitrogen layer, you can also use poultry manure (1-inch thick) or cottonseed meal (two-thirds of an inch).

Note that lawn clippings are a high-nitrogen material that may be used in place of manure, but let them and all other green materials wilt and dry a little before adding them to a compost pile. By waiting, you keep them from turning into silage. When the pile is completed, cover the top with organic mulch or burlap bags to hold the moisture in. You don't want the heap dry or soggy, just moist throughout.

Nature Balances It Out

Do you always have to add the layers of material to a compost pile exactly as given here to make it work properly? Not really. In a compost heap, you can make all kinds of mistakes by adding too little nitrogen or too much, but natural processes even out everything. If there is too little nitrogen, the composting process takes longer but still occurs. If there is too much nitrogen, the process is quicker although some nitrogen gets wasted. But whatever your method, you will end up with a finished, balanced compost with an NPK analysis of about 1-1-1 to 2-2-1. We have made many successful heaps by just adding the remains of plants from the garden. The normal time from the newly made compost heap to the half-size, finished heap is three to four months, without turning. Without putting in the layers as specified, it might take a little longer, perhaps four or five months.

OTHER THINGS YOU CAN COMPOST

Recycling everything you can is important to the environment and your food growing.

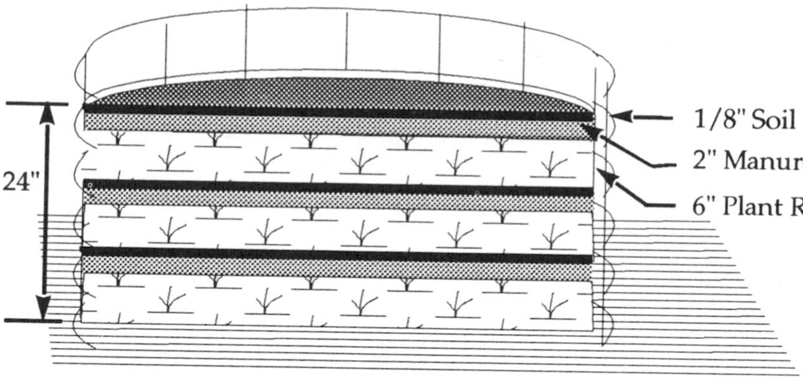

Figure 10.4 To the left is a cross-section of a newly built compost heap in a circular wire bin. Below is a photograph of an actual compost heap in its wire bin.

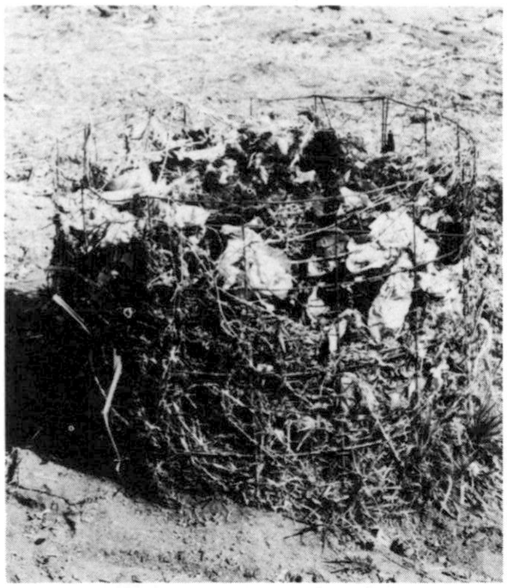

Recycle Household Wastes

Your own household generates considerable valuable organic matter that you can recycle to enrich your soil. Good items to recycle include coffee grounds, kitchen sink trimmings, hair, and other organic materials. But do not try to compost meat, bones, eggshells, or the contents of a cat's litter box.

To recycle household wastes into compost, make sure they're cut into small pieces (2-inch squares or smaller), and add them to your compost bin only after you have accumulated a small bucketful. Dig a hole in the compost pile, pour in the kitchen wastes, and cover with mulch. You can also bury household wastes in your soil. During the growing season, when all your beds are taken up, dig at the edge of your food plot a shallow pit 2 to 3 feet long, 2 feet wide, and 1 foot deep. Spread the household wastes along the bottom of this pit, and cover it with a little soil. During the non-growing season, if the ground is not frozen, you can bury household wastes in your beds. Make a trench about 8 to 12 inches deep. Start filling at one end of the trench, and cover with soil. Proceed until the trench is filled, then start on another. (See "Garbage Disposal: Wasteful" sidebar on page 124 for another method of recylcing household wastes.)

Recycle All Crop Residues

Crop residues are the inedible parts of your food-bearing crops—things such as leaves, stalks, and trimmings. Spread your lawn clippings over your food plot as mulch. When the growing season is over, put old stalks and vines in the compost bin or prepare them for mulching by chopping them up into 2-inch pieces with a hatchet and chopping block or a compost grinder.

Recycle Leaves

In the fall, save every leaf you can lay your hands on. Either shred the leaves or place them in a pen separate from the regular compost bin. You can process large amounts of leaves into valuable leaf mold by use of a wire pen. Use welded wire or a similar wire to make a bin like the one you made for the regular compost pile. Add a 12-inch layer of leaves, wet them down with a hose, trample them down, then repeat until the pen is filled to within 6 inches from the top.

Recycle Ashes

Wood ashes are the minerals left after the carbon in wood has been burned away. The ashes are alkaline minerals, mainly calcium and potassium, and can be recycled through your compost heap if you live where soils are naturally acid. These soils are usually found in the eastern and southern states, where 35 inches or more of rainfall per year is common. In other areas, especially in arid, western states, the soil is likely to have plenty of the wood ash minerals already; if that's the case by you, then keep ashes out of your compost heap.

GARBAGE DISPOSAL: WASTEFUL

The garbage disposal wastes valuable organic matter by feeding it to the sewer, which does not need it, instead of to your garden, which does need it. You can bypass the garbage disposal and bury kitchen trimmings in a continuous-process compost pile or into a trench in the soil, but there is a better way: Liquefy trimmings, and pour them onto the compost pile.

Ordinary kitchen blenders won't do this job, but there is one blender on the market that will. It is Vita Mix. Besides liquefying your trimmings, it will do a number of other useful tasks, such as bread-making. The sprouting seeds we recommend so highly would be ideal for converting into healthful loaves of whole-grain bread. We have tested Vita Mix and found that it also replaces the grain mill by grinding flour. Plus, it is a kneading machine, which makes bread-making an easier job. This machine is ruggedly built and has a seven-year guarantee. For details or a free brochure, contact Vita Mix, 8615 Usher Road, Cleveland, Ohio 44138. The company's toll-free phone number is (800) 848–2649.

COMPOST HARVESTING

Compost is not all that different from any other crop you grow. Like a row of corn or beans, compost requires water, air, temperature, and time. Both require harvesting. Your compost is finished when it sinks down about 40 percent.

When you harvest any type of compost, you will find a mixture of finished and unfinished compost. The finished material will be amorphous—that is, you cannot tell one part from another. Mixed in with the finished compost you will see pieces of partly decomposed stalks and various other materials you had put in the heap originally. These need to be separated out and either be put into the next compost heap you build or else be used as surface mulch.

When you're ready to harvest compost made in a circular wire bin, the first step is to remove the wire. You and a helper should stand at opposite sides of the bin and together lift it up and off the finished pile. Then, to harvest that or any other compost pile, use a big sieve, about 2 feet wide by 4 feet long. The frame should be made of one-by-four lumber, and the bottom should be covered with 1-inch mesh wire such as poultry netting. (See Figure 10.5.) Prop this frame up at a 45° angle near the compost heap so you can pitchfork compost onto it. Throw the compost on the top of the screen, so gravity will cause it to slide all the way to the bottom. The finished compost will fall through the screen and can be used right away. (If you are not ready to use it, then store it in plastic bags or

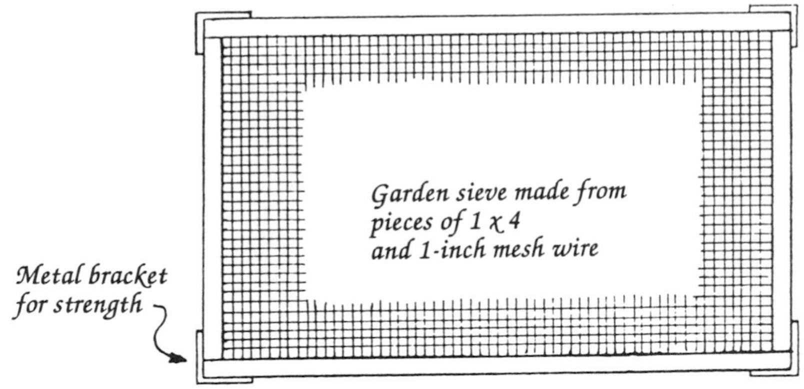

Figure 10.5 To the left is a garden sieve for compost. Photo below shows a sieve, too.

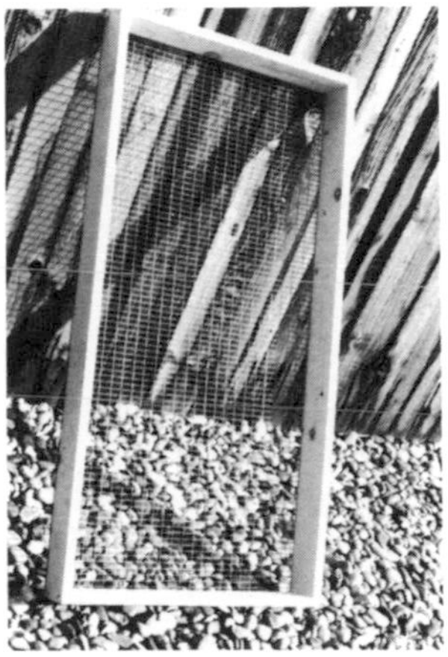

plastic garbage cans to protect it from the elements.) The parts that were too big to pass through the screen get hauled away in a wheelbarrow for mulch or recycled back into the empty compost bin.

USING COMPOST

Compost has many uses. It's great for building up soil organic matter. To make wonderful potting soil, you can use compost at full strength or mix it with an equal amount of soil. At transplanting, fill in around the rootball with compost. When you plant seeds in planting trenches, cover them with compost. Mulch your houseplants with a half-inch layer of compost and introduce a few earthworms.

11. *Common-Sense Pest Control*

A productive home food garden can come under attack and suffer severe damage by a number of pests. It can be birds. Or rabbits. Or animals burrowing underground. Or insects. Or diseases. But for every one of these problems there are safe, biologically sound solutions. For many reasons, it is important to avoid pesticides and use natural methods of pest control whenever possible.

PESTICIDES LINKED TO CANCER

While modern society has spawned many blessings, it has also brought us many environmental dangers. One danger comes from the side effects of pesticides. The National Cancer Institute did a study in 1987 on the harmful aftermath of pesticide use and reported a close link between cancer in children and pesticide use in the home. Where parents used garden pesticides, children were six-and-a-half times more likely to get childhood leukemia than in homes where pesticides were seldom used. When expectant mothers regularly used pesticides, their children were nine times more likely to develop leukemia.

The good news is there are many effective ways for the home food grower to avoid using pesticides, especially the more toxic, persistent ones. By following the entire PowerCharged method, you will be able to cut way down on all pesticides and possibly cut them out entirely.

CONTROL PESTS NATURALLY

Research has shown us that plants that receive a proper balance of all the nutrients they need over the growing season are healthier and receive less insect attack and disease than plants grown with nothing but chemical fertilizers in depleted soil. It appears from the research that insects are less attracted to strong, healthy plants than to those artificially supported with chemical fertilizers and pesticides. Pests actually seem to focus in on plants that are not truly healthy, like a virus attacks someone whose immune system is down.

It is a fact that agricultural pesticide use has tripled in the past twenty-five years, while crop losses due to pests have doubled. Pesticides have wiped out scores of beneficial natural predators while allowing harmful ones to flourish. According to the National Research Council, more than 440 insect species and more than 70 fungus species have become resistant to some pesticides, and the problem gets worse every year. In the days of our ancestors, who grew crops with no pesticides and by following nature's way of building strong plants and healthy food, pests were never the gigantic problem they are today. Where have we gone wrong?

A PHILOSOPHY OF PEST CONTROL

Is the pest problem a natural and normal part of the growing of plants, or does it result from improper cultural methods? Every once in a while, an enlightened person comes along who can look at a mass of human problems and find their common cause. As Thoreau said, "For every hundred people hacking at the branches of evil, only one is hacking at the root." One such man who hacked at the root of humankind's agricultural problems was a British agricultural scientist, Sir Albert Howard, who did forty years of research in India beginning in about 1900. In 1943, he published his findings and conclusions in *An Agricultural Testament.* Everyone really interested in a spray-free environment, organically grown food, and better health should get a copy of this classic book and study it carefully. It is available from AgAccess. (See Appendix A.) Though the book was released many years ago, the information in it is just as valid today as it was then.

Howard's book started the organic gardening and farming movement in the United States, but over the years his message has often been garbled and misinterpreted. To get the message as originally given without alteration, read his book. Howard recommends that we imitate nature in soil and crop management, which means we should always use mulch to protect the soil from the direct actions of wind, sun, and rain. Rather than plant a whole field with a single crop (monoculture), nature plants a mixture of many crops. The Law of Return is zealously followed in nature, where everything—no exceptions—is returned to the soil. Nature has neither poison-spray rigs nor vaccines to prevent disease, Howard says.

What does all this have to do with pest control? Everything. The link is this: Pest control is seated in soil fertility. Infertile soil due to mankind's mismanagement produces unhealthy plants, which seem to attract pests. This was documented by another pioneer in this field, Dr. W.A. Albrecht, former chairman of the University of Missouri soils department.

In research he did, he found that corn grown on soil with a low fertility level was more susceptible to insect damage in storage than corn grown on more fertile soil. Figure 11.1 shows an example of three ears of corn from his study. The small infested ear of corn in the center was a hybrid and grown in soil with low fertility, and it had a great deal of borer damage. The ear at the left, also a hybrid, was grown in the same soil but with added nutrients, and it was undamaged except for a few borer holes. The ear at the right, a non-hybrid, was in contact with the infested ones for five months, but it had virtually no borer damage. Good genetics and fertile soil saved it from insect attack.

The fact that insects seek out unhealthy plants is fully documented

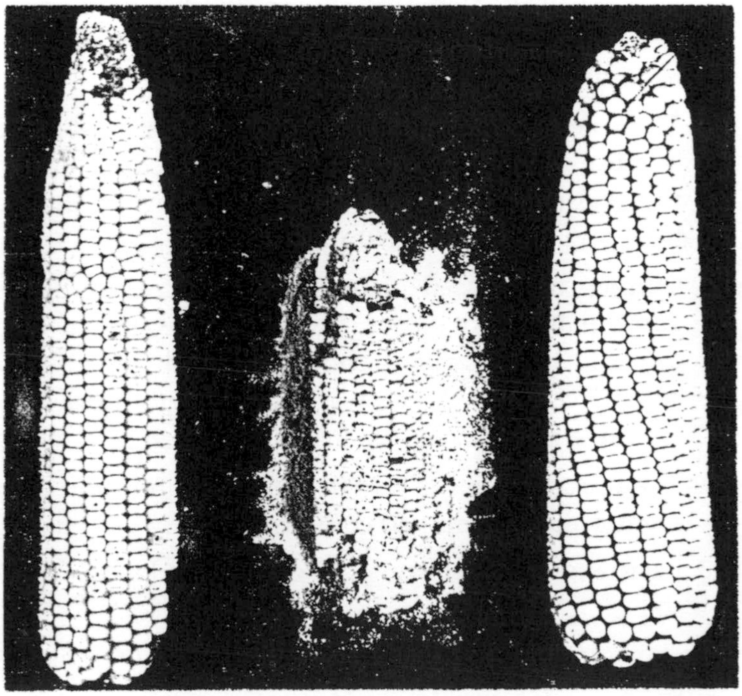

Good ear *Poor ear* *Best ear*

Figure 11.1 Corn grown in poor soil is more susceptible to insect damage than is corn grown in fertile soil. Hybrid corn is more susceptible to attack than is corn grown from non-hybrid seeds. The small, highly damaged ear in the center was grown in poor soil with hybrid seed. The ear on the left was grown in the same soil (and also with hybrid seed) but with nutrients added to the soil; that ear sustained less damage. The ear on the right was grown in good soil (and from non-hybrid seed) and had virtually no damage. (Reported circa 1950 by Dr. W.A. Albrecht, then head of the Department of Soil Science at the University of Missouri.)

in *Tuning in to Nature,* a book written by USDA entomologist Dr. Phillip Callahan and available from independent bookstores. Dr. Callahan's research found that the two bristles, or antennae, protruding from the heads of insects are more than a decoration. These antennae, he found, also receive electronic signals, functioning like the rabbit ears on a television set.

It seems that sick, unhealthy plants give off certain radio-like signals that insects can detect with their antennae. Insects follow these signals to the plants emitting them, and soon you have an insect infestation. Why does this happen? Let's see what Sir Albert Howard had to say on that question.

LEGACY OF SIR ALBERT HOWARD

In *An Agricultural Testament,* Sir Albert Howard summed up his findings on pest control as follows:

- Pests are not the real and basic cause of sick plants but only a symptom. The real and basic cause lies in unsuitable varieties or crops grown improperly. The pests that attack these sick plants are just censors pointing out crops growing on infertile soil, crops improperly nourished, crops that are unfit to survive. The insects or other pests are simply carrying out nature's law that only the fittest shall survive. This implies that if your plants have serious pest damage, the plants have "been inspected" and found unfit to survive.
- To protect plants by poison sprays is unscientific and unsound, because these poisons only serve to preserve the unfit and hide the real problem, which is how to prevent the pest problems from occurring in the first place.
- Burning of diseased plants is an unnecessary destruction of organic matter since nature never does this. In one case in England, diseased tomato plants were converted into compost in a large commercial field, which was then used to grow a second crop in the same greenhouse. No infection occurred.
- The basis of true soil fertility depends on humus or decomposed organic matter (finished compost).
- Resistance to insects and disease is conferred by humus in the soil.
- Animals need less feed if it comes from truly fertile soil.
- Food plants grown on land rich in humus are always superior in quality, taste, and keeping power to those raised by other means, but the soil must also be highly mineralized to grow food free of pests and of highest nutritional value.

THE HEREDITY FACTOR

Dr. Albrecht's research showed us that open-pollinated (non-hybrid) corn grown in fertile soil suffered no insect injury in storage while surrounding ears were almost destroyed. This suggests that it is not only soil fertility but the genetics of a plant that can give it great protection from insect damage. Nature grew most of the present-day crops in a healthy condition before they were taken over by the human race. Open-pollinated corn still retains most of those original genetics, which is why it's less susceptible to insect damage.

With apples, it is just about impossible to grow them worm-free without poisonous sprays. This might be due to an inherited defect whereby the DNA in the apple tree is not coded to resist the larvae of the codling moth without the crutch of poisonous sprays. What we need is a research program to search for apple varieties that resist the codling moth attack rather than sprays to kill the worms after they seek out the sick trees. The bottom line is, if you eat a worm-free apple today, you are almost sure to get a dose of pesticide residues.

OUR PEST PREVENTION PROGRAM

We grow an excellent food plot every year, mostly by natural methods, and avoid pest problems. We use these steps:

- Annually apply fresh dairy manure or cottonseed meal rototilled in without running it through a compost heap. There is nothing wrong with composting manure before adding it to the soil, but it is much easier just to till it in directly one to two months ahead of planting. This leads to high yields of high-quality food plants and few pests.
- Keep the soil covered with organic mulch to protect it from direct exposure to wind, rain, and sun. Why does the soil need this protection? To prevent erosion from running water and wind and to prevent the surface from drying out and baking, which wastes soil moisture by evaporation and discourages earthworms. A deep organic mulch will cover all bare soil and also give perfect weed control. No need to use a hoe, a plow, or a rototiller to keep weeds out when you use a mulch.
- Plant the right varieties at the right time at the right spacing.
- Keep the soil mineralized and balanced.
- Use permanent beds rich in organic matter, and stress the use of orgainc fertilizer rather than salt fertilizer.
- Keep a food-producing crop or a cover crop growing all the time. This will lock up nutrients, prevent leaching, and provide organic matter.

- Irrigate when it does not rain, just to refill the root zone, but avoid overirrigation and underirrigation.

HOW TO HANDLE PESTS

Because there is little money to be made in natural pest control, relatively little research has been done to perfect the methods. This means that even if you follow all the known rules for natural pest control, sometimes you'll get these unwelcome visitors. When that happens, what should you do?

Don't panic. Wait a day or two to see if beneficial insects take over. You can afford to take 10 percent damage rather than to spray.

Never spray in anticipation that pests might attack. This will kill off your beneficials and get you into a never-ending cycle of using crutches instead of prevention.

Build a "good bug" habitat. Along the food plot border or in a corner, build for beneficial insects a habitat consisting of Jerusalem artichokes (sunchokes). Stock your garden with good bugs. Mellingers (see Appendix A) carries a good line of beneficial insects and other non-toxic pest controls.

Even devoted organic gardeners have times when bugs get out of hand. Try to use the more natural non-chemical methods, such as traps and barriers. Then, if necessary, when all else fails, go to poisons that are less persistent and less toxic to people—for example, the botanical poisons, such as pyrethrum, sabadilla, and rotenone. Nicotine sulfate is not persistent but is toxic to people, so use it carefully.

Here are ways to handle various specific pests:

Aphids

These are small, soft-bodied, sucking insects, usually greenish in color. They attack the tender growing tips of vegetables by inserting their beaks and sucking out the juices. One cure is to spray the aphids off with a solution of soapy water. Use one teaspoonful of biodegradable liquid soap per gallon of water. Apply with a pump-up sprayer. Or use nicotine sulfate spray (a commercially available natural botanical insecticide). Be sure to follow the directions on the label.

Cabbage Worms

These are hungry, small green worms that love to eat the leaves of the mustard family, especially of the crucifers or brassicas, which include cabbage, broccoli, cauliflower, Brussels sprouts, kohlrabi, collard greens, turnip greens, and mustard greens. The worms are sometimes called cabbage loopers, because when they crawl they form a series of loop-like configurations. The mother is a white moth that will flit around these crops when they grow several true leaves. You can remove them by hand, but that is time-consuming. Instead, you might want to use *Bacillus thuringiensis,* which is a biological spore control sold as a powder or a liquid spray under the names Bt, Dipel, and Thuricide.

White Flies

These pests are tiny, white, flying insects that suck the life out of your plants. They love tomatoes. When a plant is infested and you go over and shake the vine, a cloud of these insects "explodes" in your face. Place yellow boards in the infested area after coating them with Tanglefoot, a moist and sticky substance. White flies love to go to yellow boards and alight. The Tanglefoot makes sure they never take off again.

You can make a yellow board by cutting a piece of plywood about 12 inches square and painting it with yellow paint. Nail it to a wood stake about a foot high, then drive the stake into the ground near the plants where you see white flies. You can make your own sticky yellow boards or buy them ready-made as "sticky stakes."

Mildew

This common disease occurs when a fungus causes the leaves of plants to turn whitish or powdery. Mildew is especially bad on cucumbers and melons. Try applying dusting sulfur or spraying with wettable sulfur.

Sow Bugs

If you make compost or use organic mulch, you will have sow bugs, literally thousands of them. These cute little insects are about a quarter-inch long and look like they are covered with armor plating. They have all their legs underneath and often will curl up into a ball if touched. The books say they live on decaying organic matter, but they also love to nibble off the tips of newly emerging shoots from seed you have just planted.

You can discourage sow bugs when you plant by raking away the mulch to expose a band of bare soil 6 inches on each side of the trench. With many plantings, that would mean raking all the mulch off the entire bed and into the walkways. That is another reason to leave mulch off or to mulch lightly until your plantings are in and the plants are up several inches tall. When plants get that big, the sow bugs will leave them alone. But raking away the mulch does not always work, so here are some other cures:

Chemical Control

We don't like to use this method, but it does work, and at least it involves one of the safest pesticides around—carbaryl, sold as Sevin. Another plus is that you can use spot treatment, which reduces the amount applied to a bare minimum. The pesticide is mixed with a bait that resembles BB pellets. The way you use it is to rake away the mulch as just described, plant your seeds, and make a note estimating when they will start emerging. Just before emergence, go out with Sevin bait in hand and thinly sprinkle the pellets along the row where your seeds are about to come up. When the seedlings have emerged and grown several inches tall, rake the mulch back to cover the bare soil.

Toads

We have a friend who swears by toads to control sow bugs, but you will have to fence in your yard to keep your toads at home. You'll also have to build a small goldfish pond and keep it full of water, since this is where toads breed. Catch some toads, bring them into your toad habitat, turn them loose, and let them feast on your bugs. (The "Toads for Insect Control" inset on page 135 explains how to do those tasks.)

Wire Insect Cages

The idea is to cage your plants, not the insects. For no matter what you do, there are times when sow bugs and other bugs can move in on you, such as in early spring when things are growing slowly and there is not much else around for the bugs to eat. Another time is in late summer when nice tender leaves from newly sown lettuce or transplants are trying to grow and, again, there's not much else around for the bugs to eat. A wire cage made of hardware cloth (one-eighth inch) is very helpful to keep out sow bugs, grasshoppers, and other pests.

This wire is quite stiff, so you can make a cage 4 or 8 feet long and it will hold its shape. Make the cage wide enough to cover the entire bed. (See Figure 11.2.) Make it about 4 inches tall. This will enable you to make it bug-proof by pushing it into the soil about 1 inch deep. If your beds are 36 inches wide, you might need to limit the cage's length to a maximum of 4 feet so it will retain its rigidity.

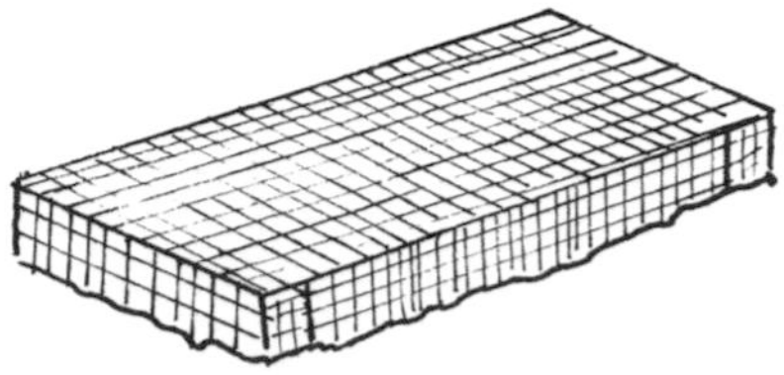

Figure 11.2 A wire insect cage made of 1/8-inch hardware cloth keeps bugs away from young plants.

Grasshoppers

These winged insects are very destructive very quickly and, because they fly, are hard to catch. If you're in a rural area, chickens and guinea fowl will take care of grasshoppers for you. In 1991, bacterial spore control (Nosema Locustae) for grasshoppers was introduced

Toads for Insect Control

Toad-keeping is a little-known secret of non-toxic, biological insect control. A fully grown toad can consume up to 10,000 insects during a single summer and is reported to be especially effective against cutworms, which, like toads, come out at night to feed. Toads are also effective against the sow bug and many other insects.

If you place shallow dishes of water in your garden where toads are found, they will sit in the water for long periods. If water is not available to them, the toads will burrow into moist soil in the heat of the day. Toads do not live submerged in water like fish, but biologically they are amphibians, which must keep a moist skin at all time. Toads also need water during their breeding season, because the female lays her eggs only in water.

Here's how to begin toad-keeping in your backyard:

1. Enclose your garden with a toad-proof fence to keep your toads home. You need this fence anyway to keep out unwanted visitors. (Include a hinged gate with a latch to allow you access.) Use poultry netting 36 inches tall with 1-inch meshes. Dig a trench about 6 inches deep along the inside of your existing fence or garden boundary, place the lower edge of the poultry netting in the bottom of the trench, fill the trench in with soil, then nail the upper portion of the netting to posts—if you already have a fence, its posts will do nicely.

2. Prepare a small sunken area that will hold water. An easy way to do this is to go to your nearest auto supply store and buy a metal, shallow, oil-changing pan. Dig a hole near your garden area, sink the pan down flush with the soil surface, and fill with water. To help your toads get into and out of the water easily, make ramps for them. Use small gravel to make ramps about 6 inches wide, starting at the edge of the pan and sloping down to its bottom. Repeat this on the other side of the pan. (See illustration below.)

3. Collect toads and stock your toad village. Toads are not available commercially, so you have to collect them yourself or have someone collect them for you. You might be able to arrange for collection by youngsters in your neighborhood. Or the biology teacher at your nearest high school might be able to set up a toad-catching project.

To find toads, pick a warm night in spring. That is their breeding season, when they are most easily collected. Put on a pair of rubber boots, get your flashlight, and look for toads gathered near ponds, streams, and road ditches, especially after rain. Toads do not cause warts, but if touching them bothers you, wear a pair of rubber gloves. Listen for their deep trilling calls and follow the sounds to their source. Distinguishing males from females is difficult, so collect half a dozen so you will more likely get a mix of males and females.

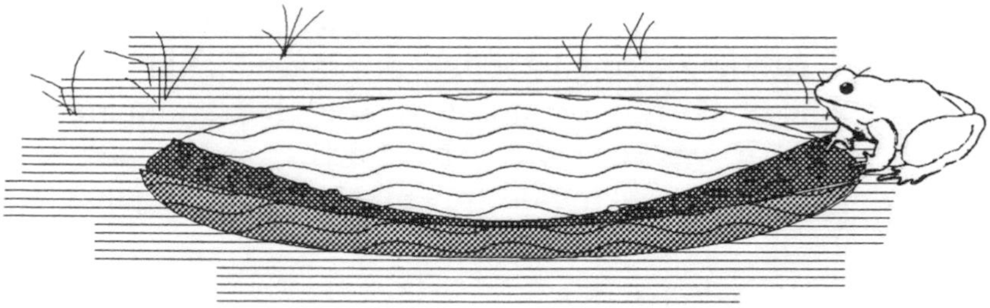

similar to Bt for cabbage worms. Your garden center should carry it under the trade name Nolo. Another way to keep them out is to build a wire insect cage for your plants.

Squash Bugs

If you don't know what a squash bug looks like, just plant a squash seed and check the plant every day when it starts to bloom. No matter where you are, even if you're away from civilization, these pests seem to find any growing squash. At first you might see a single bug, then two of them mating, and soon thereafter you will find brown egg patches on the underside of leaves. If these bugs get out of hand, your squash harvest will end. Squash bugs are among the hardest to control of all the pests we've ever encountered, but there are still a number of ways to control them. A wire insect cage is a good way when the plants are small. Another way to protect them is with a floating row cover, which is a light fabric that lets in light and air and can be placed over the plants as they grow. Seal one side of the base of the cover with a layer of soil and the other with boards. The boards are easily removed and placed back, enabling you to lift that side of the cover off for harvest while keeping the other side sealed. Floating row covers are available from Mellingers. (See Appendix A.) Here are some other things to do:

Demulching

Squash bugs are often found around the base of your squash plants and will run and hide under nearby mulch. Try mulching everything except squash plants. Rake the soil surface under your squash perfectly bare in a band 6 inches wide on each side of the plants.

Hand-Picking

This is the first line of defense. Start checking your plants every day to look for the adult bugs about the time the first flowers form. Crush the bugs or drop them in a can of soapy water. Also, look at the underside of every leaf to find and crush egg masses. This will kill a portion of the leaf, but that is far preferable to letting the eggs hatch. (In the spacing table on planning—Figure 7.1—we advised planting a single row of squash with each plant spaced about 3 feet apart. That was so you can have access to all parts of the plant for your daily search-and-destroy mission against squash bugs.)

Water Treatment

Prop up a piece of plywood 2 to 4 feet high alongside your row of squash. Then hose the plants well from top to bottom. The squash bugs will retreat from the water and look for higher ground, which will be the piece of plywood. As they crawl up, either hand-pick them or crush them with a piece of two-by-four. This will also work if your plants are growing alongside a board fence.

Sabadilla Dust

This botanical pesticide decomposes rapidly on exposure to light. It is reportedly effective for controlling the squash bug but is irritating to the eyes and respiratory system, so a mask should be worn when applying it.

Vacuum Method

If you have a tank-type vacuum, you can take the head off the end of the tube, go out to the garden, and suck up the bugs. Just make sure you haven't just irrigated.

Delayed Planting Method

The proper time to plant squash is one to four weeks after the average spring frost-free date. Squash bugs that have survived over the winter are hungry and go after the early-planted squash with gusto. Try delaying your planting to the later part of the planting period. It will throw the squash bugs off their cycle. They will be looking for their favorite food at the beginning of the planting period, but there won't be anything for them to eat, and they may leave.

Squash Bugs and Cucumbers

Squash bugs also attack cucumbers. This makes sense, because both squash and cucumber are cucurbits, or members of the gourd family. To control these bugs in cucumbers, follow the same general rules as given for squash. (Note that in Figure 7.1 we advised that in a 24-inch bed a single row of cucumbers be planted, with the plants spaced 12 inches apart.) As soon as the vines are long enough, pull them up gently with your hands and intertwine them around the trellis string. Do not allow them to run along the ground. When the vines get a little larger, pinch off any leaves that touch the ground so you can easily search for and hand-pick squash bugs. These bugs love to gather on the soil surface around the base of the plant, so if the soil there is bare and without leaves or vines, it is harder for the bugs to hide.

June Beetles

These are huge beetles that fly in and attack certain crops, especially fruits and sweet corn. Hand-pick and drop them in a can of water or oil.

Purple Martins for Insect Control

One of the greatest pleasures of gardening is watching the wild creatures that dwell in your garden where no pesticides are used. Songbirds—wild creatures that delight the eye and the ear—are one of the best of the biological controls. Dr. Peavy's choice of all the songbirds is that master of flight called the purple martin. What is so entertaining about these birds is that they live in colonies and spend a great deal of time in the most graceful flight you can imagine. Their coloring is a blue that is so dark that they appear to be black. The males are solid blue-black, and the females have white undersides.

You can attract martins to your garden by erecting a colony house with at least six compartments atop a pole about 14 feet long. The martin will come to your martin house in early spring, rear its young, then leave in the fall for its winter quarters, South America.

The natural habitat of the purple martin is the United States east of the Rocky Mountains, but these birds prefer wooded country with lots of streams and vegetation where plenty of insects can be found for food. For that reason the best martin territory is in the midwestern and eastern parts of the country.

A purple martin colony is a delight to behold. A good-sized colony house will have twelve or more compartments, with twenty-four or more occupants during the nesting season, and it is alive with activity. These birds are social and love to perch while they fill the air with their distinctive song.

To attract and enjoy purple martins, you should:

- Be located east of a north-south line that runs through Oklahoma City. For areas west of this line, especially if the annual rainfall is less than 25 inches, proceed with caution. Look around to see if anyone else has erected a martin house. Make inquiries. Consider buying and erecting a small, inexpensive birdhouse to see if you can attract these beautiful birds. If you can't, then sell the birdhouse to someone farther east.
- Buy a properly designed colony house made especially for martins and capable of being easily and quickly raised or lowered on a pole about 14 feet tall. This is usually done by having a round hole go through the center of the base and continue upward through the center of the roof, so that the colony house can slide up and down on a steel pole. You raise or lower the house by an arrangement of pulley and rope.
- Select a colony house with guardrails to prevent young birds from falling to the ground.
- Erect the pole at least 20 feet from the tips of the branches of the nearest trees. Your yard must be large enough to allow this.
- Select a house that is easily cleaned and has doorstops to keep out English sparrows when martins are not present. (Martins arrive in the spring and leave in the fall.)
- Select a house made of rot-proof, lightweight, non-porous material such as aluminum. Each nesting compartment should have a shiny interior to discourage intruding starlings.
- Protect young birds when they are learning to fly. Watch the colony house to see when the young birds venture out on the porch inside the guardrails. Keep your own house cats confined during this period, and try to get your neighbors to do the same. (They are likely to turn a deaf ear. If they do, go to your hardware store and ask for the "Hav-A-Heart" animal trap, which is simply a wire cage with a hinged door hooked up to a baited strip of metal. When a house cat goes for the bait and enters the trap, the door closes. The cat cannot escape until you open the door. This is perfectly legal. Cats, like dogs, may not trespass. This trap, which does not injure the animal in any way, enables you to catch and return the offender to its owner or the city pound.) Many of us love house cats, but these lovable pets love to catch and eat birds. Young martins that have just left the nest are still learning to fly. Their wings are weak, and they are not yet fully aware of the dangers of being on or near the ground, where prowling house cats are found. That is why we need to offer extra protection during this vulnerable period.
- Use a good pair of binoculars for bird watching of your own private colony of martins.
- Lower your colony house at the end of the season, remove all nests, and clean the compart-

ments thoroughly. Close the doors. Raise the birdhouse again next spring with the doors open.

After the birdhouse is raised in the spring, watch it for sparrow invaders. They will occupy a martin colony house and so intimidate your intended occupants that the martins might get discouraged and leave. Every week or so, lower the house, throw out the sparrow nests, and raise the house back to the top of the pole. When raising or lowering the birdhouse, you must keep it in an upright position. There may be a martin nest next door to a sparrow nest. You want to clean out and throw the sparrow nest away but not touch or disturb the martin nest. With such treatment by you, the sparrows will soon realize they're not wanted, and the martins will become aware they are wanted, so you will get all martins and no sparrows.

(For sources of martin houses, see Appendix A.)

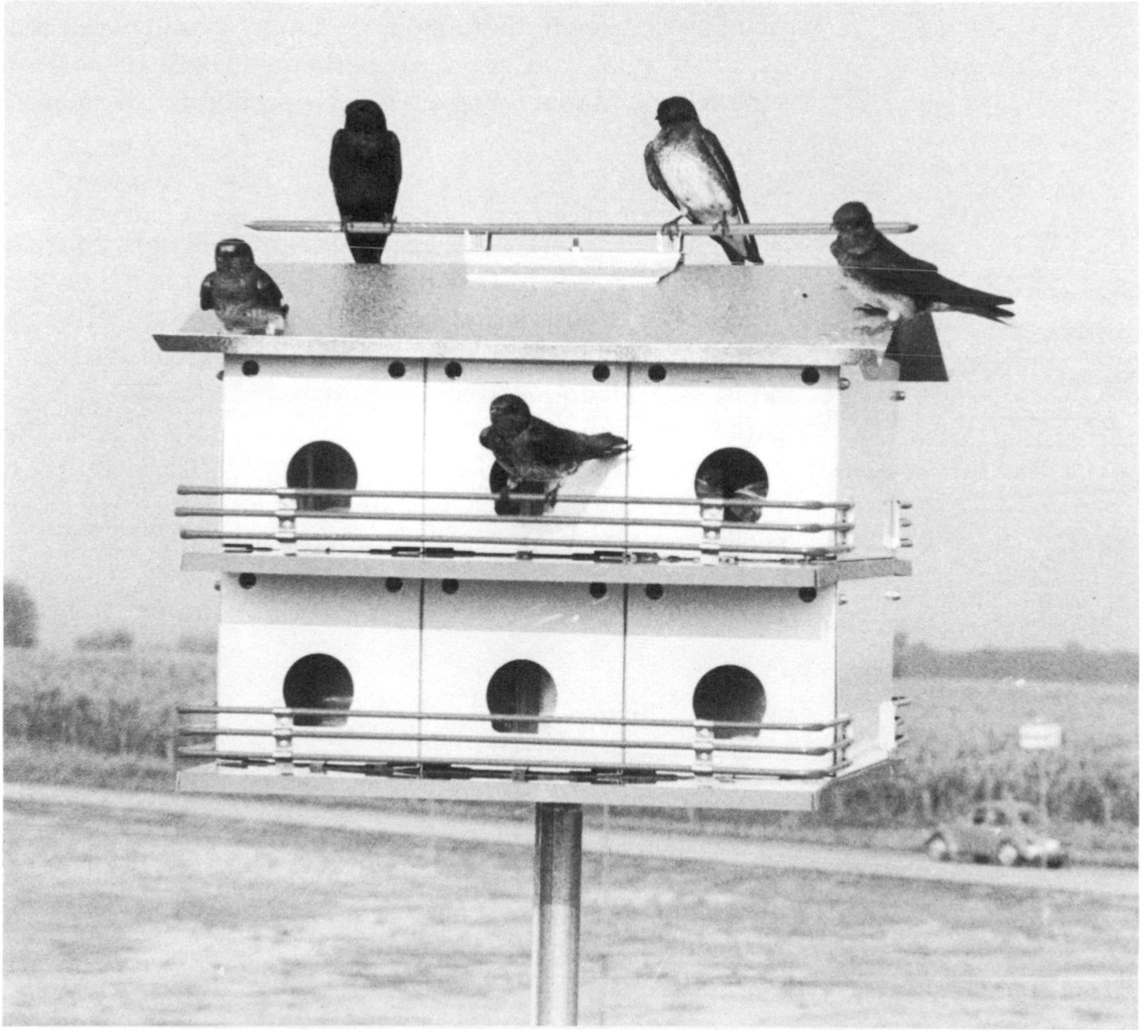

Purple martins, shown here enjoying a deluxe two-story home, eat plenty of insects that might otherwise damage your crops.

Photo courtesy of Nature House Inc., Griggsville, Illinois.

Tomato Hornworms

These monstrous worms can strip a tomato plant in a day or two. When you see holes and droppings, you might not see the worm right off, because it is green and blends in with the foliage, but it's there all right. Hunt until you find the worm, then spray your plants with the biological control Bt (*Bacillus thuringiensis*).

Snails and Slugs

These pests are found in cool, moist, shady places, especially around and in beds of perennial vines. You know you have them when you see silvery trails on the leaves. Show us a bed of English ivy on the east or north side of a house, and we'll show you some snails. Your first line of defense, then, is prevention by locating your food garden as far away as you can from permanent beds of perennial vines, where snails hide and breed. Here are six additional defenses:

Beer Traps

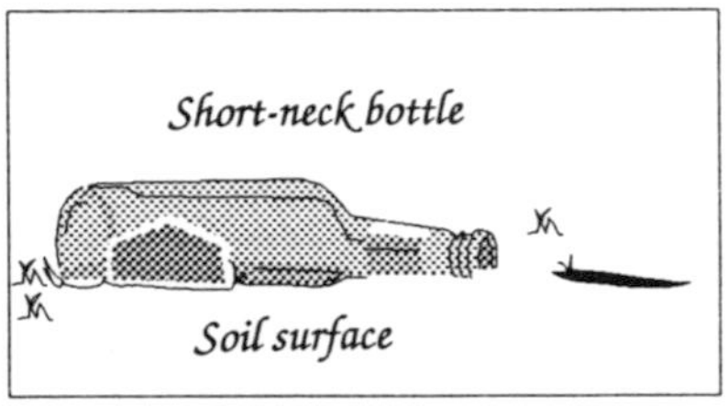

Figure 11.3 Beer trap for snails.

Snails and slugs are attracted to fermented liquids, so treat them to "happy hour" where they drink first of stale beer, then drown in it. Find the cheapest brand of beer you can find in the short-neck bottles. Empty out part of the liquid so that when you turn the bottle on its side, a depth of about two inches is left. Take this out to your garden and sink it into the soil so that the bottom lip of the bottle is about even with the soil surface. The bottle will protect the beer from wind, rain, and sun and will attract snails. When the trap is full of snails, empty it, clean it, put some more beer in it, and return it to the original site. You might need several of these traps. (See Figure 11.3.)

Poultry

If you can keep a couple of ducks or a few chickens, they will take care of your snails. Ducks are especially good at the task but require a small pond of water—the same thing needed by toads (which control sow bugs). By pond, we mean a typical goldfish pond the size of your dining room table. Ducks and toads turn a pond into a double-barreled defense against pests.

Caustic Barriers

Two things mess up the slime on which snails move around: wood ashes and diatomaceous earth. (The latter is a white powder that is like a bed of glass to crawling pests.) Place a band of either substance several inches wide around the area to be protected or across the snail trails leading into your garden.

Boards

Snails need a cool dark place to hide when the sun comes up, so scatter some boards (at least six inches wide) at the edge of your garden, prop up one end by half an inch, and mound a little earth around the edges of the boards to keep out light and heat. Go out during the day and harvest the snails.

Hand-Picking

Snails and slugs, like tomato hornworms, can be picked and dropped in a bucket of water if you can find them. Remember, snails come out only under low lighting conditions, such as very cloudy weather or early in the morning before the sun comes up or at night when the sun goes down. Go out then to look for them. Use a flashlight if necessary.

Copper Screen Barrier

In University of California tests, a fence of copper screen wire six inches high was very effective in turning away snails. When they try to climb it, they get an electric shock. Hardware stores carry copper screen or can order it for you.

Nematodes

These are microscopic roundworms that burrow into the roots of food plants, especially tomatoes, and cause root knots, which stop growth and kill the plant. They are one of the worst enemies of the food grower. They are so difficult to get rid of that you don't ever want to let them get into your garden soil. This means you should avoid acquiring plants from a garden club's flea markets, where members bring in surplus plants to trade, sell, or give away. Such "trading" plants come with soil around the roots. This soil may be infested. It's like a computer virus for plants. Always buy transplants from a reputable nursery that uses potting soils free of the pest. Cures to get rid of or control nematodes include chemical and biological methods. Chemical methods include the use of soil fumigants that are sprayed on the surface, watered in, and covered with tarps.

Organic Matter for Control

Some research has shown that adding lots of organic matter to the soil (40 to 50 tons per acre) results in control. This works out to about 240 pounds of organic matter per 100 square feet. Your charging program, including organic mulch, will go a long way toward meeting this need.

Marigolds for Nematodes

Research has also shown that the number of nematodes in the soil can be reduced by growing certain kinds of marigolds called French marigolds (Tagetes Patula). The varieties proved most effective are Tangerine, Petite Gold, Goldie, and Petite Harmony.

Marigolds will not prevent nematode attack when planted around susceptible plants in infested soil, and they do not give off substances toxic to nematodes. Instead, what they do is attract the female nematode to burrow into the root to prevent her from reproducing, thus acting as a "trap crop."

Anti-nematode marigolds to be effective have to be planted solid and allowed to grow 90 to 120 days in the same place. This means ground to be treated must be thrown out of food production for three to four months, beginning at about the spring frost-free date. Plant the marigolds in rows about a foot apart, and space the plants about a foot apart within each row. One source of these marigold seeds is the Burpee Seed Company. (See Appendix B.)

Crop Rotation

Crop rotation means you change the location of each kind of food plant every year. For example, if you planted tomatoes in Bed 1 last year, move this year's tomatoes to another bed. Moving crops around helps reduce pest problems.

CIRCUMSTANCES BEYOND YOUR CONTROL

Though Howard's and Callahan's works indicate that bugs tune into sick plants, research has not yet proven that healthy plants will repel them. It seems if there is a large population of hungry bugs that aren't being controlled by natural predators, and if yours are the only young tender plants around, the bugs will eat your plants no matter what (but probably to a greater degree if the plants were grown improperly).

12. *Irrigating and Feeding*

EVEN though every part of the United States is likely to go without natural rainfall a month or more at a time, few (if any) other garden books get down to the specifics of telling their readers how to irrigate. Yet, a good irrigation plan is needed. This chapter takes away all the unknowns and tells you when to irrigate, how much water to apply, and how often to irrigate.

Proper irrigation means applying water at the proper time and in the proper amount. This is important to maximize both the yield and nutrition of the food you grow. Overirrigation leaches nutrients out of the root zone, resulting in food with a low mineral uptake. Dr. Firman Bear's study proved this, showing food from the highly leached soils of the south and east to be low in minerals. To keep your plants growing well but also high in health-giving minerals, avoid overirrigation. By the same token, plants that do not have enough water will be highly stressed, stunted, produce less yield, and could die. You need to irrigate with the right balance. This chapter shows you how.

WATER STORAGE IN THE SOIL

A sandy soil with plants rooting 24 inches deep will, after a good rain or an irrigation, store enough water to last only three to four days in midsummer. If it does not rain within three to four days, your plants will undergo moisture stress, will stop growing, and after another day or two might die unless rain comes or you irrigate. A loam soil after a good rain or irrigation will store enough water to last about a week if the plants are rooting 24 inches deep. A clay loam with roots at the same depth will store enough water to last about a week and a half.

We lived for a couple years near beautiful Portland, Oregon, with high rainfall, big trees, and running streams all around. But one summer the rains stopped, and there was a six-week dry spell. Once a week we had to soak our garden soil with sprinklers to save the plants from dying, so location is no guarantee that you won't need irrigation.

WHEN TO IRRIGATE

The general rule is to water your plants just before they undergo moisture stress, which occurs when half the available water stored in the rooting zone has been used. The rooting zone, or active rooting depth, is where most of the feeder roots are located and where most nutrients and water are absorbed.

In midsummer, if you haven't had a good rain (an inch or more) in the past week, you will usually need to irrigate. But that will depend on the kind of soil you have and the rooting depth of your plants. A rain gauge is very helpful because it tells you exactly how much rain you've had.

Celery is the exception to the general rule. Keep your celery bed wet all the time. This usually requires daily irrigation. The next question is, how do you know when half the water stored in the soil rooting zone has been used?

Visual Symptoms

First of all, look at your plants daily, if possible. If the leaves are lightly wilted (drooping) early in the morning or late in the afternoon, there is water stress. Stress means the plant is crying out, "I'm hurting, water me quick." Get the water to your plants quickly, and make a notation on your calendar. Light wilting at midday is normal. You need to be concerned only if it occurs in the morning or late afternoon. Find out how many days pass until they go into light wilt, and write the number down. Then use that number to make plans to irrigate a day or two before the stress sets in next time. Try to prevent stress, because it cuts yields and might lead to tough vegetables of lower quality.

Moisture Meter

Another good way to head off water stress before it occurs is to check the soil moisture with an inexpensive electronic moisture meter, available by mail order or at garden centers. (See Figure 12.1.) It registers the moisture status on a dial. Our meter has numbers 1 to 8 where 1 is "dry" and 8 is "wet." To use this meter, you push its slender probe down into the soil by your plants, about 4 inches deep for shallow-rooting crops and to its full length (6 to 7 inches deep) for other crops. Shallow-rooted crops are cabbage, celery, garlic, lettuce, onion, parsley, potato, radish, and spinach. Now read the meter. For most crops, a reading of 4 means it's time to irrigate. The exceptions are pepper (irrigate when the reading goes to 5) and celery (irrigate on 7). Both of those need more moisture than most. On the flip side are melons, which should be irrigated when the reading goes down to 3. This increases their sugars.

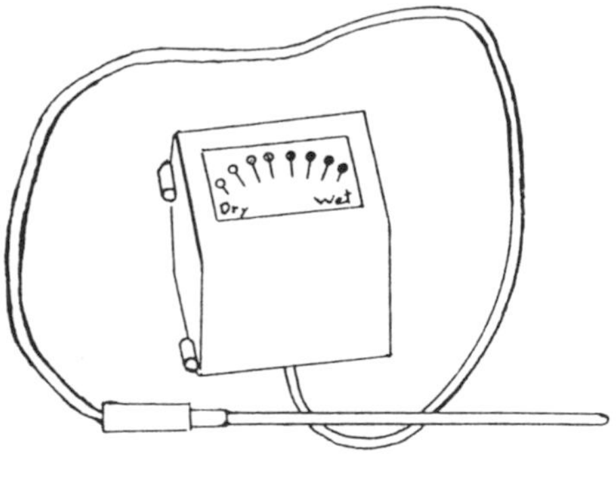

Figure 12.1 An electronic moisture meter tells you how moist or dry your soil is.

Young plants require special attention. Young plants without much height (up to 2 inches tall) have a very shallow rooting depth—the roots are around 50 percent deeper than its height. So if you measure how tall a young plant is and multiply that by 1.5, you will have the depth of its roots. Push your moisture probe down to one-third of the root depth to take your reading.

Some Plants Thirsty and Some Not?

Often you will have different kinds of plants or different ages of plants so that some need water and some do not. What do you do? Irrigate for the sake of the plants with the most shallow roots, but don't apply as much water as normal. Irrigate twice as often. This is one place a drip system (explained later this chapter) is superior to all others, since you can put a valve on each line and control the amount of water each bed gets.

HOW TO IRRIGATE

There's more than one way to irrigate a garden. You can irrigate with sprinklers, with a drip line, or by flooding.

Irrigating With Sprinklers

We prefer sprinklers whenever possible where the water is of a good quality and plentiful and the growing area consists of all beds side-by-side in a square or rectangular area.

Sprinkling the Square

To irrigate a square or rectangular growing area efficiently, the minimum size is about 16 feet square, and 24 feet square is better. Do *not* set a sprinkler in the center of the plot for irrigation. Instead, set it at one corner, adjust it to rotate in a 90° arc (a quarter of a circle), and also adjust it to throw water to the two nearest corners. (See Figure

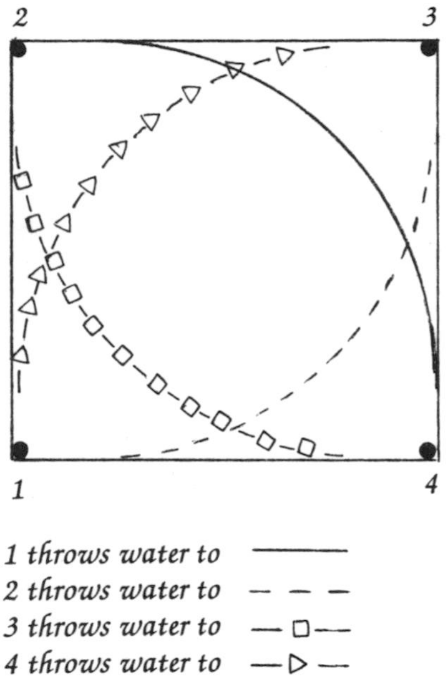

Figure 12.2 For efficient sprinkler irrigation of a square area, apply one set from each corner, with the sprinkler adjusted to rotate for a quarter-circle, giving a 50 percent overlap. Corner dots mark the sets.

12.2.) Raise the sprinkler up several feet. We have raised the sprinkler by placing it on 5-gallon buckets and on stools. Let the sprinkler run at the first corner for a set such as fifteen minutes (Set 1), cut it off, move it to the next corner (Set 2), let it run the same length of time, and so on to the remaining two corners (Sets 3 and 4).

This procedure is not guesswork. Irrigation engineers have made studies showing it is the only way to get the same amount of water applied to all parts of a growing area. Otherwise, you will wet some areas too deeply and some not deeply enough. If soil is overirrigated, valuable minerals are leached out. If underirrigated, plants won't grow well. The fifteen minutes is only an example. The actual time needed to irrigate your plot deeply enough may be up to an hour per set. (Later in this chapter, you'll find out how deeply you'll need to irrigate.)

The Solid-Set System

Using one sprinkler and four sets means you have to move the sprinkler to four different locations each time you irrigate. This is little problem if you irrigate only occasionally, but if you irrigate frequently, you can save lots of time and effort with a solid-set system. With this system, each corner has a sprinkler permanently mounted and adjusted, so no moving is necessary.

The solid-set system is easy to set up. You just dig a trench about a foot deep (see Figure 12.4), lay three-quarter-inch polyvinyl chloride (PVC) pipe in the trench, and at each corner attach a vertical piece of galvanized pipe to extend about 4 feet above the surface. At the top of the pipe, mount an impact rotary sprinkler. (Figure 12.3 shows an impact rotary sprinkler made to sit on the ground.)

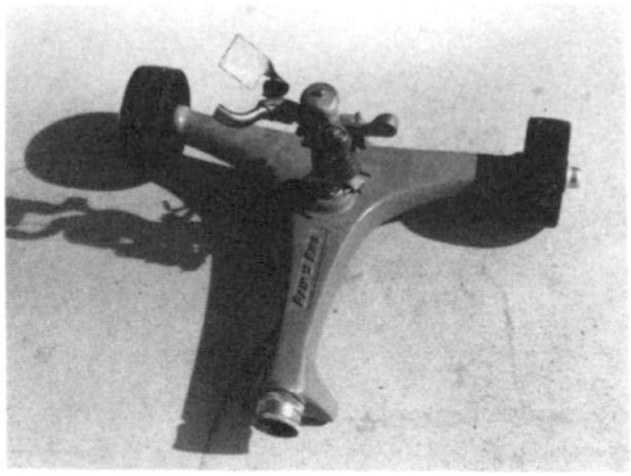

Figure 12.3 This impact rotary sprinkler has quarter-circle to full-circle adjustment and a flap to control the distance the water is thrown. It can be mounted on top of a pipe for a solid-set sprinkler system.

This sprinkler will need an adjustable pin that allows you to adjust the arc of water from 90° to 180° (a quarter- to a half-circle). It will also need a flap or adjusting screw that enables you to control the distance the water is thrown. If you have a 16-foot square, you adjust it to throw water 16 feet; if a 24-foot square, adjust it to throw water 24 feet. Be sure to put a drainage valve at the lowest point in the system to drain all water out when freezing weather comes. It's good to build a box that extends 12 inches under the surface to house the cutoff and drain valve.

Irrigating the Rectangle

Put two squares side-by-side and you have a rectangle. Now, instead of four sets of the sprinkler, you need six. (See Figure 12.5.) The four outside sprinkler sets are adjusted to a quarter-circle, and the two inner sets are adjusted to a half-circle. If you need help to design a sprinkler system for your growing plot, look in your Yellow Pages for

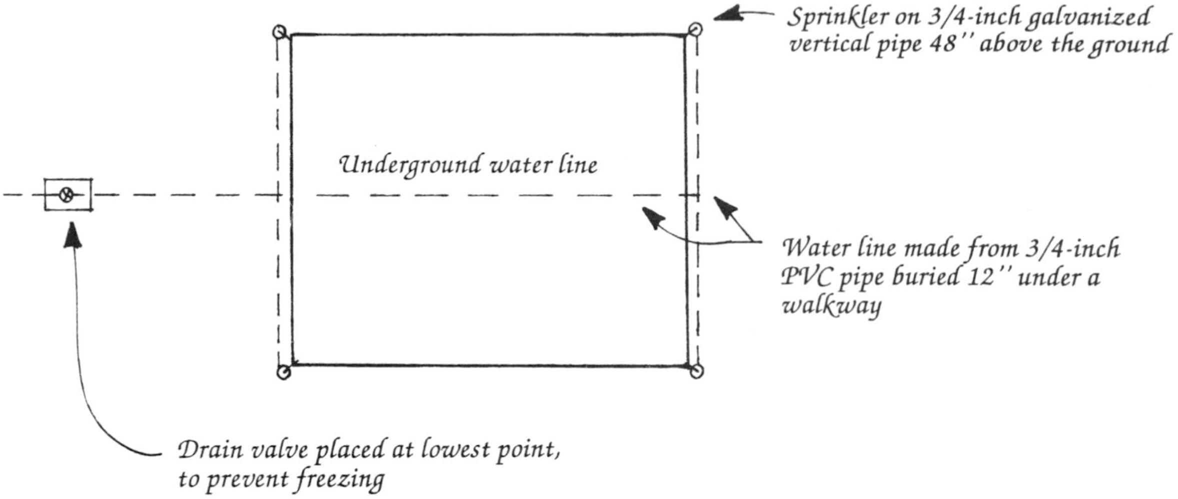

Figure 12.4 Top view of a soild-set sprinkler system.

a sprinkler irrigation company. Show them a sketch of your plot and ask for help in designing a sprinkler system.

The Can Test

To help you irrigate efficiently, you need to know about how many inches per hour your sprinkler system is applying. To find out, adjust your sprinklers as described. Then get about six straight-sided metal cans, walk diagonally from one corner to the opposite corner, and place cans evenly spaced as you go along. Take a kitchen timer with you, turn on the water, and set the timer for fifteen minutes.

When using one sprinkler to make four sets, repeat the fifteen minutes at each set while leaving the cans in place. When all sets are finished and the soil surface has dried out a bit, go out and measure the depth of the water in the cans with a ruler. The depth in all the cans should be about the same. A common depth for the full hour would be from a quarter-inch to a half-inch. In a solid-set system, with all sets running at the same time, you might get half an inch of water in fifteen minutes.

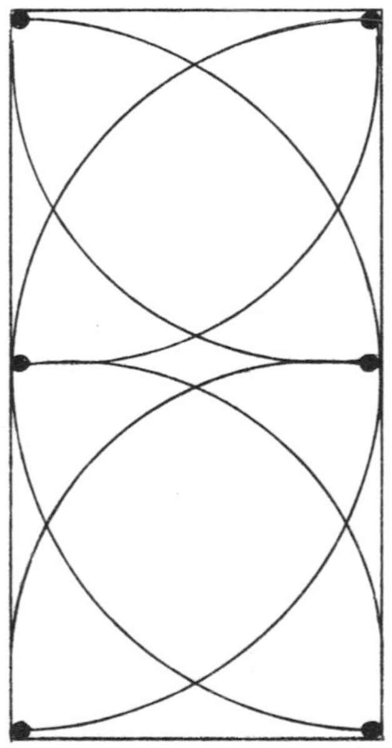

Figure 12.5 To irrigate a rectangular area properly, use six sets (marked here by dots), with the four corner sets throwing water for a quarter-circle, and the other two sets throwing water for a half-circle.

Water Application Rate

Water put out by sprinklers can be measured in inches per hour. This is called the precipitation rate. A good soil will absorb 2 to 5 inches of precipitation per hour, but irrigation engineers recommend a sprinkler system be designed to apply a quarter-inch to a half-inch per hour. Rainbird and other dealers can supply a catalog showing the precipitation rates of the sprinklers they sell. (Look in the Yellow

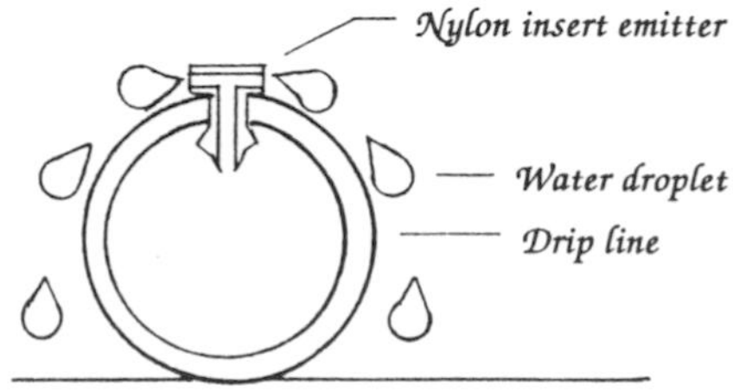

Figure 12.6 A cutaway view of the emitter in a drip line.

Pages under "Irrigation.") They usually have designers who can design a system for you or check the system you have designed.

Irrigating Scattered Beds

Scattered beds without curbs are usually along the back or side fence of the home next to a lawn and can be watered as you sprinkle the lawn. If there is no lawn, drip irrigation is probably your best bet.

Drip Irrigation

Drip irrigation applies water very slowly, drop by drop, directly to the soil surface. Water drips out of tiny holes in a small black plastic hose called a drip line, which has been laid on the soil surface. The tiny holes are usually fitted with emitters (drippers) and placed 12 to 24 inches apart along the drip line. (See Figure 12.6.)

Each emitter usually puts out only one to two gallons per hour. Because water is applied drop by drop, you have to run a drip system a long time, usually four to ten hours, to irrigate the soil. Emitters are punched into the plastic line with a special insert tool. (See Figure 12.7.)

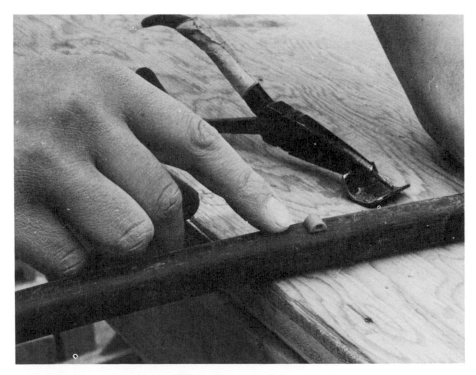

Figure 12.7 A newly inserted drip line emitter.

When to Use Drip

Drip is most useful for irrigating arid western areas, where evaporation rates are high and humidity is low; for irrigating areas where water is scarce, expensive, or salty; and for irrigating long narrow strips, including the scattered bed garden. After planting, you place the drip line or lines on the surface of the bed and leave them there all season.

How Drip Works

When an emitter-type drip system is turned on, water drips out to form small moist circles at each of the emitters. (See Figure 12.8.) Water moves out from each emitter equally in all directions by capillary action. (With flood or sprinkler irrigation, water moves into the soil by the downward pull of gravity.) As time goes on, the circles get larger and larger and finally run together to form a moist band of soil.

Black Soaker Hose Drip Line

A new kind of drip line now widely available is the black soaker hose. Made of old tires, this durable hose leaks drops of water from its entire surface, immediately moistening a narrow band of soil that gradually moves outward. With the black soaker hose, you don't have to consider emitters. They're already built in.

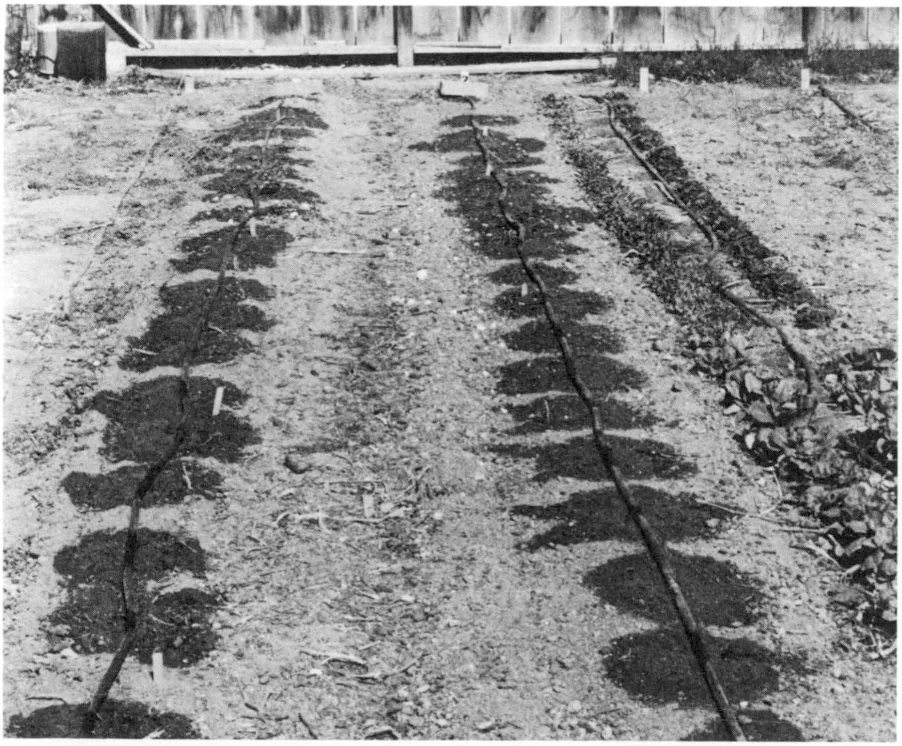

Figure 12.8 A drip system in operation. There is one drip line in each 24-inch-wide bed. The moist circles show where each emitter is. In this instance, the emitters are spaced 18 inches apart. After a few more hours, there will be a band of wet soil 24 inches wide along each drip line.

Design of the Drip System

The simplest drip system is a drip line 50 feet long used on a long narrow bed of the same length. (See Figure 12.9.) You can use the same 50-foot drip line on several shorter beds by making U-turns. (See Figure 12.10.) By using a Y-shaped fitting hose, you can run two 50-foot drip lines side-by-side. (See Figure 12.11.) You can irrigate a number of beds side-by-side by using a header line with cutoff valves for each bed. (See Figure 12.12.)

A single drip line will wet a strip of sandy soil only about 12 inches wide but will wet a strip of loam or finer soil 24 inches wide. This means that if your soil is sandy, you will need two drip lines per 24-inch bed (see Figure 12.13) or three lines per 36-inch bed.

Flood Irrigation

Flood irrigation, the most ancient way to irrigate, is the most wasteful. The only time it should be used is with raised beds with curbs. Attach a bubbler on the end of a hose.

If the curbed bed is more than 4 feet long, insert 1- by 4-inch boards into the bed every 4 feet to section it off so you can control the amount of water going to different plants. The boards are cut to fit crosswise into the bed. Place one on its edge and push it about half an inch into the soil. Place another board about 4 feet away and push it into the soil, too. Place the bubbler in the center of a section and turn the water on full force to flood the watering basin about 1 inch deep. The boards form dams so the water will be contained. After an inch or two of water of has been applied and has soaked in, move down the bed to the next 4-foot section and repeat the process.

If the curbed bed is less than 4 feet long, boards are not required.

Hand-Held Sprinkling

This is irrigation by holding a hose nozzle in your hand while you move your hand back and forth over an area. It is wasteful of time. Besides, few people have the patience to move a hand-held sprinkler over an area for the ten to thirty minutes required to irrigate properly. It is better to run a stationary sprinkler for given sets of time. Hand-sprinkling can be justified only for "spot watering" as an aid to germinating seeds.

HOW DEEP TO IRRIGATE?

Many books advise "water deeply" but never tell you just how deep is deep or tell you for sure how to find out how deeply you wetted

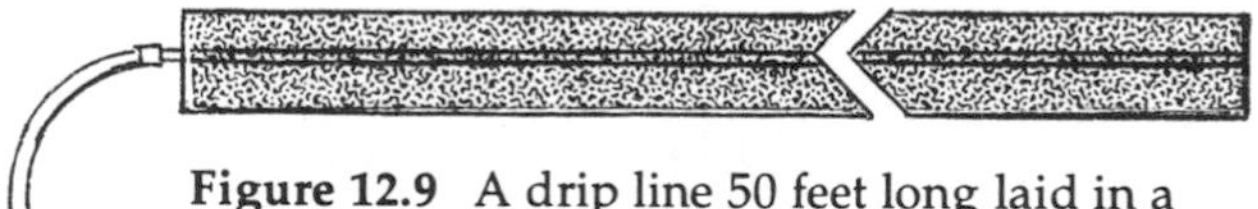

Figure 12.9 A drip line 50 feet long laid in a straight line can irrigate one long bed.

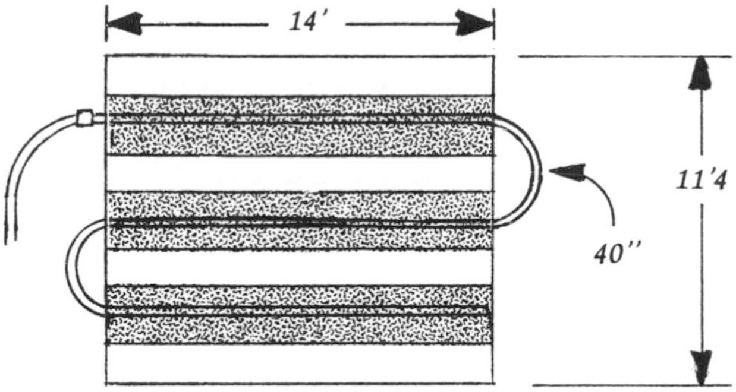

Figure 12.10 A 50-foot-long drip line with U-turns can irrigate three short beds, each 14 feet long.

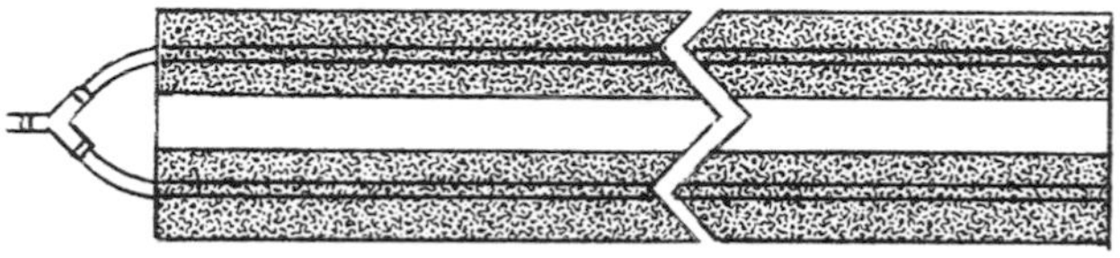

Figure 12.11 Two drip lines 50 feet long and laid in straight lines can be connected by a Y-shaped hose.

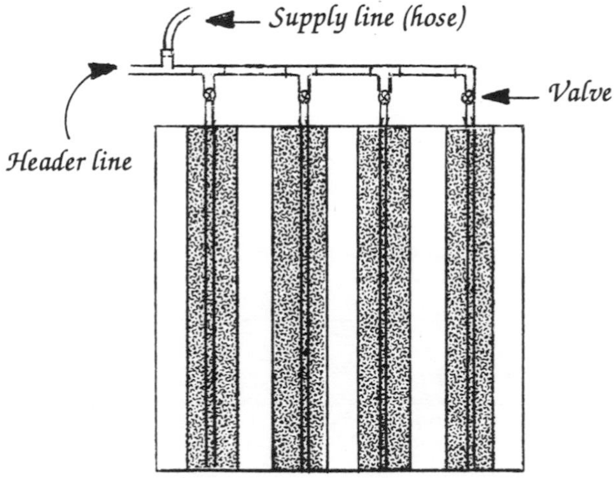

Figure 12.12 For loam, silt loam, or clay loam soils, one drip line down the center of each bed is fine, with emitters spaced 18 to 24 inches apart. The system is fed by a header line with a valve for each bed.

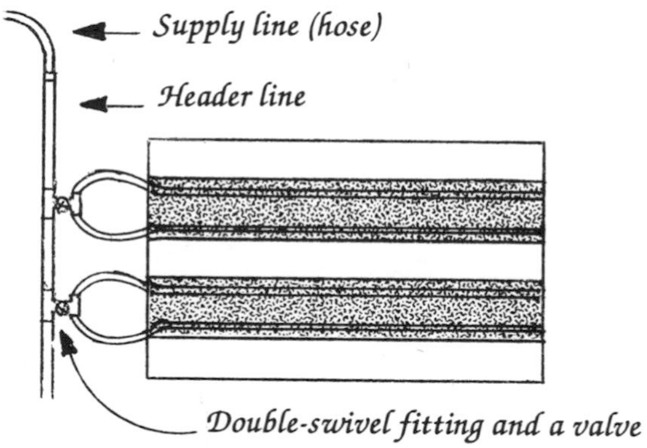

Figure 12.13 For 24-inch-wide beds with sandy soils, place two drip lines in each bed, with emitters spaced 12 inches apart.

the soil. With most crops, you will need to apply enough water to moisten the soil all the way down to 24 inches. Table 12.1 shows you how deeply each crop needs to be irrigated.

Table 12.2 shows you how much water it takes to wet soils 24 inches deep when half the water in the root zone has been used. If you are using sprinklers and you made the Can Test, you will know about how long you need to run your sprinklers to put out an inch or more of water.

To know for sure if the water went deep enough takes more than guessing. It takes testing, which you can do easily and accurately with a simple inexpensive tool called a moisture probe.

Soil Moisture Probe

This probe is simplicity itself. It does not tell you when to irrigate (use the moisture meter for that), but it will tell you how deeply you did irrigate. The moisture probe is simply a long slender steel rod about 30 inches long and three-eighths of an inch in diameter, pointed at the bottom, and with a handle welded to the top. (See Figure 12.14.)

How the Moisture Probe Works

Fully moistened soil is soft, like putty. When the moisture probe is pushed down on a moist soil surface, the probe penetrates and is

Table 12.1

How Deep to Irrigate

Kind of Plant	Depth to Irrigate* (Inches)
Lettuce	18
Onions	18
Radishes	18
Most Food Plants	24
Tomatoes	over 30
Viney Crops**	over 30

* = Based on the plant's active rooting depth, not its total rooting depth, which is merely the depth of its deepest root. But the active rooting depth is more important for irrigation, because it reflects the depth where most of the plant's roots are found, accounting for most of the plant's growth. (Refer back to Figure 5.6 for a more vivid illustration.)

** = Melons, cucumber, squash, sweet potato.

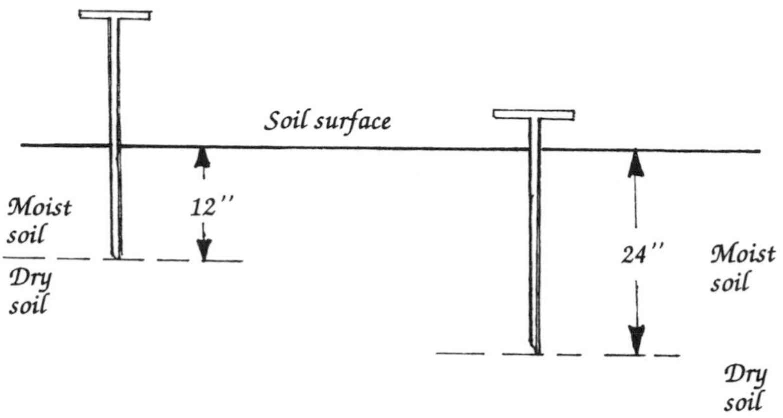

Figure 12.14 The soil moisture probe tells you how deeply you watered. It should be made of 3/8-inch-diameter spring steel. The probe on the left can be pushed down but stops at the 12-inch depth, showing where the dry soil begins. The probe on the right can be pushed down to its full 24-inch length, showing the soil is moist to at least that depth.

easily pushed down when you put your weight on it. The probe continues to go downward until it strikes dry soil, and then it suddenly stops as if you had hit solid concrete. No grower, large or small, should be without it. We file notches 12 and 18 inches from the probe's bottom so we know how deep it's going, and we paint the handle red to avoid losing it when it's pushed all the way down. Some crops need irrigation deeper than 30 inches; for those, if you can push the probe down all the way to your knuckles, you've watered deep enough. For checking shallow-rooted and young plants, a slender screwdriver with a blade about 12 inches long is good.

FEEDING YOUR PLANTS

The best way to feed your plants is to feed your soil, which then automatically feeds your plants at just the right rate at the right time. (See Chapter 6 for details on how to PowerCharge your soil.) As plants require more nutrients, the soil releases nutrients through increased

Table 12.2

How to Moisten Soil to a 24-Inch Depth

Soil Type	When Half the Root Zone Water Has Been Used, Add This Much Water
Sandy	1 inch
Loam	1.5 inches
Clay Loam	2 inches

microbial activity in response to increasing temperature. If you have followed the soil charging program, then you probably will not need to feed your plants any more in the season, except for foliar spraying, especially if your soil has a high pH.

Foliar Feeding With Seaweed

In areas where soil pH tends to be high (7.0 or above), certain trace elements, like iron, zinc, manganese, and copper, can become "locked" in the soil. Even after you balance your soil as shown in Chapter 6, in time the trace elements in the soil can become less available. The solution is to make them available to the leaves directly with a foliar spray. Using a trace-element foliar spray is a good idea even if your soil pH is not high, just to ensure that your plants, and consequently your foods, are getting plenty of micronutrients.

Your plants can absorb small amounts of trace elements through their leaves quite readily. You can use Maxicrop, a seaweed powder that dissolves in water. Mix one tablespoon of the seaweed powder with half a teaspoon of liquid soap per gallon of water, pour into a two-gallon pump-up pressure sprayer, and spray the leaves of your plants early in the morning when the wind is down and the humidity high. The little bit of liquid soap makes the solution stick to the leaves better, increasing the uptake.

POWERCHARGED FOLIAR FEED

Though seaweed is a good spray, it contains large amounts of sodium and chlorine, while plants and humans need only tiny amounts of these two elements. Because of this, we are developing a special PowerCharged foliar spray that is more in balance with the nutritional needs of food plants and humans who use these plants as food. For more information on this new foliar feed, write to us at the address given in the book's Conclusion.

Some plants form fruits from flowers. Spray such plants (tomato, cucumber, beans, squash, corn, etc.) once a week from when the flower buds form until a small fruit appears. Usually, this period lasts from four to six weeks. For foods where you eat the leaves, stems, or roots (lettuce, cabbage, celery, potato, etc.), spray once a week for four to six weeks, beginning when the first full-size leaves appear. To make your foliar feeding easier, mix up two gallons of the solution even though you might use only a quart or two of seaweed spray at one spraying, release the pressure at the end of the spraying, and leave the solution in the sprayer for next week's spraying.

Spraying the leaves of food plants with foliar feed greatly increases their nutritional value. If your garden center doesn't carry a soluble seaweed powder, you can order it yourself. (See Appendix A.)

Sonic Bloom

Sonic Bloom is a type of foliar feeding done by playing special music while spraying a "secret solution" on the leaves. Music has been found to affect plants, but no conclusive results have been proven. We strongly suspect the active ingredient in the secret solution is seaweed extract. Because of the complete lack of objective research regarding sonic bloom, we recommend you save yourself a lot of money and use a soluble seaweed powder directly to feed your plants.

Irrigation Water Quality

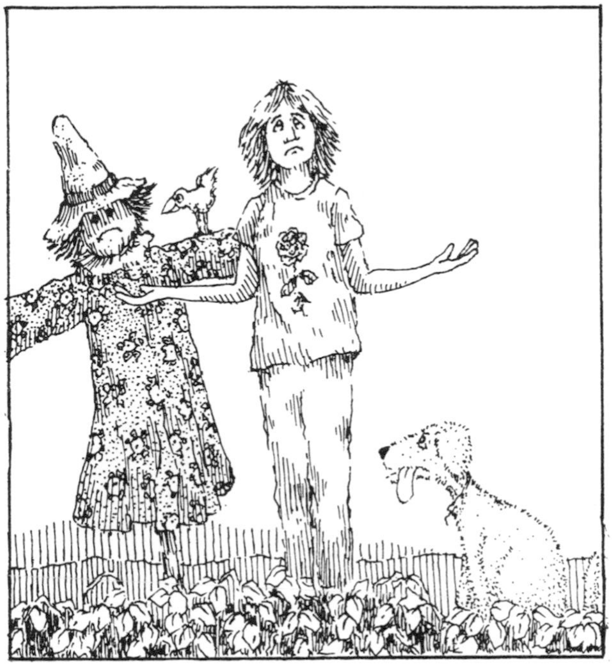

Irrigate your food garden when it fails to rain for seven days. Do you need special water? Usually not. If your tap water is drinkable, it is most likely fit for irrigation, too. But one thing to avoid like the plague is water that has been run through a water softener, because this water will have been polluted with sodium.

If you want to do some serious gardening, water quality should be an important consideration when you're thinking about buying a place. Check with the local county extension agent to find out if the water is suitable for irrigation. If you prefer, you can get an evaluation of your irrigation water by sending a one-pint sample to a good soil testing lab. (Labs are listed in Appendix A.) The cost is well worth it when you consider the importance of water when irrigation is done frequently. Several key measurements show up on the lab report. Here's how to evaluate them:

CONDUCTIVITY

The more salts the water contains, the better the water will conduct electric current. All irrigation water from wells, streams, and springs contains some salts and will give a conductivity reading. The higher the reading, the greater the amount of salts in the water.

The ideal reading for water conductivity ranges from 0.5 to 0.7 (320 to 450 parts per million). As the conductivity reading increases, plant growth and the yield of certain crops decreases. The crops most sensitive to electrical conductivity are beans, carrots, onions, radishes, and lettuce. When irrigation water conductivity increases to 1.0 to 1.4 (640 to 900 parts per million), the yield of sensitive crops decreases by about 10 percent. A yield decrease of 10 percent is not enough to worry about; however, if the electrical conductivity reading is over 1.5 (over 1,000 parts per million), it's probably getting too high.

SODIUM ABSORPTION RATIO

This ratio, often called the SAR, tells you if your irrigation water is going to cause a sodium problem in your soil. The best water will have an SAR of 3 or less, but 3 to 6 is not bad.

CHLORIDE

Should have less than 3 meq per liter (70 parts per million) if irrigating by sprinkling and less than 4 meq per liter (140 parts per million) if irrigating by flooding.

BORON

The suitable range is 0.02 to 0.5 parts per million.

NITRATE

Less than 5 parts per million is acceptable.

BICARBONATE

Less than 1.5 meq per liter is acceptable. (Meq, a chemistry term used in testing labs, is a shortened form of milliequivalents.)

Compost Tea

Even if you followed the soil charging program, special situations sometimes arise where your plants need a booster shot of nutrition, most likely in the transition period when you're building up soil fertility. How do you know when your plants need more nutrition? Let them tell you. If you have planted the right crops at the right time and your plants just sit there, not growing or growing very slowly, it probably means they are hungry. This is where a liquid fertilizer such as compost tea comes in handy.

Compost tea is not something you would want to drink, but plants love it! Compost tea is liquid compost, or compost extract—much as coffee is a water extract of the roasted coffee bean. Compost tea is a dark brown to black liquid that's full of organic colloids plus inorganic nutrient elements. It is far better than any kind of salt fertilizer solution.

You can extract and use it when plants seem to be growing too slowly, indicating they need more plant food. You shouldn't work more compost in, for fear of disturbing the plants' root systems, but you can easily apply liquid compost by sprinkling it right over the top of the plants from a sprinkler can. It is particularly useful with young plants that need a boost.

To make compost tea, fill a five-gallon bucket with four gallons of water, pour in one gallon of compost, and stir for thirty seconds. Let the mixture soak overnight, then strain out the liquid. You can do this by placing a burlap bag over an empty bucket, then pouring the contents of the first bucket onto the burlap strainer. You will end up with about four gallons of compost tea.

How much compost tea should you apply? For small plants, apply half a gallon per square foot once or twice a week until growth improves. For large plants, apply one gallon per square foot per week until growth snaps back. This way of feeding plants also irrigates them, so it is sometimes called "fertigation." The large-plant application is equal to an irrigation of about one-and-a-half inches.

If compost tea is filtered, you could also apply it by injecting it into a sprinkler system. It may even be possible to inject it through a drip system if you first run it through a fine-mesh filter. Injection is easily and commonly done with the aid of injector pumps, which force metered amounts of a fertilizer solution into a pipe leading to a set of operating sprinklers. The Porter & Sons seed cataglog offers injector pumps. (See Appendix B.)

13. *Growing Food Vertically*

SEVERAL valuable and popular food plants send out slender vines that run along the ground. This takes up a great deal of space, and you have to walk on the vines to pick the fruit. These plants include tomato, cucumber, and pole beans.

A neat way to grow these viney plants is in or on a support of some kind. This way, instead of having a row of viney plants sending out vines that cover a space ten feet wide, you induce them to grow upright. (Melons are viney crops not suitable for a support, because their fruits are too large.) Growing viney plants upright gives you several big advantages:

- You save space.
- You can stand up to harvest.
- You avoid trampling the vines.
- You prevent rotted fruit.
- You prevent sunscald.
- You improve pollination in arid climates.

TRELLISES FOR TOMATOES

A plant support, or trellis, may be made of string, wood, plastic, metal, or a combination of these. A trellis may be shaped like a fence, a box, or a cylinder. There's a large selection of trellises available for tomato plants.

Single-Stake (and Triple-Stake) Trellis

This is the most primitive form of trellis for tomato plants. A single-stake trellis consists of a stout wooden stake about 1 to 2 inches square in thickness and 5 feet long. It is driven into the ground next to the plant. The plant is then tied to the stake with soft string or strips of old cloth.

The triple-stake variation is to drive three stakes into the ground in a line, one at the tomato plant, one a foot to the left, and one a foot to the right. Then the plant is pruned to three stems, and each stem is tied to a stake.

The drawbacks to those methods are that you must prune the plant to a single (or triple) stem, which is considerable work; you have to continue to keep the stem (or all three stems) pruned; and a great deal of tying is necessary. The advantages are that the stakes are often cheap, and the pruning cuts down on the number of fruits while increasing their size.

To prune a tomato plant for a single-stake trellis, start at the bottom and pinch off from the main stem the growing points of all suckers. (See Figure 13.1.) Suckers are auxiliary stems that if not pinched off will form new stems. They arise from the crotch, where the leaf

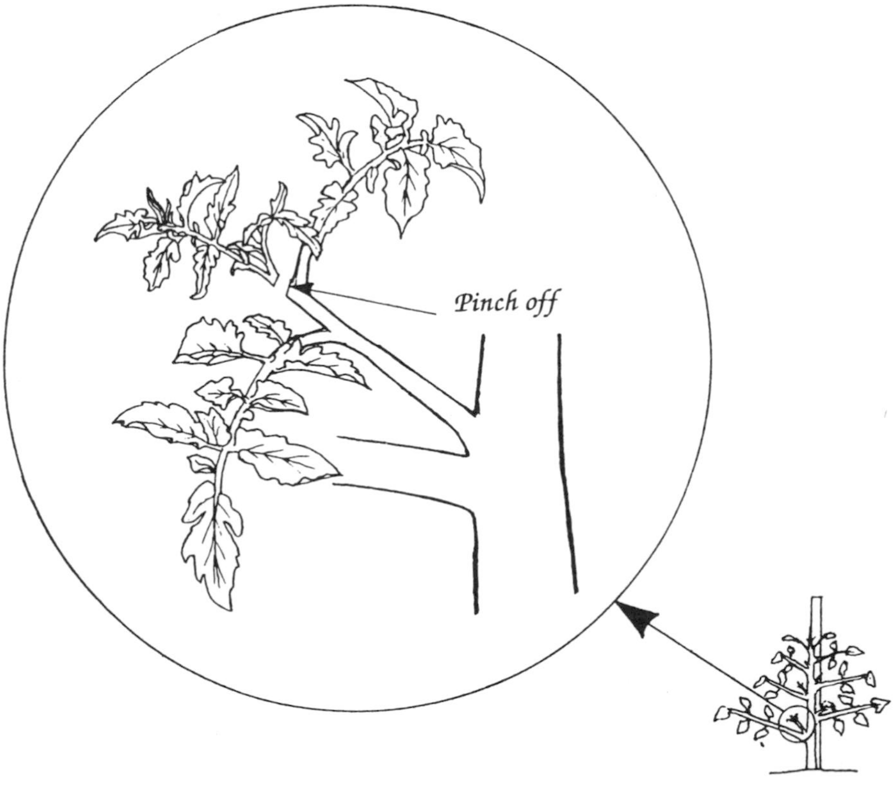

Figure 13.1 To prune a tomato plant for a single-stake trellis, start at the bottom and pinch off the growing points of all suckers from the main stem.

stems join the main stem. Continue to pinch to maintain a single stem as the plant grows.

For a triple-stake trellis, allow two suckers off the main stem to grow to form three main stems. Tie one to the center stake and the other two to the outside stakes. (See Figure 13.2.) Then pinch off all other suckers from the three main stems.

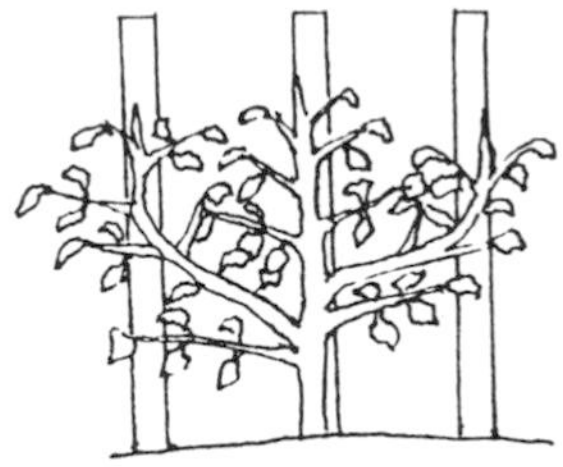

Figure 13.2 When using a triple-stake trellis, allow two suckers off the main stem to grow to form three main stems.

The Wire Cage Trellis

This is simply a piece of light-gauge concrete reinforcing wire with 6-inch meshes formed into a cylinder about 24 inches in diameter and 2 to 5 feet tall. It is placed over tomato and viney-type squash plants and makes them grow up rather than out. No posts are required, because these cages have 6-inch prongs thrust down into the soil to hold them in place. Neither pruning nor tying of tomato plants is needed in wire cages. (See Figure 13.3.)

Wire cages are the Rolls-Royces of tomato supports. They're not the easiest or cheapest kind to get, but they do the best job and last for years. The shading in the tomato wire cage results in less sunburn of fruit. Another benefit is better pollination, especially in arid climates, because the humidity around the blooms in a wire cage is higher.

Training Tomato Plants in Cages

Little or no training is needed. But when the cage is first installed, stems might already be running along the ground like a vine, and some might need to be turned upward to be contained inside the cage. From time to time, some branches try to "escape" the cage. Gently ease them back into the cage.

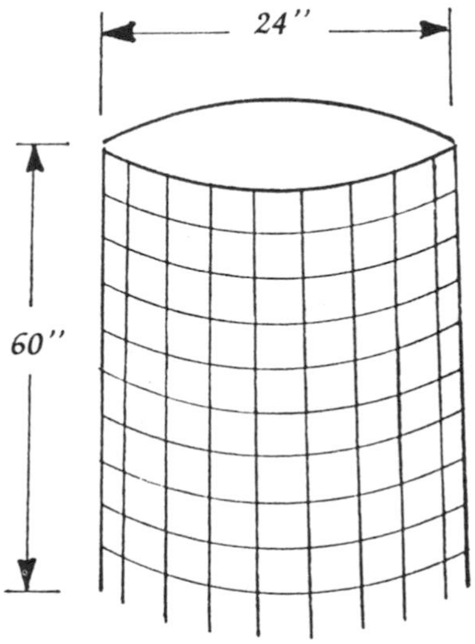

Figure 13.3 Tomato wire cage, full size.

Specs of a Good Cage

A good wire cage is constructed of stiff wire; is shaped like a cylinder, not a cone; has stiff 6-inch prongs at the bottom to thrust into the ground; and has meshes (openings) about 6 by 6 inches.

Storing Cages

At season's end, you might need to use pruning shears or a sharp knife to cut large branches of the old tomato plant. These get intertwined in the meshes of the cage. After branches are cut, simply lift the cage up and off the old plant.

The Half Cage

Some varieties of tomato such as Early Girl need only a half-height cage. To make this cage, take a completed full cage. (See "How to

How to Get Tomato Cages

They are not available in garden centers. They are made by you or someone you hire.

Tools Needed:
A pair of small bolt cutters, a pair of large pliers, a ruler, and a pair of heavy leather gloves.

Materials Needed:
Light-gauge concrete reinforcing wire with 6-inch meshes. (Be sure to use stiff wire with 6-inch by 6-inch mesh, since you will have to reach through the openings to gather the fruit. A smaller mesh won't allow this.)

Comment:
Some advise a cage 19 inches in diameter, but we find a cage about 24 inches is much better because it is less likely to blow over in high winds and because it holds a larger, more productive plant.

Procedure:
1. Put on heavy leather gloves and wear until cage is completed.
2. Lay the wire on the ground and roll it out. Measure off 75 inches of wire with the ruler, and use bolt cutters to cut. The cut should be midway across the thirteenth mesh, leaving 3-inch prongs sticking out.
3. Roll the piece of wire into a cylinder and secure with pliers by bending the 3-inch prongs and fastening them to their opposing prongs.
4. Use bolt cutters to cut out the bottom horizontal ring of the cylinder by making a cut at every vertical wire at the very bottom. This will leave 6-inch prongs all around the bottom of the cage. The prongs will get pushed into the soil to keep the cage secure. The net height of this cage is 54 inches. (See Figure 13.3.)

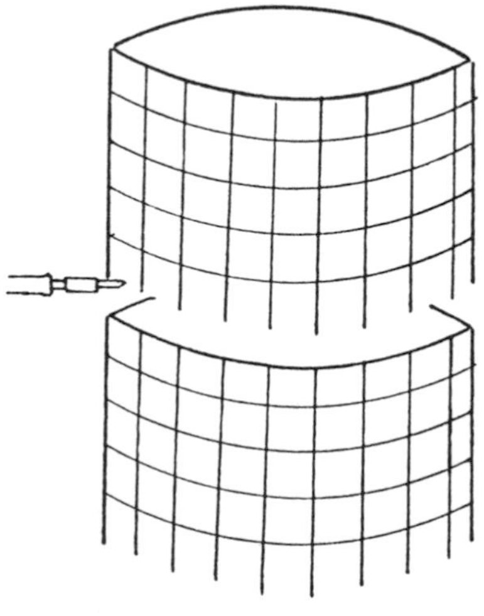

Figure 13.4 Use bolt cutters to make two half cages out of one full cage.

Get Tomato Cages" inset above.) Count down from the top of the cage to the bottom of the fifth mesh (30 inches), and make cuts all around the cage. (See Figure 13.4.) The cuts should split the cage into two identical cages, each having a net height of 24 inches plus 6-inch legs for insertion into the ground.

Precautions to Take With the Full Cage

This cage is so tall that it may get blown over during high winds after the plants have grown into into the upper areas of the cage. If that happens to your cages, straighten them back up and anchor them so they cannot blow down again. To anchor cages, get some one-by-two redwood or pine stakes that are 16 to 24 inches long. If you use pine, cover the entire length with rot-proofing paint. Make sure they're completely dry before using them. On the upwind side of the cage, drive a stake firmly down into the soil as deep as possible, with the stake touching the cage. Then just fasten the cage to the stake with twine. Or you can drive a nail into the stake about 1 inch from the top and drive the stake into the ground so that the nail catches the cage and holds it down.

The Tomato Wood Frame Trellis

Where scrap lumber is available or lumber is inexpensive, the wood frame trellis can be built for tomatoes. (See "Making the Tomato Wood Frame Trellis" inset on page 163.)

Installation

Position the frame over the bed and mark the spots where the posts go. Then dig four holes, 6 inches deep, with a shovel, trowel, or bulb planter. Drop the four legs of the trellis into the holes, backfill with soil, and tamp the soil to firm it. The bottom rail should be about 6 inches above the soil surface. This trellis holds three tomato plants, with 32 inches between each plant. (See Figure 4 on page 162.)

TRELLISES FOR POLE BEANS AND CUCUMBERS

If you're growing pole beans or cucumbers instead of tomatoes, then consider the stiff wire trellis and the wood and twine trellis.

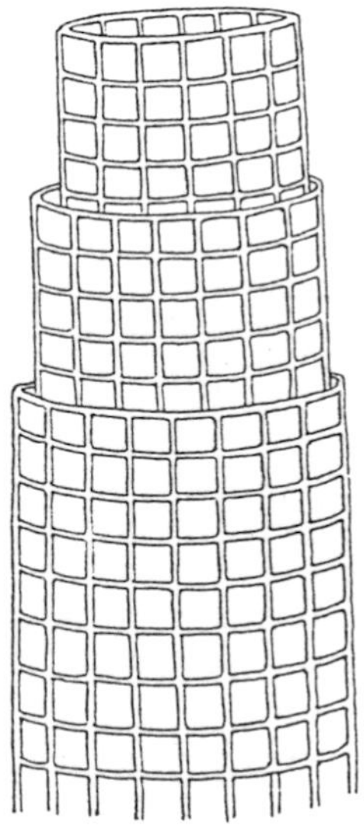

Figure 13.5 To save storage space, choose varying diameters for your tomato cages so that they can be nested together.

Nesting Cages

To save storage space, especially if you have a large area and plant lots of tomatoes, make three different sizes of cages that are about 24 inches in diameter yet fit together when not in use. (See Figure 13.5.) If you cut off a piece of wire midway through the fifteenth mesh (instead of midway through the thirteenth) and form it into a cage, the cage will be 26.7 inches in diameter. If you cut a piece of wire midway through the fourteenth mesh and form it into a cage, the cage will be 25 inches in diameter and will fit inside the larger cage. You can make as many sizes as you need.For example:

Position of Stored Cage	Diameter of Cage (Inches)	Length of Piece of Wire to Cut (Inches)	Number of Meshes (Where to Cut)
Outer	26.7	87	14.5
Middle	25.0	81	13.5
Inner	23.0	75	12.5

Tomato Wood Frame Trellis

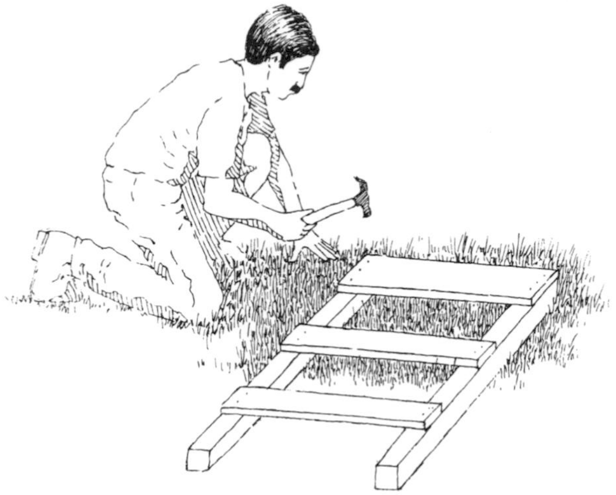

1. Make end frames first for the tomato wood frame trellis.

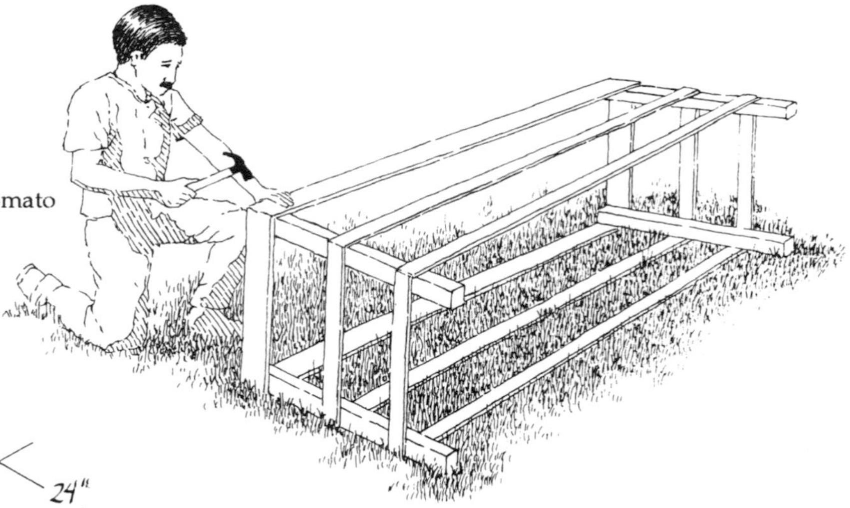

2. Nail side boards on tomato wood frame trellis.

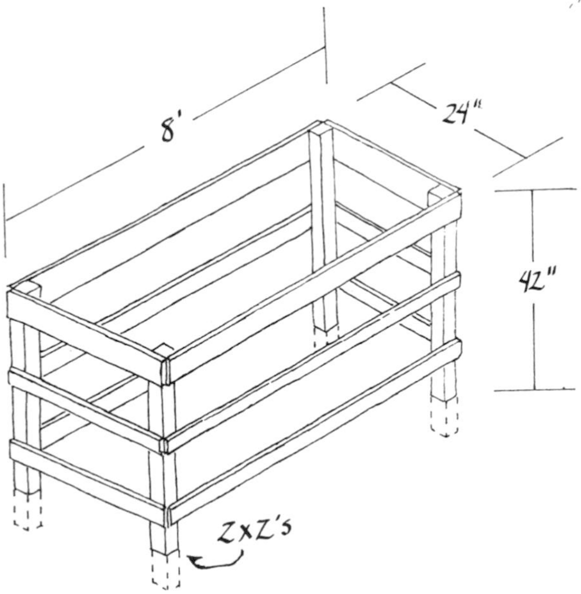

3. Angled view of finished trellis.

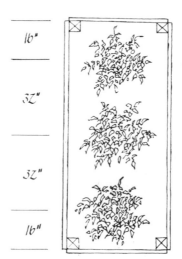

4. Top view of trellis containing three tomato plants.

Making the Tomato Wood Frame Trellis

Tools Needed:
Claw hammer, hand saw, square, 10-foot tape measure.

Materials Needed:
Quarter-pound of common nails, eightpenny size.
Four pieces of 2-by-2 redwood lumber or rot-treated pine, 4 feet long.
Two pieces of 1-by-4 pine lumber, 8 feet long.
Two pieces of 1-by-4 pine, 2 feet long.
Four pieces of 1-by-2 pine, 8 feet long.
Four pieces of 1-by-2 pine, 2 feet long.

Procedure:
1. Make the ends first by nailing the 1-by-4 and the 1-by-2 2-foot-long pieces of pine across the 2-by-2 redwood or rot-treated pine. (See Figure 1.) The bottom board should be 12 inches from the bottom.
2. Have a helper prop up one of the 2-foot ends while you hold the other and nail on the 8-foot-long boards. (See Figure 2.) Use a square to make sure the 8-foot pieces are at right angles to the 2-by-2 pieces. That is it. This trellis will support three tomato plants. It is 8 feet long and 2 feet wide, and when sunk in the ground 6 inches it stands 3.5 feet tall. (See Figure 3.)

Stiff Wire Trellis

This support is like a wire fence. It is made of a piece of light-gauge concrete reinforcing wire 5 feet tall with 6-inch meshes. It's made with exactly the same kind of wire that's used for the tomato cage. A strong top support wire supports the reinforcing wire, which, in turn, is kept taut by being connected to two posts with a turnbuckle. This kind of trellis requires some pretty good handyman skills. If you lack those skills, you can build a wood and twine trellis (described later this chapter), which is simpler. Or you can hire a handyman. Handymen can be found in the Yellow Pages under "Handy-Man Services." (The finished trellis is shown in the "Building the Stiff Wire Trellis" inset on page 164.)

The stiff wire trellis is the best choice for pole beans and cucumbers where an entire bed of 20 feet or more is to be planted with those crops. This trellis (except the end posts) can be dismantled at season's end for bed preparation, or it can be left in place permanently.

Make sure the trellis is in place before your crops are planted. A row of pole beans or cucumbers is planted about 4 inches from the trellis and would be damaged if the trellis was brought in after planting. When the growing season is over and the mass of tangled vines have died and become brittle, put on a pair of heavy gloves and pull the vines loose from the trellis.

Building the Stiff Wire Trellis

Tools Needed:
Small bolt cutters, posthole digger, pliers, hammer, carpenter's square, carpenter's level, heavy leather gloves, shovel.

Materials Needed (for trellis on bed 20 feet long):
One roll of soft (malleable) steel wire.
A quarter-pound of sixteenpenny nails.
One role of twine.
30-foot No. 9 galvanized wire or clothesline wire.
19.5 feet of light-gauge concrete reinforcing wire.
Two 4-by-4 posts, 7 feet long, made of redwood or rot-proofed wood.
One large turnbuckle.
Two bags of Sackrete concrete mix.
Water.

Procedure:

1. Dig a posthole 18 inches deep at each end of the bed. Dig the holes at the bed's centerline.
2. Place a 4-by-4 post, 7 feet long, in each hole. Be sure it protrudes 66 inches above ground level. (See below.) Fill the holes half full of soil, wet down, and tamp.
3. Mix up a bag of Sackrete with water to make concrete, then pour it around one of the posts. Fill the hole to ground level. Using a carpenter's level, plumb the post so it is straight up and down on two adjacent sides. Repeat with the second bag of Sackrete and the second post.
4. Wait a week for concrete to harden. Then use the clothesline or No. 9 galvanized wire to fasten the turnbuckle to one of the posts 5 feet above the ground. (See illustration below.)
5. At the other post, fasten the end of a piece of clothesline or wire about 22 feet long. Attach the other end of the wire to the turnbuckle while pulling it as taut as possible. Then tighten the turnbuckle to make the wire taut. This is the top support wire.
6. Cut off a piece of light-gauge concrete reinforcing wire 19.5 feet long, move it under the top support wire, and fasten it at each end to the top support wire with short pieces of soft malleable steel wire. In between, fasten it every 4 feet with twine. This makes it easy to undo at the end of the season if you wish.

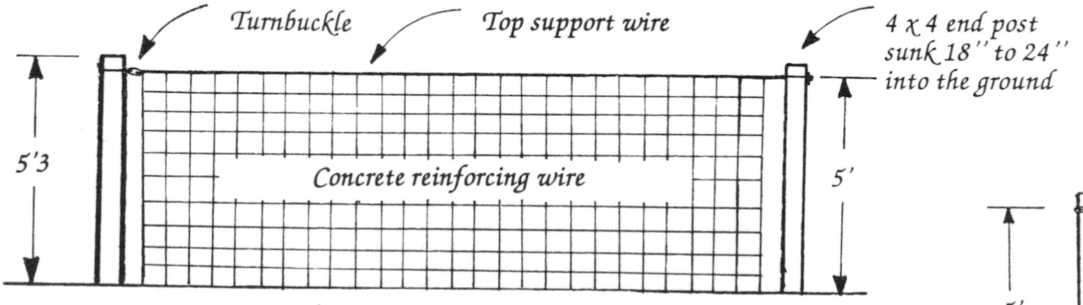

Front view of a stiff wire trellis.

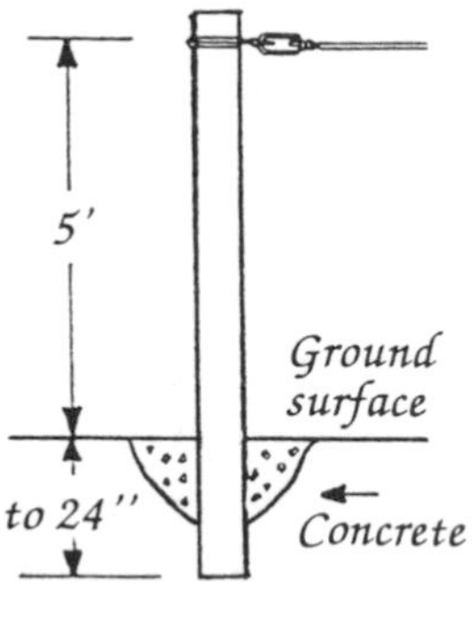

Below-ground view of end post.

How to Build the Wood and Twine Trellis

Tools Needed:
Claw hammer, hand saw, square, shovel, level.

Materials Needed:
One very straight piece of 1-by-4 pine, 8 feet long.
One very straight piece of 1-by-2 pine, 8 feet long.
Two pieces of 2-by-2 redwood, 8 feet long. (If not available in 2-by-2, then use 2-by-4 redwood, 8 feet long.)
One gallon of rot-proofing compound (if not using redwood).
A quarter-pound of 1-inch roofing nails.
A quarter-pound of eightpenny common nails.
70 feet of twine.

Procedure:

1. Use the eightpenny nails to fasten the 1-by-4 at the top of the 2-by-2 posts. Use a carpenter's square to make the angles right angles. (Posts not made of redwood should be painted or soaked with rot-proofing compound along the parts that go into the ground.)
2. At 14 inches up from the bottom of the posts, nail on the 1-by-2 at right angles.
3. Drive roofing nails 6 inches apart and half an inch deep into the top and bottom boards for lacing the twine.
4. Before planting, mark spots for the holes for the posts at the bed's centerline. Dig holes 12 inches deep.
5. Pick up the frame and drop the posts into the holes, fill half full with soil, and tamp.
6. Use a carpenter's level to plumb posts on two adjacent sides, finish filling, plumb again, and tamp the soil thoroughly around the posts.
7. Lace the twine around the nails from the bottom board to the top.

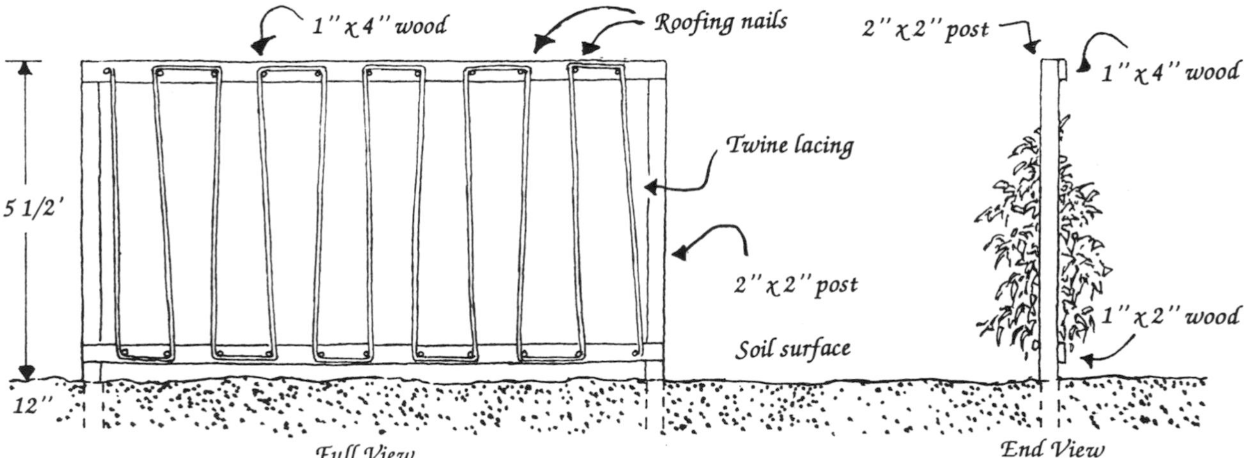

Full View
Full view of trellis shows lacing.

End View
End view of trellis, with a row of plants six inches from either side of the trellis.

Wood and Twine Trellis

This trellis for pole beans and cucumbers is ideal for the beginning gardener. It is made in modules 8 feet in length. It is simple to build, inexpensive, and does the job quite well where only a short trellis is needed. (The finished trellis is shown in the "How to Build the Wood and Twine Trellis" inset on page 165.)

If your backyard has ample storage area, you can simply nail the frame together, leave it in place until next season, or pull it up out of the ground and store it in your backyard. If you have a small electric drill and are handy with tools, you can use stove bolts with wing nuts to hold the frame together; then, for the winter, you can quickly dismantle it for compact storage and reassemble it in the spring.

Plants need help to start climbing this trellis. When the vines have grown about 6 inches long and are running along the ground, gently pull them upward and place them against an upright twine lacing. This may be all they will need to start climbing. If a vine is longer wind it around the lacing several times going upward.

At the end of the season, use a knife, scissors, pruning shears, or your gloved hands to tear or cut off the old dead or dying vines and put them in the compost pole. Remove the lacing, roll it up, and store it until the next season. You can paint the trellis to make it last longer.

THE BEST TRELLISES

We have built and used many kinds of trellises and have eliminated all except the ones listed in this chapter. It is impossible to recommend a single best trellis for everyone. What is best for you depends on a number of factors that vary with each gardener.

For gardeners with a small garden, a limited budget, and limited experience, we suggest a single-stake or triple-stake trellis (with the necessary pruning) for tomatoes and the wood and twine trellis for cucumbers and pole beans.

For the gardener with a larger garden, some experience, and more time and money to invest, we suggest wire cages for tomatoes and the stiff wire trellis for cucumbers and pole beans. This will require the purchase of a roll of concrete reinforcing wire, a small pair of bolt cutters, a posthole digger, and the usual handyman tools.

14. *Harvesting for Peak Taste and Nutrition*

THIS is it, what you've been working and waiting for: tasty, high-nutrition food grown by your own hands! What you don't want to do is mess it up by making the harvest too soon or too late. Harvest at just the right time to get superb flavor along with top nutrition.

A good example is bell pepper. Eating the green bell peppers you buy from the market is like eating green apples. What you want are red, vine-ripe bell peppers. These not only taste better but have an incredibly higher content of health-giving vitamin A. Here's the astonishing comparison: a green bell pepper contains only 42 retinol equivalents of vitamin A, while a red bell pepper contains 445! This means the red bell is ten times richer than the green in this important vitamin.

The guidelines in this chapter, if followed, will not only increase your eating pleasure but will build up your immune system through superior nutrition.

IN GENERAL

Food plants are usually ready to be harvested two to three months after planting. Some mature as soon as 35 days (radish), and some require 150 days or longer (garlic).

The part you harvest may be a root (turnip, sweet potato, carrot), a tuber (potato, sunchoke), a stem (asparagus, celery), a fruit or seed (tomato, squash, beans, peas, cucumber, etc.), buds (broccoli, cauliflower), or leaves (lettuce, cabbage, kale, etc.). In some cultures, flowers are also eaten.

There are three rules for harvesting:

- Wait until the part you are going to harvest is at its peak of quality. Avoid overmature produce that is of poor eating quality—for instance, produce that is tough or stringy or has poor flavor or poor texture.
- If in doubt, cut off or bite off a piece of the vegetable. Is it tough to cut or bite? Inspect it. Is the appearance pleasing? Taste it. Are the texture, flavor, and tenderness good? Many vegetables commonly cooked are not bad when eaten raw. Okra is one of these. Squash is another. A little practice with okra will teach you how long is too long for a pod to get before it's overmature. Bite off about an inch at the tip. If there is any difficulty in biting off a piece, it is too old. Discard it. Varieties differ as to how big they get before they get too tough.
- All foods that develop from flowers (tomato, pepper, squash, etc.) bear more produce and for a longer spell if harvested frequently. If you stop harvesting, the plant "thinks" it has done its job and will stop putting on more blooms and bearing more fruits. Some plants need harvesting daily (okra) and others every other day (squash and tomato).

When in doubt about the approximate time to begin harvesting a certain kind of vegetable, look back to Table 8.3.

WHEN TO HARVEST

Here is some advice on when to harvest your vegetables and fruits. Some tips on how to harvest are also included. The listings are alphabetical.

Asparagus

When the spears are 6 to 8 inches tall but before the tips start to open. Cut or break off the stems at the soil line or slightly below.

Beans (Lima)

When pods and seeds reach full size but are still fresh and juicy. Use the seeds only.

Beans (Pinto)

Immature pinto beans may be harvested as snap beans; nearly mature pintos may be harvested as green shell beans; or they can be left to mature on the vine and harvested as dry pinto beans.

Beans (Snap)

When the pods have grown just large enough to snap when you bend the pod double. If they are immature or too mature, they will just bend and not snap into two pieces.

Beets

As greens, when leaves are 4 to 6 inches long; as tops and small beets, when beets are 1 to 1.5 inches in diameter; as roots only, when beets are 1.5 to 3 inches in diameter.

Broccoli

When flower heads are fully developed but before individual flower buds start to open. Cut the broccoli 6 to 7 inches below the flower heads, but do not discard the small tender leaves, which are good in their own right.

Brussels Sprouts

When sprouts (buds) at the base of the plant become solid. Remove buds higher on the plant as they become firm, but do not strip the leaves from the plants, since they are necessary for further growth.

Cabbage

When the head becomes solid and firm. Excessive water uptake by the roots causes splitting of mature heads. You can stop the water uptake by twisting the plant enough to break several roots.

Cantaloupes

This is a cinch! First, squat down so you won't have to lift the melons off the ground. When the fruit is fully mature and ripe, grasp the melon in one hand and push against the attached stem with the thumb of the other hand. The stem slips off with only a slight pressure. At the place where the stem was attached to the fruit will be a smooth circular patch of tissue. This is called a "full slip," but you do not have to let the fruits get that ripe. Even a "half slip" melon will probably be mature and ripe and ready to eat.

If considerable pressure is required before the melon comes loose, then you probably have a "half slip." Pick up the melon and look at where the stem was attached. If a half slip, about half the circular area of attachment will be smooth, but the other half will have part of the stem hanging to it.

If you live where it rains during harvest, it will be advantageous for you to pick melons at half slip and store them. That's when melons are nearing maturity and their sugar content is nearing a peak. Rain would ruin the sugar content and the taste.

Carrots

When they reach three-quarters to 2 inches in diameter. Larger carrots contain more vitamin A than smaller ones. If the weather is cool and dry, carrots may be left in the ground for a later harvest.

Cauliflower

When the curds (flower heads) are full size (6 to 8 inches in diameter) but still compact, white, and smooth. Curds exposed to sunlight become cream-colored, rough in appearance, and coarse in texture. When curds are 3 to 4 inches in diameter, tie the tips of the outer leaves loosely above the curd to exclude sunlight.

Celery

When plants become 12 to 15 inches tall. While young and tender, the lowest stems (6 to 10 inches long) may be harvested.

Chard

When leaves are 6 to 8 inches long.

Chives

When young tender leaves appear.

Collard

When inner leaves are 6 to 8 inches long.

Corn (Sweet)

First, look at the silk and see if it is dry and brown. If it is, then feel the tip end of the ear. If it feels hard, peel the shuck at the tip to expose some of the kernels. Press your thumbnail against a few of them. If the kernels pop and thick juice escapes, the ear is in the "milk stage" and at the peak of quality. Soon after picking, sweet corn will rapidly lose quality unless handled properly. This is because the sugar that makes the corn taste so good begins to convert to starch. Immediately upon picking, get the ears into your kitchen or under shade. Cover with wet sacks or put the ears in the refrigerator (unless you plan to use them within an hour or two). Where large amounts of ears are to be harvested, do it in the early morning when it is cool.

Cucumber

When fruits are near full size, usually 6 to 9 inches long, but still bright green and firm. If the lemon variety, when a little yellow begins to show on the skin. For pickles, when fruits are 2 to 4 inches long.

With cucumbers on a trellis, the leaves are often so thick that it is impossible to see the fruits, especially the ones on the bottom. But if they have been growing about sixty days, you can be pretty sure some cucumber fruits will be ready to pick, so squat down, pull the vines apart, and look inside the leafy growth, especially at the bottom.

Eggplant

When fruits are near full size, about 4 to 6 inches in diameter, but still firm and bright in color.

Garlic

When foliage loses color and tops begin to fall over. Pull free, wash the roots, and place under shade to dry.

Jerusalem Artichoke

See Sunchoke.

Kale

When the outer leaves are 8 to 10 inches long, break them off. New leaves will continue to grow from the center of each plant. Harvest these newer leaves when 6 to 8 inches long.

Kohlrabi

When bulbous stems reach 2 to 3 inches in diameter.

Lettuce (Leaf)

Harvest the outer leaves when 4 to 6 inches long. The inner leaves continue to grow, providing a continuous harvest. Avoid planting head lettuce. Or, with Cos (Romaine) lettuce, cut off the entire plant at its base when 8 to 12 inches tall; with Bibb, cut off the entire plant when 4 inches in diameter; with Buttercrunch, when 6 to 8 inches in diameter.

Mustard Greens

When outer leaves are 6 to 8 inches long. Handle the same as lettuce.

Okra

Varieties differ, but generally harvest when pods are about 6 inches long. To protect yourself from the bristles on the okra plant, wear a long-sleeved shirt and cotton gloves. Harvest daily in midsummer, and cut or snap off all pods large enough for harvest.

Onions

For bulb onions, when about 75 percent of the tops have fallen over. Pull, leaving tips on, wash, and place out of the sun for drying. For immature green onions, when the base of the onion stem starts to swell slightly, to about a quarter-inch to a half-inch in diameter. The base is underground where the roots are attached.

Parsnips

In late fall, especially after early frost; and in very early spring, before growth starts.

Peas (Green)

When the pods are fully developed but still bright green. Harvest edible pod types when pods reach a length of about 3 inches but before the seeds show full enlargement.

Peas (Southern)

Like pinto beans, these peas (black-eyed, crowder, purplehull) may be harvested immature as "snap peas" or left on the plant longer to fill out the pod and be picked as "green shell peas" or left even longer to mature into dried peas. You can also sprout the dry peas and enjoy a large enzyme boost.

Pepper (Bell)

When fruits are firm. But if you wait two to three weeks, the green fruit will ripen to a bright red with a superior taste and a much higher vitamin content.

Potatoes

When the tubers are full size and the skin is firm. Immature potatoes are tasty, and a partial harvest may be made when the immature tubers are about 1.5 inches in diameter. To harvest, take a spading fork or shovel and gently dig up the ground around the vines, which will be full of potatoes.

Pumpkins

When the fruits are full size, the rind is firm and glossy, and the bottom of the fruit has a cream to orange color.

Radishes

When the roots are 1 to 1.5 inches in diameter.

Salsify

In late fall, preferably after early frost; or in early spring, before new growth starts. If you leave it over the winter in the garden row, cover the roots with 3 to 5 inches of soil to avoid freezing.

Spinach

When large leaves are 4 to 6 inches long. Harvesting just the older leaves allows new growth to develop; or harvest the plants whole.

Squash

When fruits are still small. Refer to catalog descriptions of how large a full-grown fruit is, and pick yours just before they reach full size. Harvest every other day to prevent fruits from becoming overmature.

Strawberries

Pick fruits when they turn full red. Harvest every two to three days to keep new blooms coming.

Sunchoke

Also called Jerusalem artichoke, this is actually a sunflower that not only blooms but bears edible tubers on its roots. Begin harvest after bloom is over in the fall, about the time of the first freeze. Dig up tubers with a shovel. Place the tubers in a bucket of water, wash off the soil, and place the tubers on a slab or garden sieve to drain and dry. If you prefer, you can leave most of the tubers in the ground and harvest all winter as needed, but finish harvesting a month before the spring frost-free date. When washed tubers have dried, always store them in the refrigerator to prevent sprouting.

Sweet Potatoes

When half or more of the roots are 2.5 to 3 inches in diameter and 3 to 7 inches long, usually indicated when vines begin to die. Do not allow roots to become chilled. For harvesting, clip the vines off, then take a shovel or spading fork and gently dig up the ground in the area where the vines grew. It will be full of sweet potatoes. Cure the roots by placing them in a warm humid room in slatted boxes for a week to form a thickened skin for longer storage life.

Tomatoes

When fruits are all red, with no green showing anywhere, and when the fruit comes off the stem with a light tug or twist. If grasshoppers start feeding on fruits just when a little red starts showing, pick the fruit and let it finish ripening off the vine.

Turnips

When roots are 2 to 2.5 inches in diameter but before heavy fall frosts. For greens, harvest leaves 6 to 8 inches in length.

Watermelons

This is one of the most difficult fruits to harvest at just the right maturity. Use these guidelines:

- Read the variety description to find the approximate size or weight of a mature fruit. Estimate weight by pulling a few and weighing them on a household scale.
- If melons appear to be the right size for maturity, try the old-fashioned thump test. Strike the watermelon with your fist, as if you were knocking on a door. If the fruit is unripe, there will be a high-pitched, bell-like sound. If the fruit is ripe, there will be a low-pitched dull thud, like you're thumping on a leather boot.
- A brown tendril at the stem end where the melon is attached to the vine indicates ripeness. If the tendril is still greenish, the fruit is probably not ripe.
- If the color at the bottom changes from green to white or a creamy color, it's probably time to harvest.
- Press down on the top of the fruit. A slight, subtle cracking sound indicates maturity.
- Look for a color change at the top of the melon. A dusty color that is lighter green than the young fruits indicates maturity.
- If the watermelon appears to have small wounds that look like scars that have healed, that indicates maturity.

15. *Processing and Storage*

PROCESSING vegetables means what you do to them to get them ready for the table. You will need a strong-bladed sharp knife for cutting, stainless steel bowls for washing and holding, collanders for draining, and two- to four-gallon buckets with handles for transporting picked produce from the garden to the kitchen.

THE HARVEST TABLE

A table on the back patio is a big help at harvest time when removing unwanted tops or roots or soil from vegetables. It enables you to hose off everything outside. This keeps the mess out of your kitchen.

A good harvest table should be about the same height and width as a kitchen cabinet counter (about 36 inches high by 24 inches wide). The top can be made of exterior plywood (half an inch thick), or you can even use a card table covered with a piece of plywood (three-eighths of an inch thick) that has been covered with spar varnish.

ADVANCED HARVEST TABLE

This is a specially built processing table for the serious gardener. (See Figure 15.1.) You can build it yourself if you are handy with tools. It can be made of scrap lumber and a secondhand sink. At one end is space for cutting off the tops and roots of freshly harvested vegetables. Next along the table is a round hole about 12 inches in diam-

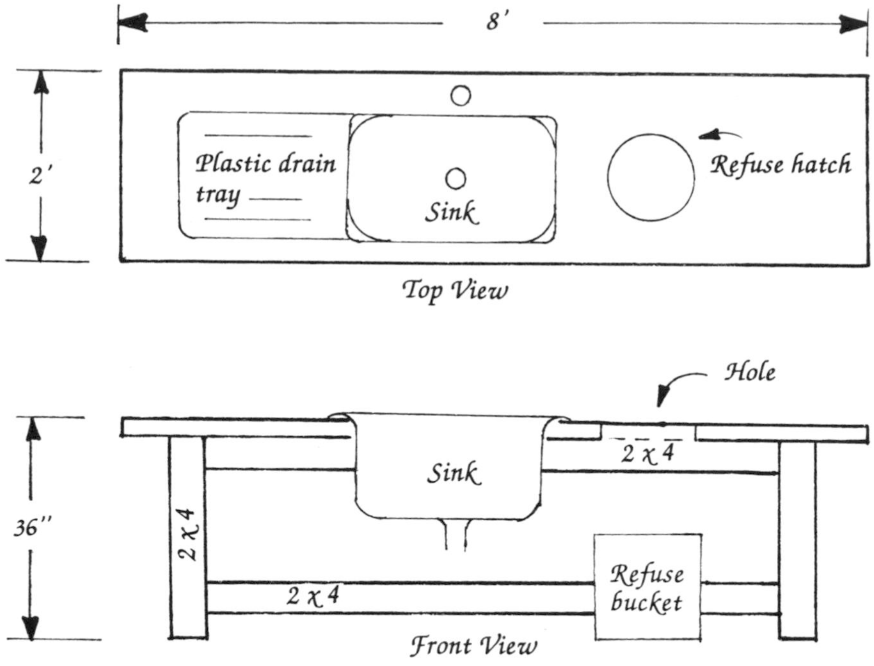

Figure 15.1 Advanced harvest table.

eter with a bucket under it. Into this hole are dropped the trimmings. The edible parts are then moved along the table for washing in the sink, and they finish their journey along the table by being placed in a drain tray.

The sink need not be fastened to the table; just set it in a hole cut for it. The four legs can be hinged so they fold and are braced at the bottom by boards set in notches in the legs. Then, when summer and harvest time is over, you can remove the sink, unscrew the hose from the sink faucet fittings, remove the leg braces, fold the table, and store it in your garage or under your patio until next season.

PROCESSING AND STORING INDIVIDUAL CROPS

Here are some tips on how to process and store beans, peas, sweet corn, onions, garlic, peanuts, sunchokes, and sweet potatoes.

Dry Beans and Southern Peas

Peas may be harvested as snaps, where the entire pod with immature peas inside is snapped, cooked, and eaten. For black-eyed peas, the usual way is to let the pods grow large and well-filled with large seeds but to harvest the pods while they're still green. When shelled, the seeds are tasty and nutritious lightly steamed. The main problem with fresh-shelled peas is the large amount of labor for hand-shelling. But a mechanical sheller can be bought at a reasonable price and is a good investment if you shell large amounts of peas. One source is Lee Manufacturing. (See Appendix A.)

After picking snap beans, wash and drain. Then snap each pod, breaking it into pieces 1 inch long. If any pods are well-filled with green, immature seeds, remove the shell of the pod and keep the seeds for cooking. These are called "green shell beans."

Processing Dry Beans and Southern Peas

Let the pods dry up on the vine, and pick them off before they shatter. If they're not completely dry, you can pull up the entire vine and hang it under a well-vented patio or shed. When the pods are well-dried, pull off the vine, and thresh the seeds out of the pods. One good way is to put pods on a clean tarp, put on a clean pair of sneakers, and walk over them in a sliding motion. Then winnow (separate out the seeds) by pouring the seeds and chaff from a bucket into another bucket when the wind or a fan is blowing. (See Figure 15.2.)

Storing Dry Beans and Southern Peas

Five-gallon buckets filled with carbon dioxide and capped with tight-fitting lids are the best way to store dry beans and peas on a long-term basis. Fill the buckets with the harvested dry beans and peas. For each bucket, put one ounce of dry ice on the produce, place the lid on loosely, and wait a few minutes. The dry ice will melt into carbon dioxide gas, which sinks downward and pushes the air out. Tighten the lids, and store in a cool place. For intermediate-term storage (up to a year), you can get by with putting dry beans and peas in sacks or jars stored in a cool dry place.

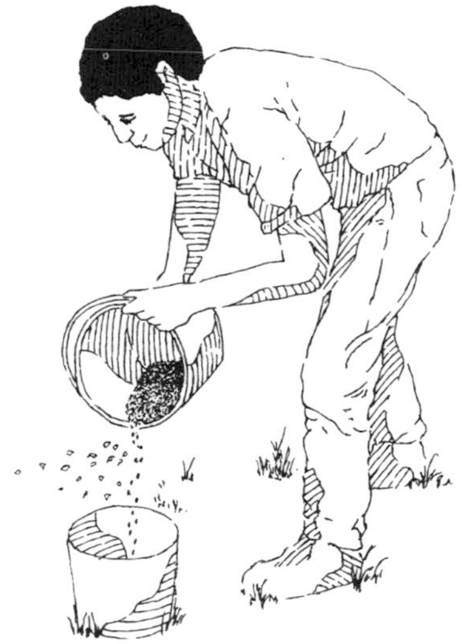

Figure 15.2 Winnowing is a breeze if there's a breeze blowing. After walking over the pods, pour the seeds and chaff from one bucket into a second bucket while the wind (or a fan) is blowing. The seeds land in the bucket; the chaff gets blown away.

Sweet Corn

After pulling an ear off the stalk, break off the stem at the bottom of the ear. Take the ears to your kitchen or harvest table and, with a sharp heavy knife, cut off the tip end and the butt end at the points where the kernels just begin. Then remove the shucks and most of the silks with your hands. Be sure to save all these trimmings for the compost pile. To get rid of the rest of the silks, hold the ear, butt end down, under a running faucet, and brush the silks off with a vegetable brush. At this point you can either cook them up or freeze or dry them for long-term storage. If you want to eat them within a week, leave the silks and shucks on, and store them in the refrigerator. They will stay fresh in the refrigerator for about eight days.

To dry without a solar-powered oven, leave the ears on the stalk until thoroughly dry. (More on solar ovens later this chapter.) Then pull off the ears, remove the shuck, put on a pair of gloves, and shell the kernels off the cob. Then store in bags or jars in a cool dry place. To use, reconstitute by soaking the kernals in water and then handle like fresh sweet corn. Or grind the dry kernels into corn meal. If you have the space, you can leave the dried grain right on the cob.

Onions and Garlic

For long-term storage, the soil needs to be removed from the bulbs, and the bulbs need to be allowed to dry. After washing the soil off, there are two ways to dry onion or garlic bulbs: tie bunches of five to ten plants together with a string around the dried tops and hang them, with the tops down, in a well-ventilated place out of the sun for a week; or cut the tops off about an inch from the bulb, place the bulbs in mesh sacks, and hang the sacks in a well-ventilated place out of the sun. An ideal place is a shed or a covered patio with rafters. Put some nails through the rafters, and attach the sacks with string.

Peanuts

Pull the seed pods off the plants by hand. A pair of cotton gloves will help. The plants with leaves make an excellent high-protein hay or high-nitrogen mulch. The peanut seeds are enclosed in a thick outer hull, or shell. If the pods are sufficiently dried, shelling the seeds out of the pods is easily done with the thumb and index finger.

Shelling Percentage

Peanuts have a shelling percentage of about 73 percent. This means that a pound of whole peanuts in the pod will yield nearly 12 ounces, or 73 percent of a pound, of edible nuts.

Roasting Peanuts

Peanuts need light roasting in an oven to increase taste and food value. After roasting, the thin, lightweight, outer skins can be winnowed away by rubbing them between the palms of your hands. If you don't mind the skins, just leave them on.

Grinding Into Butter

Roasted whole peanut seeds are tasty and may be eaten as is, but most people lack the patience or dental makeup to allow the thorough chewing necessary to promote full assimilation and to prevent gas formation. A good solution is to grind the roasted seeds into meal or peanut butter. We use a Champion juicer with a nut butter attachment. (This is available at health food stores.) Less-expensive grinders can be used, such as a heavy-duty food processor.

Sunchokes (Jerusalem Artichokes)

Dig deep under sunchoke plants to avoid cutting into tubers. A neat, efficient way is just to shovel soil, tubers and all, onto a garden sieve, then move the sieve back and forth to catch tubers on the screen and let the soil fall through. (You can use the sieve pictured in Figure 10.5.) Place the tubers in a bucket half full of water, and swish them around to loosen the soil. Remove the tubers from the bucket and place them on a raised screen (such as a garden sieve) or on a concrete slab to drain. Do not let the tubers completely dry out; just let them dry enough to get the excess water off. The key to good tubers is to keep them cool and moist at all times. Place the tubers in a plastic bag and store them in a refrigerator.

Sweet Potatoes

A refrigerator is an ideal place to store many vegetables, but not sweet potatoes. Instead, they store best at cool but not cold temperatures of 55°F to 60°F and at 85 to 95 percent humidity. (See Table 15.1 for details.)

During winter, this might be in an unheated garage or in the coolest part of the house. In the arid West, a good place during winter is in a cool part of the house in a cardboard box with a loose-fitting cover and a glass of water inside to raise the humidity.

SHORT-TERM STORAGE

The ideal is to harvest your food plot half an hour before preparing a meal and to put your food on the table within an hour after harvesting. But this is often inconvenient and is really unnecessary, since you can keep produce almost as good as new for several days in a refrigerator or under other suitable storage conditions. The first thing to do after harvesting a food crop is to get it out of the sun and into the shade in a well-ventilated place. Some foods are sensitive to solar radiation. Cover such foods, such as sweet corn ears and greens, with sacks, and wet them down in hot sunny weather.

INTERMEDIATE-TERM STORAGE

For intermediate-term storage, most foods need temperatures of 32°F to 45°F. A few others store best at 45°F to 55°F. Foods requiring either temperature range for intermediate-term storage should go into a refrigerator. Sweet potatoes, which can be stored in a cool room, are the only exception to this need for refrigeration. If you have two refrigerators, one can be kept under 40°F for those foods that need colder temperatures, and the other can be around 45°F. If you have only one refrigerator, store everything there at 40°F.

Table 15.1 shows how long each crop will last under ideal conditions. These storage temperatures are also the temperatures that will preserve vitamins the best. Keep in mind that if the ideal temperature is 32°F and your refrigerator is kept at 45°F, the food won't last quite as long.

The amount of time for which different foods can be stored under the conditions in Table 15.1 varies greatly. Some are quite short (four to seven days for ripe tomatoes), while other storage times are quite long (up to eight months for bulb onions). If you want to store a food for longer than the time shown on this table, consult the "Long-Term Storage" section beginning below.

Getting Maximum Storage Life

You need to inspect your stored produce from time to time to sort out the rots so they don't spread infection. To keep vegetables longer in your refrigerator, cover them with towels, either paper or cloth. This absorbs moisture given off by vegetables. Moisture can cause excessive humidity, leading to rot. Remove the towels frequently and replace with dry ones. You'll be surprised how much longer your produce will keep!

LONG-TERM STORAGE

You can store your home-grown produce for the long term by canning, freezing, or drying the food.

Canning

Canning is the process of sealing and sterilizing food inside airtight metal or glass containers. It is better than no preservation at all, but the heat applied during sterilization destroys much of the food value. Enzymes are all destroyed. Protein might be denatured. Vitamins are partly or wholly destroyed. Equipment can be expensive, and so can the empty cans and jars. Canning is well-suited for tomato products such as juice and sauce.

Freezing

Freezing is much better than canning, since it involves less or no heat treatment of foods but will preserve foods potentially for years. The disadvantage is that a freezer is expensive to buy and consumes a lot of energy. Some books say that before you freeze any food you must blanch it to kill the enzymes that cause spoilage. Blanching is simply a heat treatment like canning but much less severe, therefore preferable. However, we have found that blanching is not necessary. We have frozen corn, beans, tomatoes, and other vegetables without

Table 15.1

Best Conditions for Intermediate-Term Storage

Food	Storage Temperature (°F)	Relative Humidity (%)	Storage Life
Artichoke, Globe	32	90–95	1 month
Artichoke, Jerusalem	31–32	90–95	2–5 months
Asparagus	32–36	90–95	7–10 days
Bean, Snap	40–45	90–95	7–10 days
Beet (root)	32	95	3–5 months
Broccoli	32	90–95	10–14 days
Brussels Sprouts	32	90–95	3–5 weeks
Cabbage (early)	32	90–95	3–6 weeks
Cabbage (late)	32	90–95	3–4 months
Cantaloupe	32–40	85–90	5–15 days
Carrot (immature)	32	90–95	4–6 weeks
Carrot (mature)	32	90–95	4–5 months
Casaba Melon	45–50	85–90	4–6 weeks
Cauliflower	32	90–95	2–4 weeks
Celery	32	90–95	2–3 months
Collards	32	90–95	10–14 days
Corn, Sweet	32	90–95	4–8 days
Cucumber	45–50	90–95	10–14 days
Eggplant	45–50	90	7 days
Garlic	32	65–70	6–7 months
Kale	32	90–95	10–14 days
Kohlrabi	32	65–70	2–4 weeks
Lettuce	32	95	2–3 weeks
Okra	45–50	90–95	7–10 days
Onion, Bulb	32	65–70	1–8 months
Pea, Black-Eyed (green shell)	40–45	90–95	7–10 days
Pea, Green	32	90–95	1–3 weeks
Pepper (green)	45–50	90–95	2–3 weeks
Pepper (red ripe)	40–45	90–95	7 days
Potato	40	90	2–3 weeks
Radish	32	90–95	3–4 weeks
Spinach	32	90–95	10–14 days
Squash, Summer	32–50	90	5–14 days
Squash, Winter	50–55	50–75	2–6 months*
Sweet Potato	55–60	85–90	4–6 month
Tomato (ripe)	45–50	85–90	4–7 days
Turnip (greens)	32	90–95	10–14 days
Turnip (roots)	32	90–95	4–5 months
Watermelon	40–50	80–85	4–6 weeks

Source: USDA Agricultural Handbook. No. 66

* = Table Queen, 55–65 days; Butternut, 60–90 days; Hubbard, 180 days.

blanching and found nothing wrong with the taste when we cooked and ate them.

Drying

This is our choice for preserving most foods. Foods properly dried and stored in airtight jars in a dark place will last several years with no problem. The best food dehydrator is solar powered. Even in a low-sun area like the Pacific Northwest, electricity is cheap and wood is plentiful, so those energy sources can be used along with solar for drying foods.

We have been involved in the design and operation of several solar food dryers, and the best of the lot is also the simplest. It is just a shallow black box with a hinged top and is covered with plastic and air holes at the top and bottom. A screened tray inside the box holds the fresh produce to be dried. The oven is 4 feet long by 2 feet wide by 6 inches deep. (See Figure 15.3.) It will operate at about 140°F; however, raw food enzymes are deactivated at temperatures over 118°F. If you want to dry your produce while preserving the enzymes, partially shade the top of the oven to cut down on the solar energy as much as necessary to reach the temperature you want.

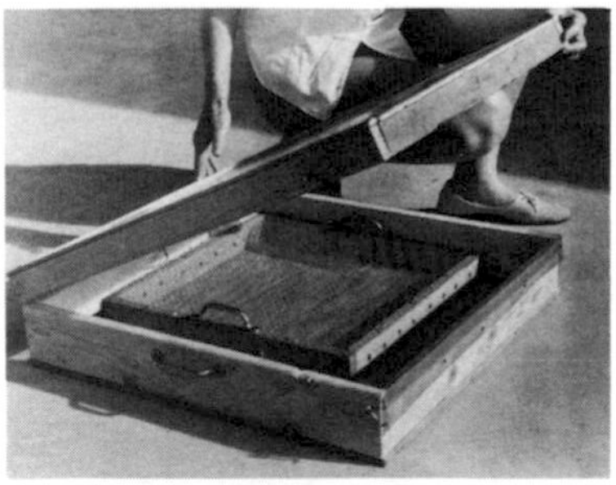

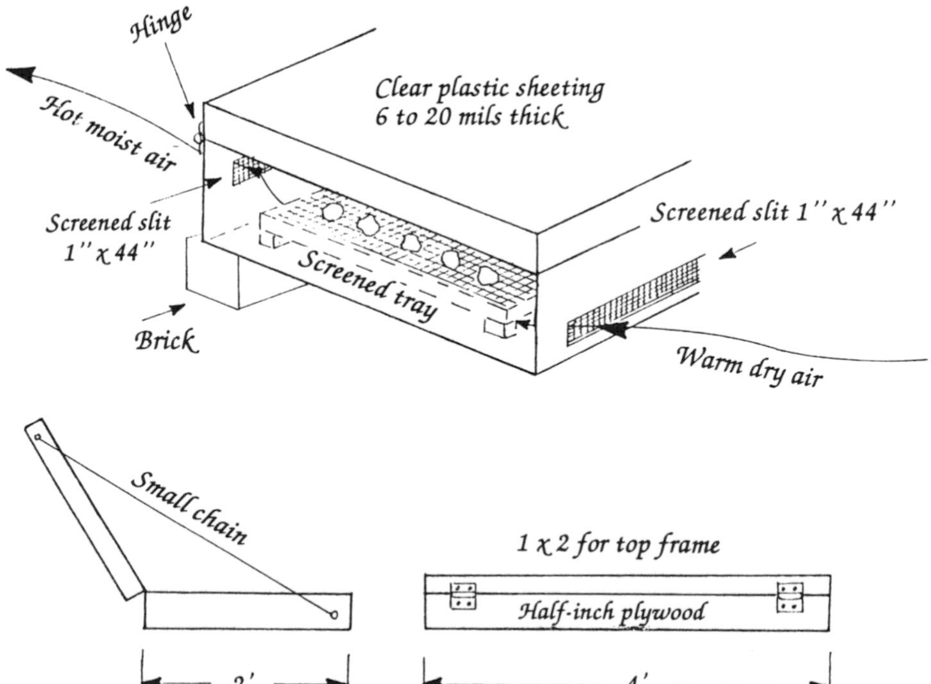

Figure 15.3 Top illustration shows a cutaway view of a solar food oven in use. Below it and to the left is a side view of the oven ready for loading. The small chain is 38 inches long and is fastened with no. 8 screws to the inside of the top and the inside of the bottom of the oven. Bottom right illustration shows a back view of the oven, showing two hinges. The above photograph shows an actual solar oven.

(You will need to place a thermometer inside the oven to monitor its temperature.)

It might be more practical just to let the solar oven operate at top temperature and sacrifice some enzymes. You can get them instead from fresh vegetables from either a cold frame (an unheated box for plants, usually made of wood with a glass or plastic top to admit solar radiation) or a greenhouse during offseason or, best of all, from sprouts.

Drying Procedure

Select produce of high quality and clean it thoroughly. Do not dry overripe fruit or wilted vegetables. Dried fruits and vegetables are said to keep their color better if they first undergo an anti-oxidant treatment. Make a solution of one-third a cup of pure crystalline ascorbic acid per quart of water or a solution of one tablespoonful of salt per quart of water. As soon as a piece of fruit or vegetable is cut, drop it in the solution. Whenever you're ready, place the cut pieces on the screened tray, let them drain, then place the tray in the solar oven.

Here are some tips for drying certain types of produce.

- Tree Fruits: Core them, cut in halves, then fourths, then eighths, or cut into rings a quarter-inch thick.
- Vegetable Fruits: Cut into wedges, with the wide side not over an inch wide.
- Herb Leaves: Cut and tie in bunches and hang on strings in the shade. Or place on wire-bottomed trays in the shade under the roof of a wall-less structure (such as a covered patio) that provides protection from rain but does not impede air movement.
- Beans, Peas: Let the pods dry on the vine to the point where they're tan-colored but not brittle, then harvest the pods and dry them in the solar oven. After they're dried, the seeds will be easy to separate from the husks and winnow away.
- Thick, Fleshy Vegetables (Squash, Celery, Onion, Carrot): Cut into slices an eighth to a quarter of an inch thick and up to about 1.5 inches in diameter.
- Sweet Corn: For fastest drying, let the ears mostly dry on the vine, harvest, and put them in the dryer to finish drying. You can also shuck the ears as if you were going to eat them, and then place them in the dryer as regular corn on the cob. That way just takes longer. Whichever method you use, you can store the dried corn on the cob in a cool dry place if you have the room, or you can shell the kernels and store in bags or jars.

Drying Time

High-moisture produce such as fruits might take several days in the solar oven, but other produce such as carrot might take only six hours. After four hours, check the solar oven for drying progress, then check again every hour thereafter when the sun is shining. When pieces are leathery and you see no moisture when you cut or squeeze them, drying is completed. Store cut produce in an airtight container in a cool dry place.

16. *Growing Choice Foods*

THE most commonly grown kinds of food crops are not only popular but high in nutrition and easy to grow. They tend to give you the most eating for the least space and work, with the exception of sweet corn. Here are our secrets for growing the most frequently grown crops successfully.

DRY BEANS AND PEAS

Beans and peas, also called legumes, are high in most of the minerals, including iron and zinc. Also important is that they are a wonderful source of protein, have virtually no fat or cholesterol, and have fiber that will lower blood cholesterol and keep your digestive tract healthy.

Pintos and Other Common Beans

Pinto and other common beans may be grown and harvested as snap beans (immature stage), as green shell beans (pods filled but still green), or left to mature on the vine until the pods are dry. Plant and care for these beans just like snap beans.

Southern Pea

This is an old favorite of the South but is a winner anywhere it will grow. Like the pinto, it may be harvested and used at three different stages. In addition, dry seeds make excellent sprouts, delicious when lightly cooked. Southern peas are also called cowpeas and include the well-known black-eyed variety, sometimes called the blackeye bean, and the lesser-known Mississippi Silver, a high-yielding crowder pea.

Southern peas love warm weather. Plant them two to ten weeks after the spring freeze-free date. Plant each row in the middle of its own 24-inch bed. Open a planting trench with the corner of a regular hoe or a V-hoe, drop the seeds 1 inch apart, cover 1 inch deep with covering mix, then mulch. After insects, weather, and bad seeds have taken their toll, thin to 3 inches between plants. You can also plant two rows per bed. (See Chapter 7.)

Maximum Yields

It might be possible to get a much higher yield of food from each square foot of peas if you make multiple harvests, including one or more harvests of green shell peas followed by the final dry pea harvest. Harvest black-eyed peas when the first pods mature and are firm and filled out but still green. This harvest allows the small unfilled pods to grow faster and more blooms to appear. After waiting a week or two, go back for a second green pea harvest; again, young pods will fill out and more blooms will appear. The third and final harvest comes much later, when all the remaining pods have matured and dried up on the stalk. The vines (stalks left after harvest) are high in protein and good for mulch, compost, and hay.

BEANS (SNAP)

Snap beans are a good source of calcium, magnesium, and iron.

Bush or Pole?

Bush snap beans grow as a short, bushy, self-supporting plant; the pole type makes long vines, which must have a trellis to climb. Which should you have? Both. The bush beans bear earlier, and just as they stop bearing, the pole beans start. Planting both kinds keeps you in fresh snap beans longer.

For example, say you plant both bush and pole beans May 1. You could expect this to happen:

Type of Bean	Planting Date	Start Bearing	End Bearing
Bush	May 1	June 20	July 4
Pole	May 1	July 4	Sept 4

You'll need to plant three bush beans for every pole bean to get the same amount of harvest. During planning, allow about 15 linear feet of row per person for bush beans and 5 linear feet per person for pole beans. This is because the harvest for pole beans lasts twice as long and the yield per linear foot is greater. Pole beans also taste better and are the clear choice of the gardener if only one type is to be planted. The advantages of the bush bean are that it needs no trellis and matures earlier.

BEET, CARROT, COLLARD, TURNIP

Among these four, you have a powerhouse of every mineral and vitamin known to man. Beet greens are packed with magnesium, iron, zinc, and copper; collard and turnip greens are packed with calcium, magnesium, B-6, and folacin; and nothing beats carrots for vitamin A.

All four are early-season crops planted two to six weeks before the average spring freeze-free date, and all are planted in double rows. The range of suitable growing temperature is 45°F to 75°F, with 60°F to 65°F the optimum.

Sow all these at the rate of about twelve seeds per linear foot. Turnips emerge in about only three days, but carrots and beets need about ten days. (There is no data for collard emergence time.) It is often a little difficult to get a good stand of carrots or beets, so mulch the soil surface over newly seeded rows by covering with old burlap bags or cloth strips, and sprinkle lightly with water every one to three days. Thin the beets and turnips to one plant every 3 inches, carrots to every 2 inches, and collard to every 12 inches. Turnips and beets mature rather quickly, in forty to fifty-five days; collard takes sixty days; and carrots require about seventy-five.

SWEET CORN

Few foods in the home garden can equal the taste of freshly picked sweet corn. And few are so widely grown. Corn is high in vitamin B-6 and potassium and, being a grain, will be a top source of selenium if grown properly. Though corn grows best at 60°F to 75°F, its full range for growth is 50°F to 95°F. The spring crop should be planted between the average freeze-free date and six weeks afterward; the fall crop should be planted twelve to fourteen weeks before the average fall freeze date.

Hilling

Corn needs "hilling," which is mounding soil around the stalks from each side to keep the plants from blowing over during thunderstorms. It is much easier to hill corn where there is 18 to 24 inches between rows. This is easily done where beds are 36 inches wide; double rows of corn can be planted with 18 inches between rows and 10 inches between plants within a row. (See Appendix E for spacing on 36-inch-wide beds.) But double rows in a 24-inch bed would make it difficult to maneuver the soil for hilling; if that's the width of your bed, then it's better to use a single row, with the plants spaced 6 inches apart.

Leave Suckers

Corn has a bothersome habit of growing extra, miniature stalks arising from the base of the plant. It is a big temptation to remove them, but don't. Scientific studies show this practice not only wastes your time but might injure the corn plant. You may want to make your own studies to see if this holds true in your food plot. Some varieties are much worse at suckering than others, especially the Golden Bantam and Country Gentleman, open-pollinated varieties.

Block Plantings Necessary

Don't plant just a single row of corn or two rows side-by-side if you want corn to eat. Those methods lead to poorly pollinated ears, which will not fill out properly. Corn is cross-pollinated as wind blows the pollen about, so adjacent rows pollinate each other. So be sure to plant a block of three or four rows parallel and adjacent to each other at any single planting.

Succession Planting

If four rows of corn all the way through your garden are too much at one planting, then don't plant the full length of the bed. Plant four rows side-by-side, but plant only a portion of each row. For example, let's say your garden planning shows you need 20 linear feet of corn coming off the same week and your beds are 20 feet long. Mark off 5 feet on four rows alongside each other and plant those. Then, ten to fourteen days later, mark off the next 5 feet of those rows and plant another 5 feet.

Varieties

Try Merit, Golden Cross, Bantam, and Aristogold Bantam.

CUCUMBER, PEPPER, SQUASH

All these are heat-loving, growing best from 60°F to 90°F, with an optimal temperature of 65°F to 75°F. All are planted about a week after the average spring freeze-free date.

Cucumber

Cucumber is high in magnesium, potassium, and folacin. Cucumber in a small garden needs a trellis so the vines can be trained up rather than grow outward. The trellis should be installed first, and then a single row should be planted per 24-inch bed alongside the trellis several inches out. (See Chapter 13 for our advice on trellises.) The proper spacing between plants is 12 inches, but for insurance plant two seeds every 6 inches and later thin back the plants. Cover the seeds about half an inch deep with soil or compost. Emergence occurs in about a week.

Cucumber is quick to bear, needing only about two months, and bears for quite a long while (one month). For a continuous supply, make a second planting three to four weeks after the first.

Fresh cucumbers are so good to eat it seems a pity to pickle them, but some folks want to. They should plant a "pickling" type instead of a "slicing" (fresh use) type of cucumber. Slicing types, while regularly cut to serve on a salad plate or in a tossed salad, can be eaten whole. The Straight 8 variety is common in supermarkets. The Poinsett is a popular slicing cucumber. The hybrid variety, Sweet Salad, is said to be top quality. Don't overlook the Lemon variety. It is shaped like a lemon and looks like a lemon, but it is one of the tastiest cucumbers you will find. It's our favorite. Look at your seed catalog for variety descriptions or check your local nursery.

Sweet Pepper

There is sweet, or bell, pepper; and there is hot, or chili, pepper. The chili pepper is really a spice used as a condiment because it is so hot that a little goes a long way. But bell peppers, especially when red ripe, are a wonderfully sweet vegetable that can be eaten in quantity. This is the type we're talking about. It is extremely high in vitamins C, A, and B-6.

Pepper is a heat-loving plant, but you can start it indoors eight weeks before the outdoor planting date and get a harvest much sooner. Space the peppers 12 inches apart in the row. Pepper and squash are so widely spaced in the row that you don't need many plants, so it is wise to grow transplants rather than direct-seed.

Pepper requires about seventy-five days to mature to the green stage and perhaps another two weeks to progress to the red, ripe stage. Instead of harvesting the green (unripe) peppers, leave them on the stalk to ripen to a full red. The red ripe bells are sweet and far richer in vitamin content. If you pick the peppers as they mature to the red, ripe stage, the plants will continue to bear for up to eight weeks.

Squash

If grown properly, squash is rich in calcium, magnesium, potassium, zinc, vitamin A, vitamin B-6, and folacin. Plant squash in one row per 24-inch bed. Space the plants 36 inches apart. Plant three seeds in each hole, then thin later to one plant. Vine squash, such as Hubbard, may be planted the same as bush squash if you provide a trellis. If there's no trellis, space rows of vine squash 6 to 7 feet apart. The wide spacing between plants helps control the pesty squash bug by allowing you easy access for hand-picking.

Summer Squash

This type is the highest in calcium, magnesium, and zinc. It includes varieties such as Yellow Crookneck (also called Yellow Straightneck) and Zucchini. These must be harvested and eaten before the seeds ripen or else the rinds harden. They require fifty to sixty days to mature for harvest.

Winter Squash

This type is the highest in vitamins A and C. It includes varieties such as Hubbard, Butternut, and Acorn. These are planted the same time as the summer squash but require eighty-five to a hundred days to mature and are not harvested until the rind hardens. This means they come off late in the season and have a hard skin resistant to bruising. This makes them a good variety to store in a cool place for winter eating.

LETTUCE

Looseleaf lettuce is one of the most nutritious foods you can grow. It is particularly rich in calcium, magnesium, potassium, iron, zinc, folacin, and vitamins C, A, and B-6.

Lettuce is a cool-season crop. It is generally planted from six weeks before the average spring frost-free date to two weeks after. This is about the same time other cool-season crops are planted, such as cabbage, kohlrabi, and turnip. The suitable growing temperature ranges from 45°F to 75°F, similar to green peas and potatoes, with 60°F to 65°F the optimum.

Small varieties like Bibb and Buttercrunch are best planted in four rows per bed with a final spacing of 6 inches between plants. Large varieties like Romaine are best spaced in two rows per bed with a final spacing of 12 inches between plants. If you use transplants, set the plants at the final spacing. But in our experience, it is easier and more practical to direct seed, then make several thinnings to get to the final spacing. (For details on thinning, see Chapter 8.)

Varieties

The only way to get a really nutritious salad lettuce is to use green looseleaf lettuce, not the anemic, bleached-out head lettuce, which is low in nutrition. Some of the best varieties of looseleaf lettuce for the home garden are Bibb, Buttercrunch, and Romaine. Bibb and Romaine are especially tasty and nutritious. Bibb is rarely found in the supermarket.

ONIONS

If you grow onions, you'll need to know the difference between green onions and bulb onions.

Green vs. Bulb Onions

Green onions are small immature onions (scallions), ready to eat sixty-three to seventy-seven days after planting. Any onion eaten when small can be called a green onion, which is mainly used in salads. Harvest begins when the stem of the onion, just under the soil surface, begins to swell. This harvest can continue for many weeks.

Bulb onions are the familiar large onions, 2 to 4 inches in diameter, used largely in cooking. They require 150 days to mature. In their early stages of growth, bulb onions can also be used as green onions by simply thinning the stand and eating the thinnings, especially the green top, which is incredibly high in vitamin A.

Planting and Harvesting

Onions for bulbs should be planted six to eight weeks before the average spring freeze-free date. The most common and least expensive way is to plant the seed. Onions may also be planted by onion transplants grown from seed in a greenhouse. That gives you a slightly quicker harvest.

In the home food plot, seven rows of onions can be planted in a bed 24 inches wide. The final spacing between onions in the rows should be 3 inches. With seeds, try to sow one every quarter-inch or four every inch, and thin them several times to arrive at the final spacing. (See Chapter 8 for details on thinning.) It is better to plant too thickly and to thin rather than have skips in the rows. With transplants, just plant them at the final spacing.

You can begin harvesting "baby" onions as scallions within nine to eleven weeks after planting by thinning and eating the thinnings. You can grow scallions by planting green bunching onions anytime during the growing season right up to the fall freeze date. Succession planting of green bunching onions about thirty days apart will keep you in green onions all season.

Varieties

In middle and southern latitudes, good varieties for bulbs are Yellow Sweet Spanish and White Sweet Spanish. For bulbs in northern latitudes, try Southport White Globe and Early Harvest. For scallions, try Southport White Globe, Evergreen Long White Bunching, and Crystal White Wax Bermuda. A good source of green onion varieties is the Stokes Seeds catalog. (See Appendix B.)

GREEN PEAS

The green pea, sometimes called the English pea, is unlike the Southern pea, which was examined earlier this chapter under the "Dry Beans and Peas" heading. The green pea is a cool-season plant planted very early in the spring. Both kinds of peas have a place in your garden. Both are high in magnesium, zinc, and iron. (Green peas are particularly high in iron.)

Spacing

Peas do well in double rows in beds 24 inches wide, with plants spaced 2 inches apart in the row. There are tall varieties and short varieties. The tall ones need a trellis for support. A half-height vertical wire trellis (24 to 30 inches tall) works well and can be held in place by driving stakes into the ground.

Planting Considerations

Green peas need to be planted and brought to maturity under cool conditions. They will grow when the temperature is 45°F to 75°F but for best growth prefer 60°F to 65°F. Peas require two to three months to mature, depending on the variety and the weather.

Pea-planting time lasts from eight to two weeks before the spring freeze-free date. At a soil temperature of 50°F, fourteen days are required for emergence; at 59°F, nine days; and at 77°F, six days. No germination occurs when the soil temperature is much over 86°F. Likewise, if you try to start your crop at the earliest planting date, you might find the soil too cold for germination.

One way to decide when to plant is to use a soil thermometer and take the soil temperature every morning. Continually compute three-day averages. (Add the temperatures of the three most recent days, then divide by three.) Try seeding when the average three-day soil temperature at 2 inches deep is 60°F or above. This should give you germination and emergence in about a week. To aid this process you can do the following:

- Pre-germinate the seeds. (Use the sprouting techniques explained in Chapter 3.) Plant the sprouted pea seeds when they have tiny sprouts about a quarter-inch long.
- Plant your seeds 1 to 1.5 inches deep.

- Keep your row of seeded peas warm. If days are sunny, keep mulch off your soil so it can absorb as much solar energy as possible. At night, insulate the soil or it will lose its warmth. To do this, lay boards over the top of the rows in the late afternoon, and remove them the next morning if the day is sunny. If it's not sunny, just leave the boards on.
- Sow the seed thickly, about every half-inch, even though you need to end up with a plant every 2 inches. Some seedlings are less vigorous than others, and some don't even make it out of the ground; but if you plant thickly you can choose from the seedlings, making it more likely you'll get a good stand.
- Use row covers to cover the top of the bed. These can be floating row covers or tunnels of wire-supported plastic hoops. You could also try planting your row of seeds in a depression about 2 inches deep, then covering the top with a piece of clear plastic.

SUNCHOKE (JERUSALEM ARTICHOKE)

This is an unusual food crop. It is an ornamental you can eat. It makes huge yields, and the white tubers are delicious eaten raw. It is high in iron and potassium. The sunchoke plant is actually a sunflower (Helianthus tuberosum) that is covered with lovely yellow flowers during the summer. As autumn sets in and your other produce is killed by cold, the sunchoke provides a rich harvest of food. Under each sunchoke plant you will find a nest of white tubers waiting to be dug up, washed, and taken to the kitchen. Even in cold regions, if you mulch the surface you can just leave the tubers in the ground and harvest them as needed. The mulch insulates them from freezing. Or they can be dug up and stored in the refrigerator or root cellar. Just be sure they're kept moist so they won't shrivel.

Cultural Methods

Sunchokes should be planted from four weeks before to four weeks after the spring freeze-free date or from the fall freeze date to four weeks after. Sunchokes planted in the fall will be ready to harvest the next summer, giving you a jump on the year's harvest. Use one row per 24-inch bed. Plant the sunchokes 12 inches apart in the row and 4 inches deep. Since these plantings stay in for years, plant them on one side of your garden. The sunchoke comes back year after year from tubers formed the year before. In fact, it is best to harvest all the tubers each year, then replant some of the best tubers for next year's crop. If you fail to harvest all the tubers, the ones you leave will send up shoots so crowded that only small tubers will result.

Varieties and Sources

Sunchoke is a specialty item, and not all seed houses carry them. The best variety we know is Stampede, which bears a very large tuber. It is available from Johnny's Selected Seeds. (See Appendix B for sources.)

Yields

Sunchokes have been suggested for use in fuel alcohol production because of their ultrahigh yields. You can get 50 to 60 pounds of sunchokes from a 20-foot row. In addition, the large amount of stalks produced are a valuable source of compost and mulch material.

TOMATO

The favorite of home food growers, tomatoes grown properly are high in vitamin C, vitamin A, magnesium, and copper.

Adaptation

The tomato is a tropical and grows as a perennial in frost-free areas and in greenhouses. In other areas, it grows as an annual. It originated in South America (Peru or Ecuador) and likes warm weather. Fruit will not form unless the daily temperature reaches 59°F or higher. But tomatoes grow poorly in the summer in very hot places such as Phoenix, where daily temperatures can reach 120°F. In such hot-summer areas, fall and winter might work with tomatoes. Temperatures for best growth and quality are 65°F to 85°F, with the optimal range at 70°F to 75°F.

Spacing

Use 24-inch beds with 16-inch walkways, and space your plants 3 feet apart in the row. That gives you just the right space per plant. Avoid double rows of tomatoes where you have access to only one side of the cage. Without full access, you might grow lots of tomatoes but be unable to harvest them.

When to Plant

Tomatoes can be transplanted outdoors from the spring freeze-free date to eight weeks after. If the odds fall your way, tomatoes transplanted outdoors on the freeze-free date will do well, and you will end up with a nice early crop. But that might not happen. Instead, you might lose your plants to a late freeze. If you plant on the freeze-free date, make sure you have on hand enough buckets to cover your plants in case a freeze is predicted; or place hotkaps over your transplants when setting them outdoors; or when you set each plant, cover it with an empty 3-quart coffee can with the plastic lid on top and the bottom cut out. If you do not protect your tomato plants, then wait until three weeks after the freeze-free date to set your plants outdoors. By that time, chances of damage from cold are almost nil.

Varieties

There are dozens of varieties, and you might need to ask knowledgeable local gardeners which varieties do best. You might want to test different varieties in your own garden, especially Early Girl, Fantastic, Sweet 100, and Celebrity.

Grow Your Own Transplants

Quite often you cannot get the varieties you want or they do not arrive at your local garden center at the right time. If that is the case, consider growing your own transplants. This means you must select the proper varieties, order the seeds far in advance (usually in January), and plant the seeds indoors about six weeks prior to your planned outdoor transplant date.

Wind Protection

Tomatoes are often set outdoors when spring winds are at their worst. At transplanting, place a cylindrical wind shield around each plant. A good wind shield is an empty 3-quart coffee can with the bottom cut out. (These cans are about 7 inches tall and 6 inches in diameter.) With the plastic top in place, your wind shield will double as a frost-protection device as well. Contact some office workers near you where lots of coffee is consumed, and ask them to save their empty cans for you.

To install the can-type wind shield, place it on the soil with the plant in its center and push it down into the soil about half an inch to anchor it. Then, to anchor the shield further, use a trowel to mound the soil 2 inches high on the outside. When the plant is well-established and wind has abated, gently remove the can and store until next season.

Wire Cage Wind Shield

This is even better than the coffee can, since it is a dual-purpose device that protects from the wind early in the season and then doubles as a vertical wire cage trellis. It also admits more light to the plant and removes the need for lifting cans off the plant.

To make the wire cage wind shield, first construct a wire cage. (See Chapter 13.) Then wrap asphalt-saturated felt (sometimes called tar felt builders paper) or thick plastic around the outside of the bottom 18 inches of the aboveground part of the cage and secure with twine. Place the wire cage on the soil surface with the plant in the center at transplanting and push the prongs into the ground. The felt or plastic may be removed from the cage after the plants are well-established.

Pollination Problems

During hot dry weather when humidity is low, tomatoes might not "set fruit" (a term that refers to the pollen grain's fertilizing the egg to create a tiny, marble-shaped fruit). You can tell by watching the fruiting clusters. When things are normal, each bloom will set fruit, and you can see a tiny green tomato where the bloom was. But if, instead of a tiny ball, you see a bare, knob-like projection, the bloom has not set fruit, natural abortion has occurred, and no tomato fruit will be produced. Why is that? Each bloom has a center stem with an ovary at the bottom. The top of the stem is called the stigma, which has a sticky substance on it that catches and holds the pollen from the stamen (the male part of the flower), which is also inside the flower. When the weather is hot and the humidity is low around the tomato flowers, the stigmas dry out, so there is no sticky substance to catch and trap the pollen grains.

One solution is to spray the stigmas with a hormone solution that fools them into thinking they have been fertilized by pollen grains, so they go ahead and set fruits. These fruits will be seedless but good to eat. However, you will find the application of the spray a chore, and it might not work.

A better solution is to increase the humidity around the flower clusters naturally by placing wire cages over your tomato plants. The cages soon are filled with foliage, which gives off water vapor. We have measured humidity with a hygrometer and have found it to be considerably more humid inside a cage filled with tomato foliage than outside the cage.

STRAWBERRIES

There is nothing that tastes better and is higher in vitamin C then fresh red-ripe strawberries.

What Strawberries Like

If you want lots of red-ripe strawberries as soon as possible after planting, then do the following:

- Build a well-drained soil high in organic matter and slightly acid (pH of 6.0 to 6.5).
- Keep the soil around the roots cool and moist at all times.
- Build and maintain a soil low in salts.
- Plant in early spring, from about four weeks before to four weeks after the spring freeze-free date—about the same time as cool-season vegetables like lettuce.
- Use adapted, ever-bearing varieties, such as Sweet California Giant, Selva, Tristar, and Tribute.
- Use close spacing, disbud for six weeks, and cut off runners the first year.

Beds for Strawberries

You can use several bed systems, but the two best are the narrow, 12-inch, 2-row bed and the wide, 24-inch, 4-row bed. (See Figure 16.1.) In both systems, plants are spaced 5 to 6 inches apart in a staggered pattern. A narrow bed 10 feet long will hold 40 plants, and a wide bed the same length accommodates 80 plants.

Soil Preparation

Strawberries need permanent beds made with a special raised-bed soil mix. (See Chapter 5.) Since you can plant so many plants in a small amount of space, it's worth doing a good job of soil building.

Your soil might not need phosphorus, but it is so important to flowering and fruiting that it is a good idea to apply a little, just in

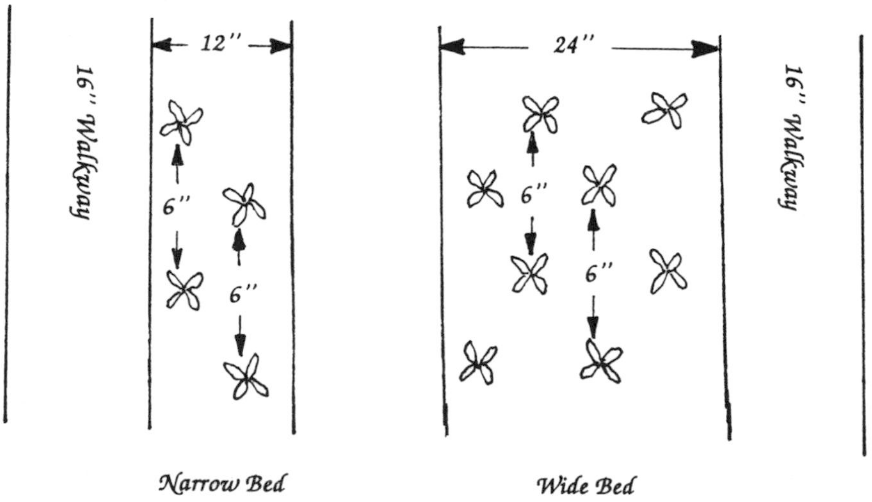

Figure 16.1 Strawberries should be planted 5 to 6 inches apart in a staggered pattern. A narrow bed 10 feet long will hold forty plants; a wide bed the same length will hold eighty.

case. Phosphorus does not move far from where you place it, so it should be placed in the bottom of the planting hole, not worked into the surface. Colloidal phosphate is probably the best, but you can also use superphosphate. Whichever, apply 0.1 to 0.2 pound per 10 square feet, which figures out to about half a teaspoonful of phosphate fertilizer per plant.

After you've worked in the raised-bed soil mix, wet the bed and let it dry a little, stretch garden lines on top of the bed to mark rows, then use a bulb planter to remove a core of soil every 6 inches where a plant is to be set. Dig each hole 2 inches deeper than the plant needs, drop the half a teaspoonful of phosphate fertilizer in the bottom of each hole, cover with 2 inches of soil, then set the plant.

After plants are set, place a drip line or a soaker hose between each two rows of plants, then cover the soil between the plants with a 2-inch layer of mulch such as straw. In warm weather, irrigate every two days for sandy soil and twice weekly for other soils.

Disbudding

When flowers appear, pinch all of them off for six weeks; when runners appear, cut all of them off for an entire year. That forces growth into the mother plant for berries.

17. *What You're Going to Need*

ONLY a few basic tools, supplies, and pieces of equipment are necessary to grow PowerCharged food. We have listed these in what we feel is their order of importance. The essentials are listed under "Basic Equipment and Supplies." When you start to collect these tools and supplies, start from the top and work your way down.

After you have collected the basics and have the money to invest, you can buy another set of items to make food growing easier and more efficient. We have listed these items in descending order of importance under "Helpful Equipment."

BASIC EQUIPMENT AND SUPPLIES

These are the absolute essentials for growing your own PowerCharged food and efficiently working your land.

Sprouting Kit

This is the most important of all Super Nutrition food-growing equipment, because it will return your family more outstanding nutrition for the least cost and effort. A good kit will make it easy to keep a continuous supply of fresh sprouts coming. It consists of sprouting jars, lids, netting, and a rack to hold the jars. (For sources of the sprouting kit, see Appendix A.)

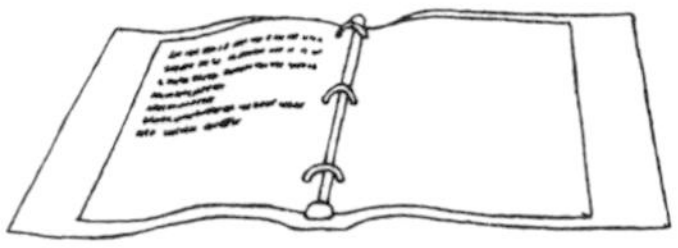

Notebook

Looseleaf Notebook

A good-quality three-ring notebook (1-inch rings) with dividers and ruled paper will enable you to plan, store information, and keep a simple diary of your food-growing activities. This notebook provides a quick and ready reference to your outdoor garden. It will show your planting plan, your seed inventory, and other valuable records.

Sprayer (For Foliar Feeding)

To PowerCharge your outdoor food crops fully, you will need to spray liquid fertilizer on the leaves of your plants. (See "Foliar Feeding With Seaweed" in Chapter 12.) This will let you be certain your plants have the eleven trace elements they need, as well as the six trace elements needed by humans but not by plants.

Get a sprayer with a capacity of one to two gallons. A two-gallon, pump-up, compression-type sprayer is best, but for starting out you can even use an inexpensive, lever-operated, one-quart sprayer. If Roundup or some other herbicide is to be applied, use a separate sprayer, one from which you spray nothing else.

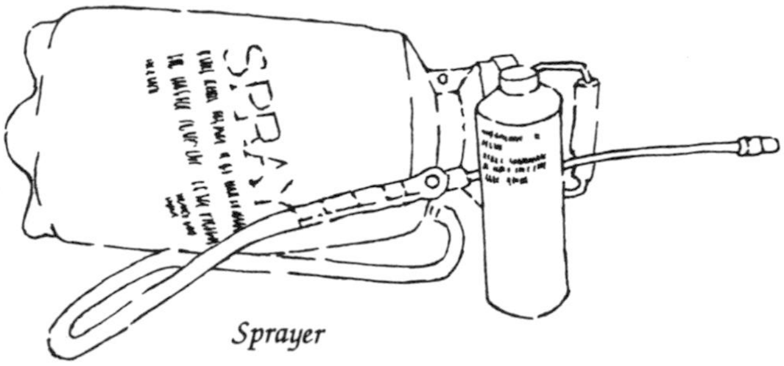

Sprayer

Foliar Feed Concentrate

This is for use with the just-described sprayer to PowerCharge fully the food you grow. Liquid seaweed is good but has far too much sodium and chloride to be ideal. A new, improved foliar feed product being developed and tested promises to be far superior to seaweed. (For information, write to the authors at the address given at the end of the book's Conclusion.)

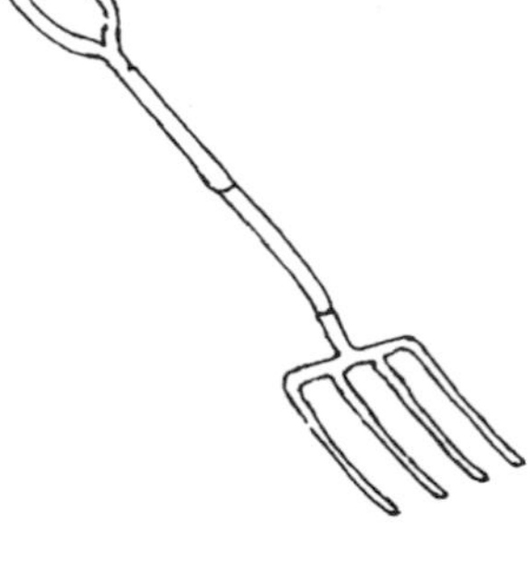

Spading fork

Spading Fork (Short Handled)

This important basic tool replaces the rototiller for small plots. It is somewhat similar to the pitchfork, except the spading fork's four tines are very thick and sturdy and 10 inches long. It is used for loosening the soil (spading) to prepare beds and mix in soil charging materials. Avoid the long-handled type, which allows too much leverage that may bend or break the fork.

Garden Rake

This is used for leveling beds after spading, for raking off the surface of beds just before planting, and for raking up debris in a general cleanup. This tool has fourteen teeth 2 inches long and rakes a swath 14 inches wide.

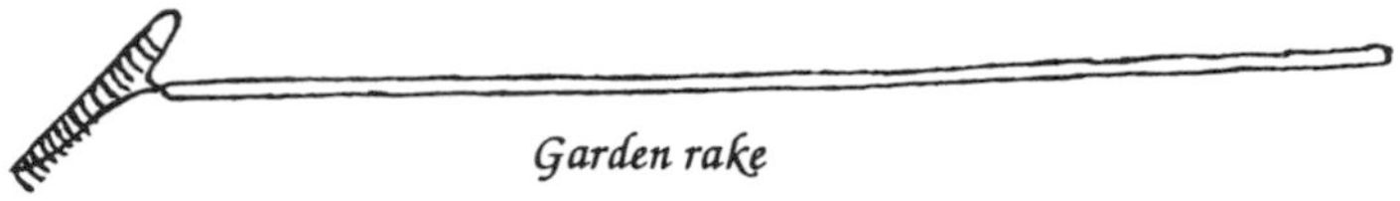

Garden rake

Nursery Hoe

This is used for weed control (by cutting off weeds at the soil surface) and for making planting trenches. The nursery hoe has a wide, slim blade about 7 inches long and 2 inches wide, which enables it to get between plants to remove weeds. Avoid the short, stubby field hoe, which has a 4-inch square blade. If you can't find the nursery hoe locally, look in mail-order catalogs under "hoe" or "rake."

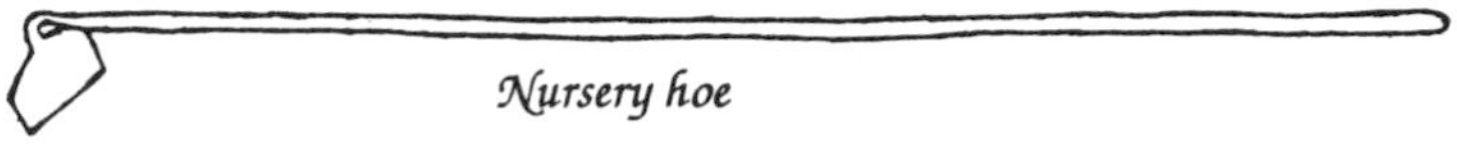

Nursery hoe

Twine

Twine is simply a tiny but very strong rope, about a sixteenth of an inch thick and made of nylon, cotton, jute, or sisal. Use it to lace up the wood-and-twine trellis, to stretch around the four corners of your garden plot, to mark the centerlines of beds, and for a dozen and one other uses. Your best buy is a roll of sisal or jute twine large enough to last a lifetime. For a 500-foot roll of nylon twine, you might pay as much as you would for a 2,500-foot roll of jute or sisal twine.

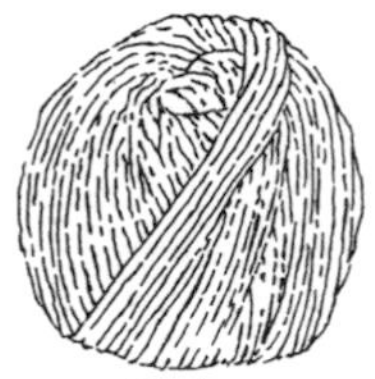

Twine

Wood Preservative

This is a thin, paint-like liquid found in the paint department of stores. It is used to prevent wooden posts and stakes from rotting when they come in contact with soil. The best compound is Green Copper Napthanate, available in one-gallon cans.

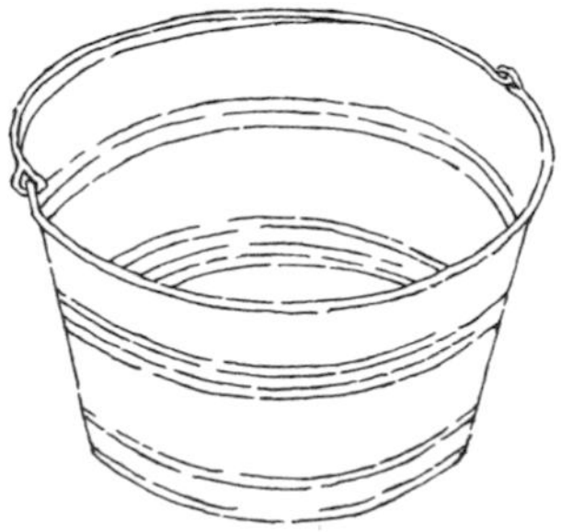

Bucket

Bucket (Metal, Four-Gallon)

This durable, sturdy bucket is good for transporting tools, compost, soil, and food you have just harvested. You really need two of these buckets, with one reserved for "clean" work like tool transport or harvesting.

Spikes (Steel, 12 Inches)

Use these king-size nails for staking off your food plot and marking the centerlines of beds. Get two spikes per bed.

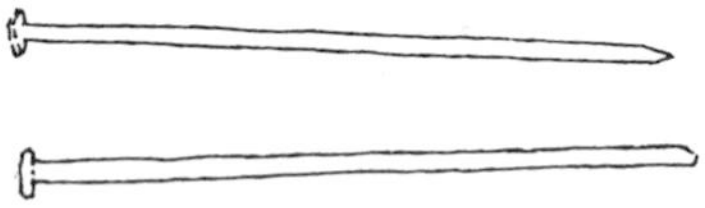

Spikes

Lumber (For Wood-and-Twine Trellis)

See Chapter 13 for the amount and type of lumber you'll need to get.

File

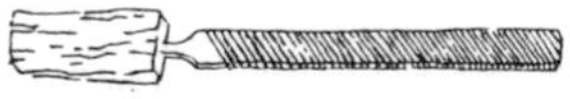

File

Use a king-size fingernail file to sharpen hoes and other tools. Get a mill file 10 inches long.

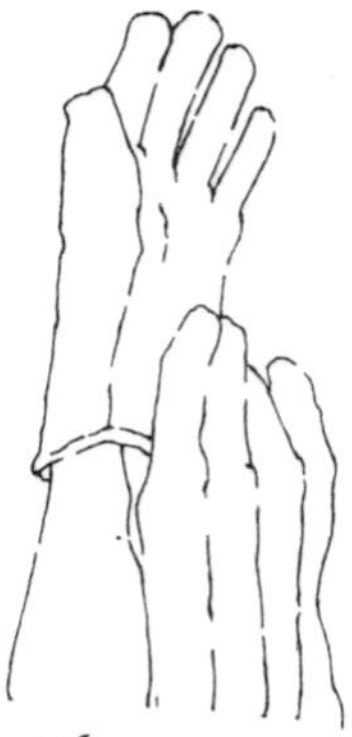

Gloves

Gloves

Wear these to protect your hands when doing heavy work. We prefer cloth gloves, because they are lightweight and flexible; but for really heavy work, you may need leather gloves.

Welded Wire (1-Inch by 2-Inch Mesh)

Use this when making the circular wire compost bin. (See Chapter 10.) Get your local hardware store to cut off 14 feet of the 24-inch-wide wire mesh. Put on your gloves, form the mesh into a circle, fasten the ends together securely, and place it in a corner of your yard to start your compost pile.

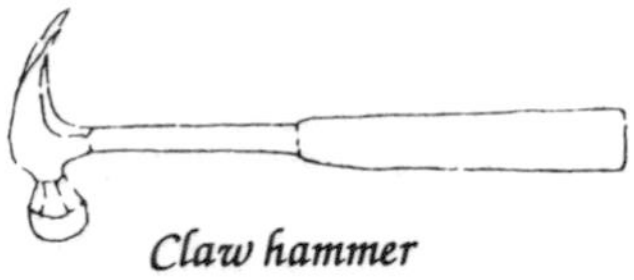

Claw hammer

Claw Hammer

No household should be without this basic hand tool. Use it to drive nails into wooden boards. Use the claw part of the hammer to pull nails out. The least expensive hammer you can find will probably fit your needs. Be sure it is standard size, with a handle about 10 inches long and a nail-driving head about 1 inch in diameter.

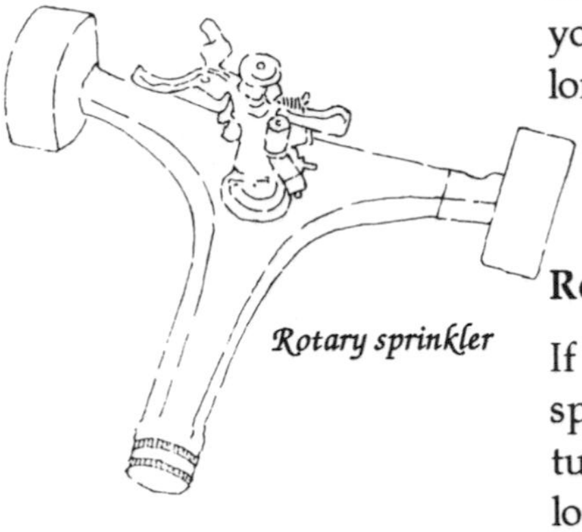

Rotary sprinkler

Rotary Sprinkler (Impact)

If rain has not fallen for seven days, you will need to irrigate. The sprinkler you need will rotate in a circle with audible impulses as it turns and sits on a metal base. Be sure it is all metal, has pins that allow adjusting the water to a quarter-circle arc, and has a flap or other device you can adjust to determine how far the water is thrown. The Rainbird brand is one of the best.

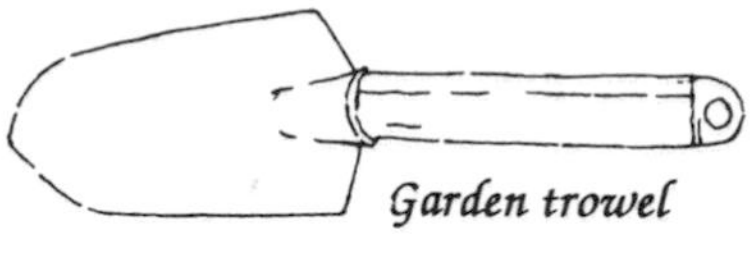

Garden trowel

Garden Trowel

This is really a miniature shovel, with a short, 6-inch handle. The trowel is useful for moving small amounts of soil around when transplanting.

Yardstick

A slim ruler 36 inches long by three-sixteenths of an inch thick is useful for measuring short distances and for making planting trenches for small seeds. Hardware stores usually provide yardsticks for free.

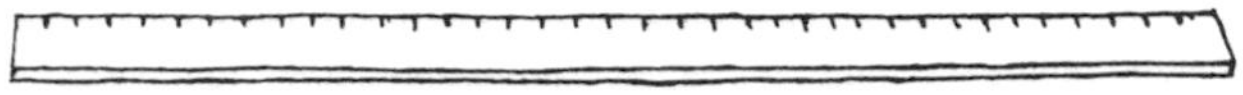

Yardstick

Sliding Hoe

This cleverly designed hoe is moved back and forth across the soil surface to shave off weeds without digging into the soil. It is especially good for beginning growers who cannot afford to buy the considerable amount of organic surface mulch needed to control weeds. The sliding hoe is not suitable for very rocky soil, since this makes it difficult or impossible for the blade to move smoothly along the soil surface. It is sometimes called a "hula" hoe or a swing-head hoe.

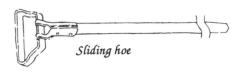

Sliding hoe

HELPFUL EQUIPMENT

Beyond the basic equipment is some helpful equipment, which are items that are not necessary but make gardening more efficient and easy.

Bulb Planter

This is used for extracting a round plug of soil out of a bed to make a perfect planting hole for tomato plants or other transplants.

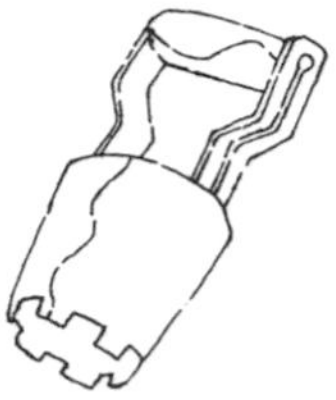

Bulb planter

Soil Sieve

When you make the covering mix (described in Chapter 8), you will need to get the lumps out of the ingredients you're mixing. Use a soil sieve for this purpose. It is not available in stores, so you'll have to make it yourself or hire a handyman to do so. It's easy to build. It's just a wooden frame of one-by-four lumber with a piece of quarter-inch mesh hardware cloth nailed on one side.

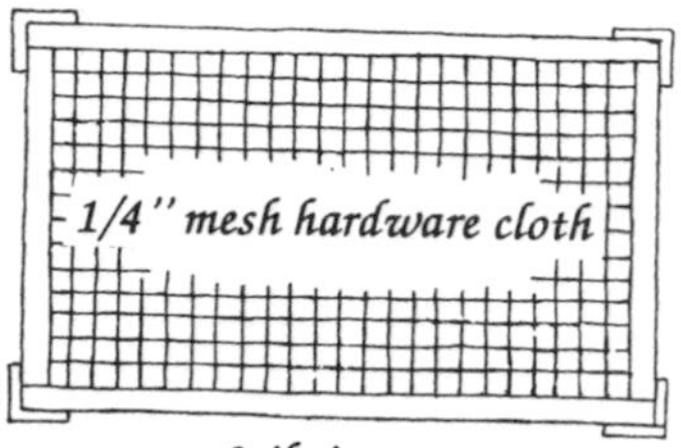

Soil sieve

Pruning Shears

These are heavy-duty scissors with a stout cutting blade only 2 inches long. It is used for pruning small limbs, for food growing, and for cutting large, long stalks of old plants into smaller pieces so they will fit into your compost pile for recycling. Get a good-quality scissor-type that has one blade passing by the second blade, creating a

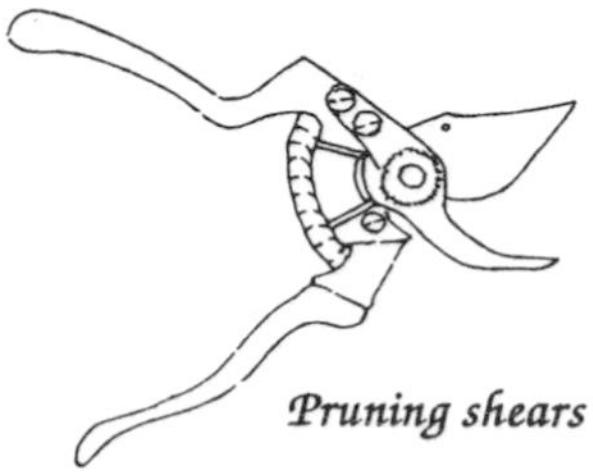

Pruning shears

shearing action. Avoid the type where the blade moves down against a flat plate. The best use for pruning shears is to cut tomato vines so they can be removed from the wood stake trellis or wire cage and be recycled.

Garden Reel

A garden reel keeps twine handy and untangled. This is another handy, build-it-yourself project. To construct, start with a short piece of one-by-four lumber (about 6 inches long), then use a saw and a chisel to make the depicted notches. When finished, wind 50 feet of strong twine on the reel. The attached twine is known as the line.

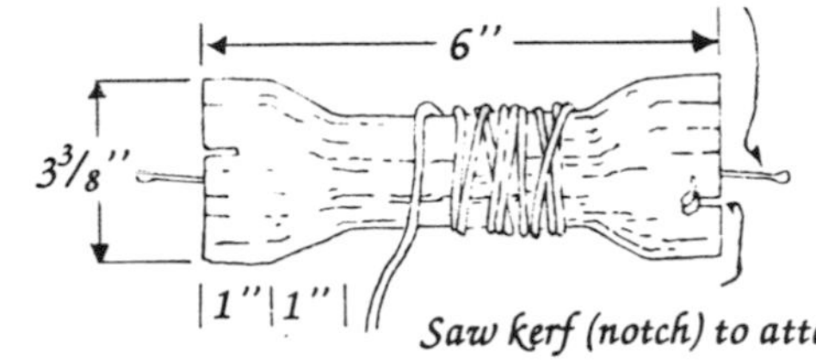

Hatchet

This is a combination tool for driving stakes into the ground. If the stake is made of wood, the hatchet blade can also sharpen it. Like the pruning shears, it, too, can be used to cut long stalks into smaller pieces so they will fit into the compost pile. The hatchet is a miniature, short-handled ax designed for light-duty cutting and chopping jobs.

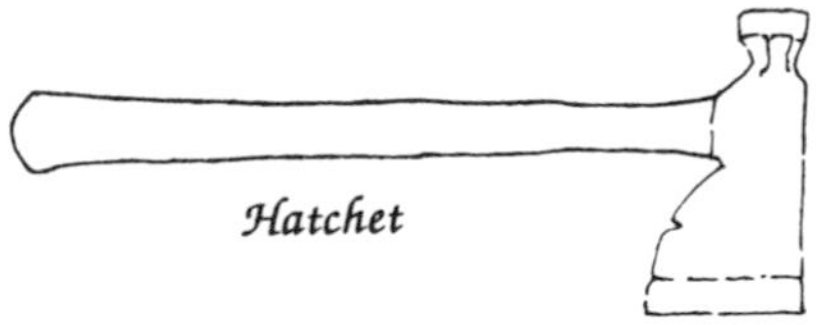
Hatchet

Square-Point Shovel

This is a shovel with a blade shaped like a dustpan—flat and wide at the bottom. It is useful for mixing soil with amendment on a flat, hard surface (such as a concrete slab) and is also useful for cleaning up.

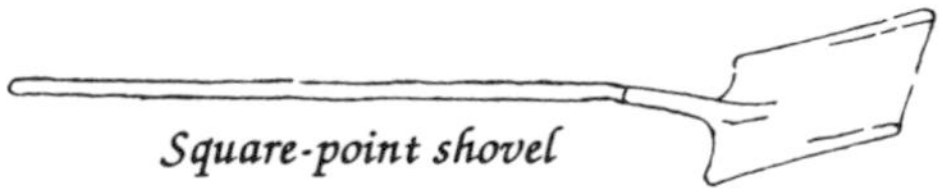
Square-point shovel

Wheelbarrow

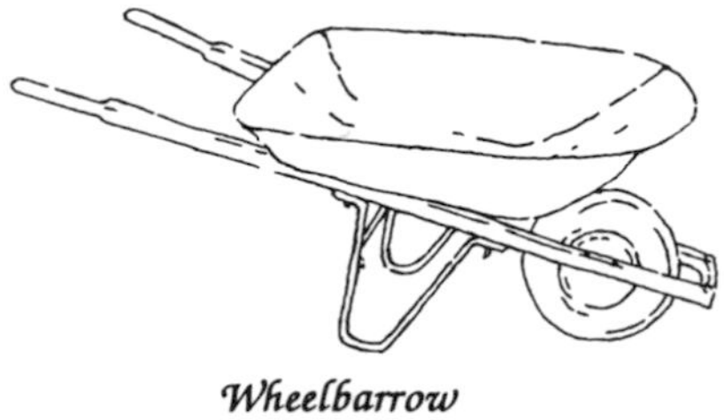
Wheelbarrow

This is useful during harvest and for transporting large amounts of soil or compost. It is also a good place for mixing small batches of soil with amendment, such as the seed covering mix, or for mixing small batches of concrete. It replaces buckets on big jobs. Get the type with hard rubber tires that are non-inflatable and puncture-proof.

Posthole Digger

This is for digging holes 6 to 24 inches deep, such as holes for setting posts for the stiff wire trellis.

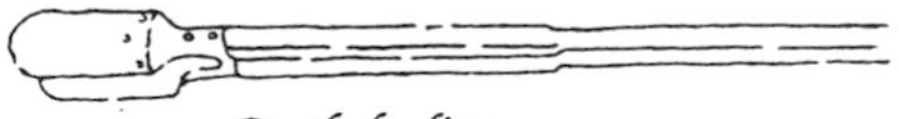

Posthole digger

Compost Shredder

We'd rather have this than a rototiller for the small outdoor garden because you can use a compost shredder many times during the year to make mulch. It also comes at a fraction of the cost of a good, standard-size, rear-tine tiller. One good small shredder is a 3-horsepower gasoline engine model called the Mighty Mac, available for about $600 from Amerind-Mackissic (P.O. Box 111, Parker Ford, Penn., 19457).

Vita Mix Machine

This rugged, heavy-duty blender is useful for natural living. It liquefies kitchen trimmings for quick breakdown in the compost pile. It converts surplus tomatoes into tomato sauce. It even grinds whole grains into flour, and it mixes and kneads the dough for baking whole-grain bread. (See Chapter 10 for details.)

Electric Fence

Dogs and gardens don't mix. An electric fence gives a painful but harmless jolt of electrical energy, which is very effective for keeping dogs out of planted areas. "Fido Fence" is one brand of electric fence usually available at feed stores in outlying areas, and it sells for about $50.

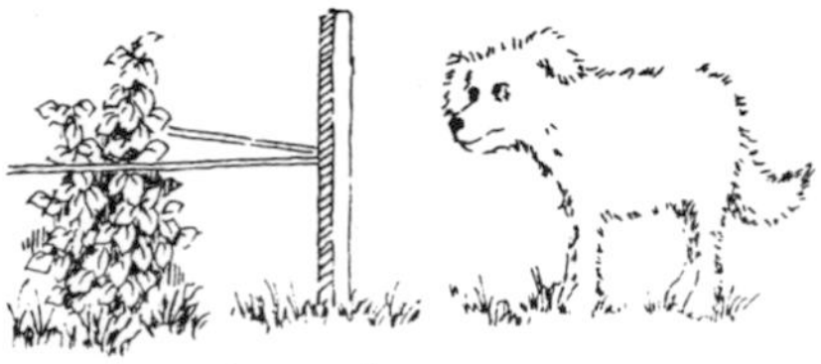

Electric fence

Metal-Cutting Snips

This can be used when cutting wire to make the soil sieve or compost sieve and when cutting sheet metal.

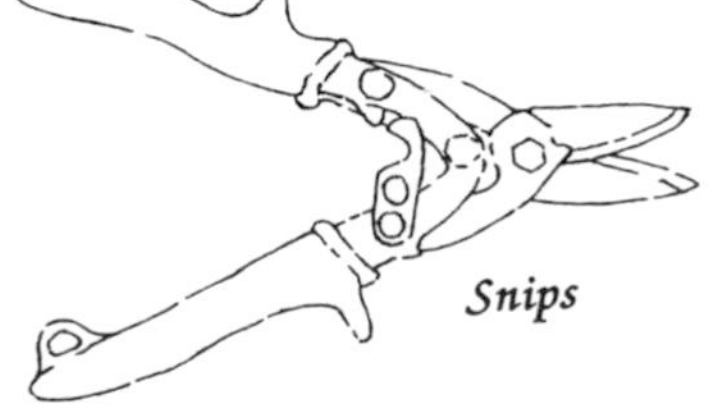

Snips

Motor Vehicle Adapted to Food Growing

The usual sedan is not well suited to the one-car family that wants to grow some of its own food from an outdoor garden. What you need is a vehicle that has a box-like shape for hauling lots of cargo, has a

Table 17.1

Costs of What You'll Need for Super Nutrition Gardening

(Based on a 20-Foot by 20-Foot Model Garden)

Basic Equipment and Tools

Sprouting Kit	$49
Looseleaf Notebook	3
Two-Gallon Sprayer	17
Spading Fork (Short-Handled)	25
Garden Rake	21
Nursery Hoe	22
Metal Bucket (Four Gallon)	5
12-Inch Steel Spikes (Set of 12)	6
Wood Preservative (One Quart)	5
Twine (300 Feet)	5
Lumber (for Wood and String Trellis)	6
Mill File (10 Inches)	5
Gloves	5
Welded Wire (14 Feet of 1- by 2-Inch Mesh)	20
Claw Hammer	15
Garden Trowel	2
Yardstick	0
Rotary Sprinkler (Impact)	25
Sliding Hoe	12
Subtotal	$248

Basic Supplies

Plants and Seed	$20
Organic Soil Amendment (2-Inch Layer)	40*
Mulch (Lawn Clippings in Vicinity)	0
6-Inch to 7-Inch Tomato Stakes (Set of 4)	8
Organic Fertilizer (Cottonseed Meal, 50 Pounds)	10
Soil Test	12
Soil Balancing Service	15
Minerals for Soil Balancing	10
Foliar Feed Concentrate	10
Subtotal	$125

* = A 3-inch layer, costing about $60, would work better, but the 2-inch layer is the basic amount needed.

Helpful But Not Required Equipment, Tools, and Supplies

Bulb Planter	$3
Soil Sieve	5
Garden Reel	1
Pruning Shears	25
Hatchet	20
Shovel (Square-Point)	21
Garden Wheelbarrow	30
Posthole Digger	22
Electric Fence	(if circumstances warrant)
Compost Shredder	(if circumstances warrant)
Rototiller	(if circumstances warrant)
Motor Vehicle	(if circumstances warrant)
Metal-Cutting Snips	15
Moisture Probe	20
Wood Preservative (One Gallon)	13
Subtotal	$175

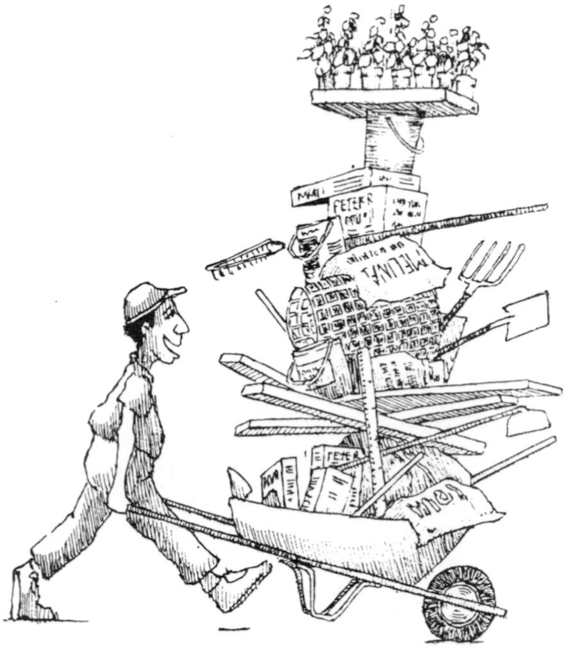

rear door that opens down to floor level, has enough power but is not so big and powerful that it is a gas hog, and can be used for many family activities. This is the mini-van.

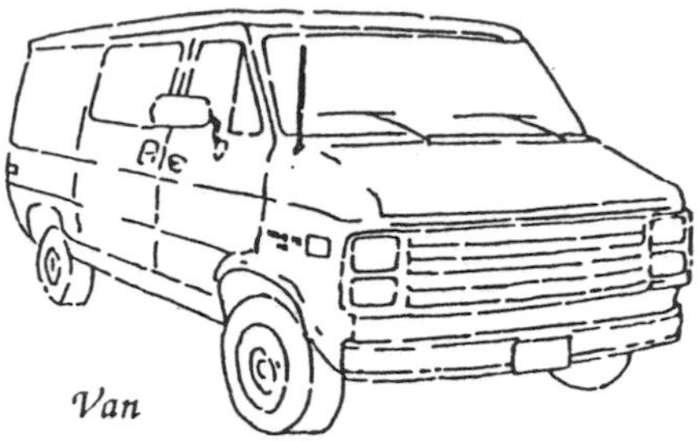

Van

The two-car family can get by fine with an ordinary sedan if it has a pickup truck to go with it. The pickup truck is great because it is a large box on wheels with the top open, so you can go to a commercial composting yard, order a yard of compost, and have them drive up with a big power loader and drop it all into your truck from the top. Because the bed of the truck is separated from the cab, you can keep the bed messy without fouling your seats or clothes. Your best bet is a mini-pickup such as the Chevy, Ford, or Dodge. Avoid the Japanese imports, since they lack the vertical wells that enable you to install sideboards on your mini-pickup for hauling large amounts of light, fluffy, organic materials.

Rototiller

This is for the outdoor food-growing plot, but in most cases it may be better to rent than to buy. The exceptions are when people have very large gardens or live too far away from a town where tillers can be rented. If you do buy, be sure to get a good-quality tiller that cuts a swath 18 inches wide and has its tines at the rear. Avoid the cheaper types, with the engine mounted above the tines (teeth). New machines sell for $1,500 to $2,000—a big investment, unless you have a huge garden. Look around for a good used tiller or rent one. A compost shredder is probably a better investment.

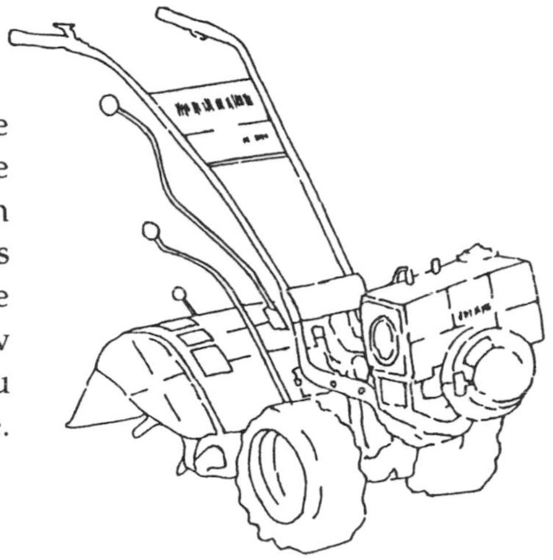

Rototiller

Moisture Probe

This long slender steel rod lets you know how deeply you irrigated your plants.

QUALITY

There is no substitute for well-designed and well-built equipment and high-quality supplies. If properly cared for, well-built equipment will last a lifetime and be a one-time cost.

Be wary of plastic tools (except sprayers). Nothing lasts like steel. For tools with handles, check to see if the handle can be replaced. Beware of cheap imports that can't be repaired. Two good brands are Ace and True Temper.

SOURCES OF TOOLS

Check your local hardware stores first and write down their prices. Be sure the tools meet our stated specs. Compare prices. Then look for mail-order sources. (See Appendix A.) Of all these, we prefer Mellingers. You can start gathering equipment during winter when it's too cold to do any gardening outdoors.

You may be able to shop around and find better buys. You can try to find good used tools at garage sales, but get there early. Good tools are snapped up quickly.

COSTS

How much does all the equipment and tools and supplies cost the beginning gardener? Table 17.1 shows current prices. Keep in mind that equipment and tools are one-time, non-recurring costs, while supplies have to be replenished periodically.

For basic equipment, tools, and supplies, the cost is about $373. Of course, that number will vary from state to state and is subject to inflation. Plus, a person who purchases the items that are helpful but not required would end up paying more.

Conclusion

A chain is only as strong as its weakest link. In today's world, the quality of the food you eat is likely to be the weakest link in the chain of health. Your long-term health will be only as good as the quality of the food you eat. Even if you're eating the right foods, if they are grown in nutrient-poor soil you are depriving yourself of a healthy diet.

You have seen why the nutritional quality of the food you buy in stores is substandard. Even food sold as organic can be low in essential minerals and vitamins. Our food is grown in soils that have been depleted of mineral nutrients for decades by erosion and nutrient uptake due to highly intensive commercial farming practices. These nutrients are not replaced by the billions of pounds of chemical salt fertilizers used every year.

While chemical fertilizers keep the yields high and make our food look big and beautiful, this food is deficient in the nutrition required for good long-term health. Some of the most key elements, such as calcium, magnesium, iron, copper, zinc, and selenium, are widely deficient or unavailable in our soils and, as a consequence, in our food. Huge vitamin losses also occur during the harvesting, processing, shipping, storing, and displaying of food. As a consequence, deficiencies of minerals and vitamins are widespread throughout our population. And supplements are not a lasting solution.

FOOD IS THE BEST SOURCE OF NUTRIENTS

Supplements are a temporary remedy and a poor substitute for high-quality food. In food, minerals and vitamins are found in organic compounds with enzymes and with other co-nutrients and have the highest biological value for your body. This means your body will make the greatest use of that mineral or vitamin. No supplement contains all the co-nutrients known to have important health-promoting and disease-preventing properties, such as phytochemicals and trace-element-containing enzymes. And none contain co-nutrients that aren't yet known to exist but are still needed.

To get the full function of the vitamin or mineral, you need all the co-nutrients working together. And beyond that, remember that highly concentrated forms of vitamins and minerals may overload your system and become waste products, which have to be eliminated from your body through the use of enzymes. The bottom line is that while supplements can be beneficial therapeutic agents, food is the best source of nutrients for long-term health. But not just any food. You need some high-quality, high-nutrition PowerCharged food in your diet for optimal health.

PowerCharged food is food that is grown in properly mineralized and balanced soil. It contains optimal amounts of all twenty-three mineral nutrients needed for human life and the highest vitamin content possible. The minerals and vitamins in PowerCharged food are in a form that offer the highest biological value to your body. These nutrients are put to maximum use in the enzymes, hormones, and other systems of your body to regenerate and detoxify the cells, give you energy, boost your immune system, and keep your whole body healthy and free of disease.

THE FOUNDATION IS THE SOIL

The foundation of *Super Nutrition Gardening* rests in the soil. The seven-step soil charging program taught you how to balance the soil to make an optimal amount of mineral nutrients available to your food plants and, thereby, boost their nutritional value. You learned how to provide optimal amounts of nitrogen to your food plants through slow-release natural sources. Then you learned how to ensure that your plants are getting optimal amounts of trace elements. Those methods, along with high levels of organic matter in the soil to hold nutrients and feed microbes, produce high-nutrition PowerCharged food.

PowerCharged methods also produce healthy plants, which resist insect and disease attack without pesticides. What small problems there are can be handled by simple, biologically sound methods without poison sprays. Modern agriculture, by ignoring the foundation of the soil, has created a crisis of increased dependence on chemicals, salt fertilizers, and poisonous sprays, leaving a legacy of pollution and depleted soil. Yet, the problems these quick-fix solutions are supposed to solve keep getting bigger. Soil erosion; the declining response to increased fertilizer use; the increased application of pesticides while more and more pests become resistant; the pollution of the soil and water; and finally, depleted food—all those are consequences of our abandonment of the soil.

A WAY OF LIVING

Super Nutrition Gardening is not just a way of growing food, it is a way of living. It is a way each of us can pay homage to the glorious Web of Life, from the lowliest microbe to the plants to the most magnificent creation of nature, our own human body. *Super Nutrition Gardening* is caring for the soil and the environment. It is being a good steward, not only of our own health, but of the entire Earth. It is a way each one of us can contribute as individuals to the healing of the planet, whose life-support systems are in jeopardy.

With all the attention over the alarming rate of disease in this country and the soaring costs of the health-care crisis, the answer to human health may be simply to eat fresh food grown in fertile soil that is mineralized, balanced, and rich in organic matter as laid out in this book.

Everyone interested in good health should grow some of their own food—and the more, the better. If you live in an apartment you can have a sprout garden right on your kitchen counter and seek out a source of food grown the PowerCharged way. Form a food co-op and hire a local grower to grow your food that way. If you have outdoor growing space, even a 20-foot by 20-foot food garden, you can grow an astonishing amount of super-nutrition, PowerCharged food to go along with your sprout garden.

Happy gardening, and may good health always be yours!

OFFER TO READERS

You have made a quantum leap toward saving your health and the Earth by buying this book. We congratulate you! If you would like to get on our mailing list to learn about new developments from our ongoing research program into the links between soil, food, and health, plus other startling discoveries in the new science of electroculture and subtle energy, just write us a postcard and say "Put me on your mailing list." Write to:

Dr. William Peavy
c/o Avery Publishing Group
120 Old Broadway
Garden City Park, New York 11040

Notes

Chapter One

1. Geoffrey H. Bourne, ed., *Impact of Nutrition on Health and Disease*, Vol. 59 of *World Review of Nutrition and Dietetics* (Basel, Switzerland: S. Karger, 1989), 29.

M.S. Chaney and M.L. Ross, *Nutrition* (New York: Houghton Mifflin Co., 1966), 435.

Stephen Davies, M.D., and Alan Stewart, M.D., *Nutritional Medicine* (New York: Avon Books, 1987), xviii.

Ivor E. Dreosti and Richard M. Smith, eds., *Neurobiology of the Trace Elements* (Clifton, NJ: Humana Press, 1983), 156.

Y.H. Hui, *Essentials of Nutrition and Diet Therapy* (Monterey, CA: Wadsworth Health Sciences Div., 1985), 83.

Z.A. Karcioglu, M.D., and R.M. Sarper, Ph.D., *Zinc and Copper in Medicine* (Springfield, IL: Charles C. Thomas Publishing, 1980), 229.

J.P. Mareschi, "Mineral and Trace Element Status: Problems and Solutions," *Medecine et Nutrition*, Vol. 25 (1989): 93–107.

Walter Mertz, ed., *Trace Elements in Human and Animal Nutrition*, Vol. 1, 5th ed. (New York: Academic Press, 1987) 304.

Richard A. Passwater, Ph.D., *Selenium as Food and Medicine* (New Canaan, CT: Keats Publishing, 1980), 9, 167–168.

Jean A. Pennington, Ph.D., R.D., *Dietary Nutrient Guide* (Wesport, CT: Avi Publishing Co., 1976), 42.

Marshall Phillips and Albert Baetz, eds., *Diet and Resistance to Disease*, Advances in Experimental Medicine and Biology, Vol. 135 (New York: Plenum Press, 1981), 107.

Ananda S. Prasad and Donald Oberleas, eds., *Trace Elements in Human Health and Disease*, Vol. 1 (New York: Academic Press, 1976), 16.

Bruno Quebedeaux and Frederick A. Bliss, eds., *Horticulture and Human Health: Contributions of Fruits and Vegetables* (Englewood Cliffs, NJ: Prentice-Hall, 1988), 15.

J.I. Rodale, et al., *The Complete Book of Minerals for Health* (Emmaus, PA: Rodale Books, 1976), 10, 91, 144.

H.E. Sauberlich, Ph.D., R.P. Dowdy, Ph.D., and J.H. Skala, Ph.D, *Laboratory Tests for the Assessment of Nutritional Status* (Boca Raton, FL: CRC Press, 1981), 4.

Maurice E. Shills, M.D., and Vernon R. Young, Ph.D., eds., *Modern Nutrition in Health and Disease* (Philadelphia: Lea & Febiger, 1988), 152, 194.

Eric J. Underwood, *Trace Elements in Human and Animal Nutrition* (New York: Academic Press, 1977), 327.

U.S. Department of Health and Human Services and U.S. Department of Agriculture, *Nutrition Monitoring in the United States*, a Progress Report From the Joint Nutrition Monitoring Evaluation Committee (Hyattsville, MD: USGPO, July 1986), 8–11.

U.S. Department of Health and Human Services and U.S. Department of Agriculture, *Nutrition Monitoring in the United States: an Update Report on Nutrition Monitoring*, 1989, xxxi.

Ronald R. Watson, Ph.D., ed., *Nutrition and Heart Disease*, Vol. II (Boca Raton, FL: CRC Press, 1987), 63–65.

Eleanor Whitney and Eva Hamilton, *Understanding Nutrition* (New York: West Publishing Co., 1984), 329, 417, 466–467.

Sue Williams, Ph.D., M.P.H., R.D., and Bonnie Worthington, Ph.D., R.D., *Nutrition Throughout the Life Cycle* (St. Louis: Times Mirror/Mosby College Publishing, 1988), 269, 423.

Eva Wilson, Katherine Fisher, and Mary Fuqua, *Principles of Nutrition* (New York: John Wiley & Sons, 1967), 162, 253, 434.

Myron Winick, M.D., *Nutrition in Health and Disease* (New York: John Wiley & Sons, 1980), 102.

Myron Winick, M.D., ed., *Nutrition in the 20th Century* (New York: John Wiley & Sons, 1984), 161.

2. Shills & Young, *Modern Nutrition in Health and Disease*, 271–288.

3. Stephen Seely, et al., *Diet-Related Diseases: The Modern Epidemic* (Westport, CT: Avi Publishing, 1985), 1.

4. John Rose, ed., *Nutrition and Killer Diseases: The Effects of Dietary Factors on Fatal Chronic Disease* (Park Ridge, NJ: Noyes Publishing, 1982), xi, 148.

5. Myron Winick, M.D., *Nutrition and Cancer* (New York: John Wiley & Sons, 1977), 55.

Chapter One Inset on "Why Food Is Better Than Supplements"

1. Vivian Cody, Middleton, and Harborne, eds., *Plant Flavonoids in Biology and Medicine II: Biochemical, Cellular, and Medicinal Properties* (New York: Alan R. Liss Inc., 1986), 1–15.

C. Regnault Roger, "The Nutritional Incidence of Flavonoids: Some Physiological and Metabolic Considerations," *Experientia* 15 Sept. (1988): 725–804.

2. Cody, Middleton, and Harborne, eds., *Plant Flavonoids in Biology and Medicine I*, 243–247, 395–410, 437, 511–520.

Cody, et al., eds., *Plant Flavonoids II*, xix, 157–171, 173–182, 313–316.

3. Charles A. Owen Jr., M.D., Ph.D., D.Sc., *Biochemical Aspects of Copper* (Park Ridge, NJ: Noyes Publishing, 1982), 17–18.

Jack Peisach, Philip Aisen, and William F. Blumberg, eds., *The Biochemistry of Copper* (New York: Academic Press, 1966), 305–306.

David S. Robinson, *Food—Biochemistry and Nutritional Value* (Essex, England: Longman Scientific and Technical, 1987), 469–470, 477–480.

Maurice E. Shills, M.D., and Vernon R. Young, Ph.D., eds., *Modern Nutrition in Health and Disease* (Philadelphia: Lea & Febiger, 1988), 253.

4. Walter Mertz, ed., *Trace Elements in Human and Animal Nutrition*, Vol. 1, 5th ed. (New York: Academic Press, 1987), 240.

John Rose, ed., *Nutrition and Killer Diseases* (Park Ridge, NJ: Noyes Publications, 1982), 148–149.

World Health Organization, R. Masironi, ed., *Trace Elements in Relation to Cardiovascular Disease* (Geneva: WHO, 1974), 28–29.

5. Shills and Young, eds., *Modern Nutrition*, 216.

E.R. Williams and M.A. Caliendo, *Nutrition* (New York: McGraw-Hill, 1984), 369.

6. O.A. Levander and Loraine Cheng, *Micronutrient Interactions: Vitamins, Minerals, and Hazardous Elements*, Annals of the New York Academy of Sciences, Vol. 355 (New York: The NY Academy of Sciences, 1980), 30.

7. Richard A. Passwater, Ph.D., *Selenium as Food and Medicine* (New Canaan, CT: Keats Publishing, 1980), 185–195.

Robinson, *Food—Biochemistry and Nutrtional Value*, 326.

8. Bonnie Liebman, "Getting Your Vitamins?" *Nutrition Action Health Letter*, 17, no. 5, June (1990): 1, 5–7.

Chapter Two

1. J.I. Rodale, et al., *The Complete Book of Minerals for Health* (Emmaus, PA: Rodale Books, 1976), 255.

John Rose, ed., *Nutrition and Killer Diseases* (Park Ridge, NJ: Noyes Publications, 1982), 148.

Samuel L. Tisdale, Werner L. Nelson, and James D. Beaton, *Soil Fertility and Fertilizers* (New York: Macmillan, 1985), 382.

2. Maurice E. Shills, M.D., and Vernon R. Young, Ph.D., eds., *Modern Nutrition in Health and Disease* (Philadelphia: Lea & Febiger, 1988), 243.

3. Julian Spallholz, Ph.D., John L. Martin, Ph.D., and Howard E. Ganther, Ph.D., eds., *Selenium in Biology and Medicine* (Westport, CT: Avi Publishing, 1981), 178.

4. J. Kubota, Ph.D., et al., "Selenium in Crops in the United States . . ." *Journal of Agricultural and Food Chemistry* 15 (1967): 448–453.

5. Rodale, et al., *Book of Minerals*, xviii.

Tisdale, Nelson, and Beaton, *Soil Fertility and Fertilizers*, 366.

6. National Research Council, Board on Agriculture, John Pesek, et al., *Alternative Agriculture* (Washington D.C.: National Academy Press, 1989), 35, 115–117.

7. Ibid., 116–117.

8. National Research Council, Board on Agriculture, Pesek, et al., *Alternative Agriculture*, 116.

9. Don Ankerman, B.S., and Richard Large, Ph.D., eds., *Agronomy Handbook* (Memphis, TN: A&L Agricultural Laboratories, 1990), 10.

O.A. Lorenz and D.N. Maynard, *Knott's Handbook for Vegetable Growers* (New York: John Wiley & Sons, 1980).

Based on nutrient removal studies, if the nutrients are available and present in the soil, plants will remove an average of one pound of iron per acre, three-quarters of a pound of manganese, one-third of a pound of zinc, one-quarter of a pound of boron, and one-tenth of a pound of copper, plus twelve other trace elements that may exist in the soil, for an estimated total of 2.5 pounds of trace elements removed per acre that are not replaced by the nitrogen, phosphorus, potassium, and sulfur that are usually supplied by fertilizers. Calcium and magnesium are supplied in some areas by farmers who put lime on their soil; otherwise it's taken out of the soil and not replaced. Removal of 2.5 pounds of trace elements per acre over 300 million acres results in 750 million pounds of nutrient removal for the above 17 trace elements, plus some removal of calcium and magnesium. This rate of removal represents ideal soil conditions. Because of depletion in most areas, the actual removal is likely to be less, resulting in deficient food.

10. National Research Council, John Pesek, et al., *Alternative Agriculture*, 40.

11. Don Ankerman, B.S., and Richard Large, Ph.D., eds., *Agronomy Handbook* (Memphis, TN: A&L Agricultural Laboratories, 1990), 31.

12. World Health Organization, R. Masironi, ed., *Trace Elements in Relation to Cardiovascular Disease* (Geneva: WHO, 1974), 40.

13. WHO, R. Masironi, ed., *Trace Elements*, 40.

14. National Research Council, Board on Agriculture, John Pesek, et al., *Alternative Agriculture* (Washington D.C.: National Academy Press, 1989), 40–42.

Dr. Charles M. Benbrook of the National Research Council quoted in "U.S. Farming Practices Reap Pollution," Alston Chase, *Albuquerque Journal* Feb. 26, 1990.

15. This is known in the field of agronomy and documented in the following books and papers:

Firman E. Bear, "The Inorganic Side of Life," reprint from *Better Crops With Plant Food*, March 4, 1952.

Harry O. Buckman and Nyle C. Brady, *The Nature and Properties of Soils* (New York: The Macmillan Co., 1969), 437–443.

Gabriel Hocman, "Prevention of Cancer: Vegetables and Plants," *Comparative Biochemistry and Physiology*, 93B, no. 2 (1989): 201.

National Research Council, John Pesek, et al., *Alternative Agriculture*, 127.

J.I. Rodale, et al., *The Complete Book of Minerals for Health* (Emmaus, PA: Rodale Books, 1976), 608.

Philip L. White, Sc.D., and Nancy Selvey, R.D., *Nutritional Qualities of Fresh Fruits and Vegetables* (Mount Kisco, NY: Futura Publishing, 1974), 140.

16. Buckman and Brady, *Nature and Properties of Soils*, 437–443.

17. Buckman and Brady, *Nature and Properties of Soils*, 520.

Samuel L. Tisdale, Werner L. Nelson, and James D. Beaton, *Soil Fertility and Fertilizers* (New York: Macmillan, 1985), 386–387.

18. Tisdale, Nelson, and Beaton, *Soil Fertility and Fertilizers*, 268, 336.

19. This is well known in the field of agronomy and documented in the following study by the USDA:

J.F. Hodgson, R.M. Leach Jr., W.H. Allaway, U.S. Plant, Soil, and Nutrition Laboratory, U.S. Department of Agriculture, "Micronutrients in Soils and Plants in Relation to Animal Nutrition," *Journal of Agricultural and Food Chemicals* 10, no. 3 (1962): 171–174.

20. Dr. William A. Albrecht, *Soil Fertility and Animal Health* (Webster City, IA: Fred Hahne Printing, 1958), 152.

21. Firman E. Bear, et al., "Variation in Mineral Composition of Vegetables," *Soil Science Society Proceedings* 13 (1948): 380–384.

22. U.S. Department of Agriculture, prepared by Bernice Watt and Annabel Merrill, *Handbook of the Nutritional Content of Foods*, Handbook 8 (New York: Dover Publications, 1975), 175.

23. USDA, Watt and Merrill, *Handbook of the Nutritional Content of Foods*, 44.

24. Jean A. Pennington, Ph.D., R.D., *Dietary Nutrient Guide* (Westport, CT: Avi Publishing, 1976), 30.

25. C.E. Pantos and P. Markakis, "Ascorbic Acid Content of Artificially Ripened Tomatoes," *Journal of Food Science* 38 (1973): 550.

26. Philip L. White, Sc.D., and Nancy Selvey, R.D., *Nutritional Qualities of Fresh Fruits and Vegetables* (Mount Kisco, NY: Futura Publishing, 1974), 139.

27. Bruno Quebedeaux and Frederick A. Bliss, eds., *Horticulture and Human Health* (Englewood Cliffs, NJ: Prentice-Hall, 1988), 22.

28. Michael Colgan, Ph.D., *Your Personal Vitamin Profile* (New York: William Morrow & Co., 1982), 35.

Quebedeaux and Bliss, eds., *Horticulture and Human Health*, 22.

Rodale, et al., *Book of Minerals*, 589.

29. Quebedeaux and Bliss, eds., *Horticulture and Human Health*, 22.

White and Selvey, eds., *Nutritional Quality of Fresh Fruits and Vegetables*, 54.

30. Pantos and Markakis, "Ascorbic Acid Content . . ." 550.

31. Colgan, *Vitamin Profile*, 31.

32. USDA, Watt and Merrill, *Handbook of Nutritional Content of Foods*, 175.

White and Selvey, eds., *Nutritional Quality of Fresh Fruits and Vegetables*, 35–36, 53.

33. Ian Brighthope, "AIDS—Remissions Using Nutrient Therapies . . ." *International Clinical Nutrition Review* 7, no. 2 (1987): 58.

Marshall Phillips and Albert Baetz, eds., *Diet and Resistance to Disease*, Advances in Experimental Medicine and Biology, Vol. 135 (New York: Plenum Press, 1981), 1–4.

Shills and Young, eds., *Modern Nutrition in Health and Disease*, 424.

Rich Wentzler, *The Vitamin Book* (New York: Gramercy Publishing Co., 1980), 147.

34. Reprinted from *The Complete Book of Minerals for Health*, ©1972 by Rodale Press Inc. Permission granted by Rodale Press Inc., Emmaus, PA 18098. xvii, 595.

35. Stephen Davies, M.D., and Alan Stewart, M.D., *Nutritional Medicine* (New York: Avon Books, 1987), xxiv.

36. Reprinted with permission from *Health Secrets You Were Never Supposed to Have* by Dr. David G. Williams from *Alternatives for the Health Conscious Individual*, ©1989 by Mountain Home Publishing, P.O. Box 829, Ingram, TX 78025. 39.

Chapter Two Inset on "Deficiencies in Animal Foods"

1. J. Spallholz, J.L. Martin, and H.E. Ganther, eds., *Selenium in Biology and Medicine* (Westport, CT: Avi Publishing, 1981), 186.

Eric J. Underwood, *Trace Elements in Human and Animal Nutrition* (New York: Academic Press, 1977), 328.

World Health Organization, R. Masironi, ed., *Trace Elements in Relation to Cardiovascular Disease* (Geneva: WHO, 1974), 28.

2. Underwood, *Trace Elements in Human and Animal Nutrition*, 327.

3. Spallholz, Martin, and Ganther, *Selenium in Biology and Medicine*, 179.

4. G. Patrias and O. Olson, "Selenium Contents of Samples of Corn . . ." *Feedstuffs*, Vol. 41, Oct. 25 (1969): 33.

5. Underwood, *Trace Elements in Human and Animal Nutrition*, 328.

6. Spallholz, Martin, and Ganther, *Selenium in Biology and Medicine*, 185–187.

Underwood, *Trace Elements in Human and Animal Nutrition*, 304, 326.

7. Spallholz, et al., *Selenium in Biology and Medicine*, 179, 192, 195.

Underwood, *Trace Elements in Human and Animal Nutrition*, 329.

8. Underwood, *Trace Elements in Human and Animal Nutrition* (1971), 473.

Chapter Three

1. J.K. Chavan and S.S. Kadam, "Nutritional Improvement of Cereals by Sprouting," *CRC Critical Reviews in Food Science and Nutrition* 28, no. 5 (1989): 401–437.

M.L. Fernandez and J.W. Berry, "Nutritional Evaluation of Chickpea and Germinated Chickpea Flours," *Plant Foods for Human Nutrition* 38, no. 2 (1988): 127–134.

Abdus Sattar, et al., "Effect of Soaking and Germination Temperatures on Selected Nutrients and Antinutrients of Mung Beans," *Food Chemistry* 34, no. 2 (1989): 111–120.

2. U.S. Department of Agriculture, prepared by Bernice Watt and Annabel Merrill, *Handbook of the Nutritional Content of Foods* (New York: Dover Publications, 1975), 10, 58–59.

3. Ibid, 10.

4. M.H.A. El-Aal, "Changes in Gross Chemical Composition . . . During Germination of Fenugreek Seeds," *Food Chemistry* 22, no. 3 (1986): 193–207.

S.S. Kadam, et al., "Effects of Heat Treatments of Antinutritional Factors and Quality of Protein in Winged Bean," *Journal of Food Science and Agriculture* 39, no. 3 (1987): 267–275.

A. Kataria and B.M. Chauhan, "Contents and Digestibility of Carbohydrates of Mung Beans," *Plant Foods for Human Nutrition* 39, no. 4 (1989): 325–330.

S. Jood, B.M. Chauhan, and A.C. Kapoor, "Contents and Digestibility of Carbohydrates of Chickpea and Black Gram . . ." *Food Chemistry* 30, no. 2 (1988): 113–127.

M.J. Moron Jimenez, et al., "Biochemical and Nutritional Studies of Germinated Soybeans," *Archivos Latinoamericanos de Nutricion* 35, no. 3 (1985): 480–490.

M.L. Romo-Parada, et al., "Influence of Germination on the Nutritional Value of Sorghum Protein," *Microbiologie-Aliments-Nutrition* 3, no. 2 (1985): 125–132.

5. M.A. Akpapunam and S.C. Achinewhu, "Effects Of Cooking, Germination, and Fermentation on . . . Cowpeas," *Qualitas Plantarum: Plant Foods for Human Nutrition* 35, no. 4 (1985): 353–358.

V.S. Babar, J.K. Chavan, and S.S. Kadam, "Effects of Heat Treatments and Germination on Trypsin Inhibitor Activity," *Plant Foods for Human Nutrition* 38, no. 3 (1988): 319–324.

V.I.P. Batra, "Effects of Cooking and Germination on Hemagglutinin Activity in Lentil," *Indian Journal of Nutrition and Dietetics* 24, no. 1 (1987): 15–19.

S. Jood, B.M. Chauhan, and A.C. Kapoor, "Polyphenols of Chickpea and Black Gram . . ." *Journal of Food Science and Agriculture* 39, (1987): 145–149.

S. Jood, B.M. Chauhan, and A.C. Kapoor, "Saponin Content of Chickpea and Black Gram," *Journal of Food Science and Agriculture* 37 (1986): 1,121–1,124.

S.A.R. Kabbara, et al., "Soaking and Cooking Parameters of Tepary Beans . . ." *Qualitas Plantarum: Plant Foods for Human Nutrition* 36, no. 4 (1987): 295–307.

S.S. Kadam, et al., "Trypsin Inhibitor in Moth Bean . . ." *Qualitas Plantarum: Plant Foods in Human Nutrition* 36, no. 1 (1986): 43–46.

A. Kataria, B.M. Chauhan, and S. Gandhi, "Effect of Domestic Processing . . . on the Antinutrients of Black Gram," *Food Chemistry* 30, no. 2 (1988): 149–156.

L.A. Shekib, S.M. El-Iraqui, and T.M. Abo-Bakr, "Studies on Amylase Inhibitors . . ." *Plant Foods for Human Nutrition* 38, no. 3 (1988): 325–332.

V. Ravindran and G. Ravindran, "Nutritional and Antinutritional Characteristics of Mucona Bean Seeds," *Journal of Food Science and Agriculture* 46, no. 1 (1988): 71–79.

6. Dr. Edward Howell, *Enzyme Nutrition* (Wayne, NJ: Avery Publishing Group, 1985), 125.

7. Howell, *Enzyme Nutrition*, 34–39.

W. Bednarske, et al., "Processing Suitability and Nutritive Value of Field Bean Seeds After Germination," *Journal of Food Science and Agriculture* 36, no. 8 (1985): 745–751.

8. Reprinted with permission from "Health Secrets You Were Never Supposed to Have" by Dr. David G. Williams from *Alternatives for the Health Conscious Individual*, ©1989 by Mountain Home Publishing, P.O. Box 829, Ingram, TX 78025. 39.

9. Ibid, 72.

Chapter Four

1. National Research Council, Board on Agriculture, Committee on Scientific and Regulatory Issues Underlying Pesticide Use Patterns, *Regulating Pesticides in Food* (Washington, D.C.: National Academy Press, 1987), 4.

National Research Council, Board on Agriculture, John Pesek, et al., *Alternative Agriculture* (Washington, D.C.: National Academy Press, 1989), 45.

2. "Warning, Your Food Nutritious and Delicious May be Hazardous to Your Health," *Newsweek*, March 27 (1989): 18.

3. National Research Council, *Regulating Pesticides in Food*, 11–12.

4. Ibid., 36.

5. G.A. Beall, C.M. Bruhn, A.L. Craigmill, and C.K. Winter, "Pesticides and Your Food: How Safe Is 'Safe'?" *California Agriculture*, Vol. 45, no. 4 (July–August 1991): 8.

6. National Research Council, *Regulating Pesticides in Food*, 34.

7. C.K. Winter, J.N. Seiber, and C.F. Nuckton, *Chemicals in the Human Food Chain* (New York: Van Nostrand Reinhold, 1990), 13.

8. World Health Organization, G. Vettorazzi, P. Miles-Vettorazzi, *Safety Evaluation of Chemicals in Food: Toxicological Data Profiles for Pesticides* (Geneva: World Health Organization, 1975), 6.

9. Reprinted with permission from *Alternative Agriculture*, ©1989 by the National Academy of Sciences. Published by National Academy Press, Washington D.C., 83.

10. Winter, et. al., *Chemicals in the Human Food Chain*, 10.

11. Wayland J. Hayes Jr. and Edward R. Laws Jr., eds., *Handbook of Pesticide Toxicology*, Vol. 1 (New York: Academic Press Inc., 1991), 251.

12. Reprinted with permission from *Alternative Agriculture*, ©1989 by the National Academy of Sciences. Published by National Academy Press, Washington, D.C., 84.

13. William H. Hallenbeck and Kathleen M. Cunningham-Burns, *Pesticides and Human Health* (New York: Springer-Verlag, 1985), 3.

14. Reprinted with permission from *Alternative Agriculture*, ©1989 by the National Academy of Sciences. Published by National Academy Press, Washington, D.C., 84.

15. Hayes and Laws, eds., *Handbook of Pesticide Toxicology*, 312.

16. Ibid., 312.

17. Reprinted with permission from *Alternative Agriculture*, ©1989 by the National Academy of Sciences. Published by National Academy Press, Washington, D.C., 84.

18. Hayes and Laws, eds., *Handbook of Pesticide Toxicology*, 312.

19. "Warning, Your Food Nutritious and Delicious . . ." 18.

20. Sheldon L. Wagner, M.D., *Clinical Toxicology of Agricultural Chemicals* (Park Ridge, NJ: Noyes Data Corp., 1983), 82–83.

21. National Research Council, *Alternative Agriculture*, 126.

22. Janice E. Chambers, Ph.D., and James D. Yarbough, Ph.D., *Effects of Chronic Exposures to Pesticides on Animal Systems* (New York: Raven Press, 1982), v.

23. Sheldon, *Clinical Toxicology of Agricultural Chemicals*, 70.

24. Hayes and Laws, eds., *Handbook of Pesticide Toxicology*, 255.

25. Ibid., 246.

26. National Research Council, *Regulating Pesticides in Food*, 119.

27. Hayes and Laws, eds., *Handbook of Pesticide Toxicology*, 313.

28. Ibid., 248.

Chapter Four Inset on "A New Pesticide Menace"

1. Clive A. Edwards, *Persistent Pesticides in the Environment* (Cleveland: CRC Press, 1970), i, 33, 48.

Chapter Six

1. E.N. Whitney and E.M.N. Hamilton, *Understanding Nutrition* (New York: West Publishing Co., 1987), 311, 313.

E.R. Williams and M.A. Caliendo, *Nutrition* (New York: McGraw-Hill Book Co., 1984), 304.

2. California Fertilizer Association, *Western Fertilizer Handbook* (Danville, IL: Interstate Printers & Publishers Inc., 1985), 269.

APPENDIX A:
Sources of Gardening Supplies and Services

From years of hands-on gardening and sifting through many local and mail-order sources of supplies and services, we have gleaned the following list for recommendation.

BOOKS

AgAccess
P.O. Box 2008
Davis, CA 95617

Rodale Press
33 East Minor Street
Emmaus, PA 18098

Storey Communications
Schoolhouse Road
Pownal, VT 05261

EARTHWORMS

Carter Fishworm Farm
Plains, GA 31780

GROW LIGHTS (INDOOR)

Parks Seed Co.
Cokesbury Road
Greenwood, SC 29647

HOTKAPS, ROW COVERS, HARVESTING KNEE PADS, MULCHING

Mellingers
Department SNG
2310 South Range Road
North Lima, OH 49452

MARTIN HOUSES

Mac Industries
8125 South I–35
Oklahoma City, OK 73149

Sears Roebuck
(see catalogue in retail stores)

PEST CONTROL, BIOLOGICAL

Mellingers
Department SNG
2310 South Range Road
North Lima, OH 49452

PLANTING EQUIPMENT

Mellingers
Department SNG
2310 South Range Road
North Lima, OH 49452

PROCESSING

Lee Manufacturing Co.
P.O. Box 29153
Dallas, TX 75229

SALT METER

Myron L Co.
P.O. Box 876
Encinitas, CA 92024

SEAWEED

Mellingers
Department SNG
2310 South Range Road
North Lima, OH 49452

SEEDS

(see Appendix B)

SOIL PH KITS

Forestry Suppliers
P.O. Box 8397
Jackson, MS 39284

SOIL TESTING LABS

East (acid soils and rainfall over 35 inches):

Brookside Farms Labs
New Knoxville, OH 45871

West (alkaline soils, rainfall 25 inches or less):

A&L Labs
P.O. Box 1590
Lubbock, TX 79408

A&L Labs
1311 Woodland Avenue
Modesto, CA 95350

SPROUTING KITS

Dr. William Peavy
c/o Avery Publishing Group
120 Old Broadway
Garden City Park, NY 11040

SUSTAINABLE AGRICULTURE

(See Books)

WEED CONTROL

Nasco (nursery hoe)
901 Janesville Avenue
Fort Atkinson, WI 53538

Mellingers (sliding hoe)
Department SNG
2310 South Range Road
North Lima, OH 49452

APPENDIX B
Mail-Order Seed Companies

There are literally dozens of mail-order seed companies out there. We have scanned them to select what we consider the best, based on the following criteria: good selections of food crops that are basic; good prices; high-quality viable seeds; orderly arrangement of kinds of seeds (such as an alphabetical listing or putting all tomatoes in one place in the catalog); sources of open-pollinated seeds; and hard-to-find equipment and seeds of special varieties.

Bountiful Gardens
5798 Ridgewood Road
Willits, CA 95490
(Good source of non-hybrid, open-pollinated seeds so you can save your own seeds.)

Burpee Seed Co.
300 Park Avenue
Warminster, PA 18974
(Puts out a big, colorful catalog with forty pages on vegetable seeds. Vegetables arranged in alphabetical order so you don't have to hunt around for what you want.)

Johnny's Selected Seeds
Foss Hill Road
Albion, ME 04910
(Carries some special, hard-to-find varieties.)

Porter & Sons
P.O. Box 104
Stephenville, TX 76401
(Black-and-white catalog but good seeds at inexpensive prices. Good drip irrigation supplies.)

Seed Savers Exchange
P.O. Box 70
Decorah, IA 52101
(An organization of vegetable gardeners who grow and exchange non-hybrid seeds. Many good, old-fashioned varieties are preserved this way.)

Stokes Seeds
P.O. Box 548
Buffalo, NY 14240
(Carries a good selection of onion varieties, greenhouse varieties, and hard-to-find equipment.)

Westwind Seeds
2509 North Campbell Avenue—#139
Tucson, AZ 85719
(Specializes in open-pollinated seeds for the southwestern United States.)

APPENDIX C

Letter to Soils Lab With Soil Sample

When you mail out a soil sample to a soils lab, you must enclose a short but complete note showing your name and address and specifying what test you want done. Also include your check as payment. Here is a sample note:

(Date)

TO: (name of soils lab)

FROM: (your name and address)

Enclosed is a one-cup sample of soil from my garden. Please do your soil test (S-1, S-2, etc.) at (cost of test). My check for $__________ is enclosed.

APPENDIX D

*Composition of Organic Materials**

(Dry Weight Basis)

For the proper use of any fertilizer, you need to know what's in the fertilizer, especially the nitrogen content. Knowing the nitrogen content will guide you on how much fertilizer to use in your beds or compost pile. This table lists the most common organic fertilizers.

Organic Material	**Nitrogen**	**Phosphorus****	**Potassium*****
Bat Guano	13.0%	5.0%	2.0%
Blood (Dried)	12.0%	1.5%	0.0%
Cottonseed Meal	6.5%	3.0%	1.5%
Compost	1.0%	1.0%	1.0%
Fish Emulsion	5.0%	2.0%	2.0%
Grass Clippings	2.4%	no data	no data
Kitchen Trimmings	1.0%	no data	no data
Leaves	0.3%	no data	no data
Manure, Cattle	2.0%	1.9%	2.8%
Manure, Poultry	3.4%	2.0%	2.0%
Manure, Rabbit	2.0%	1.5%	1.5%
Manure, Sheep	2.0%	1.8%	1.7%
Sawdust (Aged)	0.25%	0.0%	0.0%
Sawdust (Fresh)	0.1%	0.0%	0.0%

* = Average values. Organic materials vary widely in composition.
** = As P_2O_5, or phosphorus oxide.
*** = As K_2O, or potassium oxide.

Sources of data:

1. University of California, Berkeley, CA, "California Agriculture." July–August 1981.
2. Texas A&M University, College Station, TX: Texas Agriculture Extension, Service Fact Sheet L-1220, 1974.
3. World Health Organization, Geneva, Switzerland, book, *Composting* by Gotaas, 1956.
4. Peavy, W.S., 1979, *Southern Gardeners Soil Handbook*, Gulf Publishing Co., Houston, TX.

APPENDIX E
Spacing on 36-Inch Beds

The 24-inch bed width is good, but so is the 36-inch bed width. The spacing charts in Chapter 7 were all based on the 24-inch bed, but if you want to use the 36-inch bed you will need different spacings, shown here.

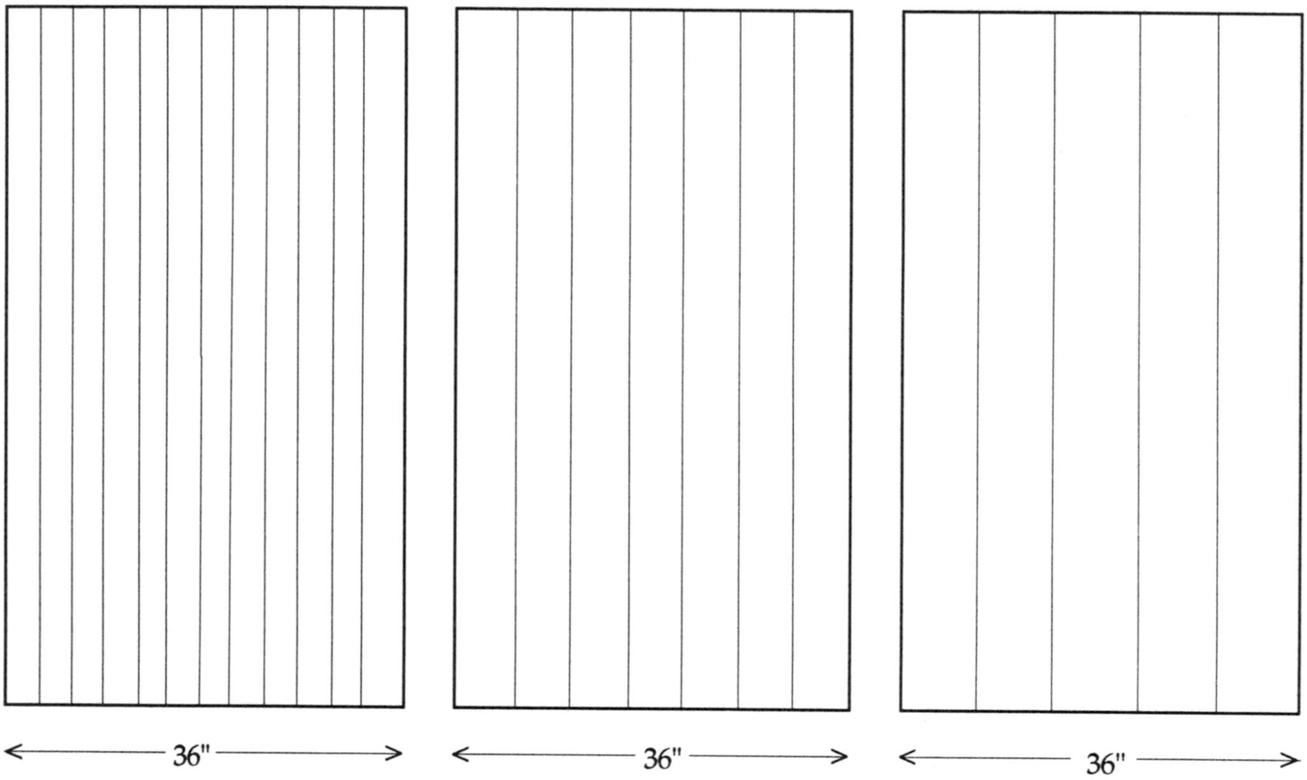

A. 11 ROWS
Plant first row on centerline and other rows 3 inches apart.

Distance between plants in row:
Onion—3 inches
Radish—1 inch

B. 6 ROWS
Plant two center rows each 3 inches off centerline and other rows 6 inches apart.

Distance between plants in row:
Lettuce, Bibb—6 inches

C. 4 ROWS
Plant two center rows each 5 inches off centerline and other rows 10 inches apart.

Distance between plants in row:
Lettuce, Romaine—10 inches
Celery—6 inches

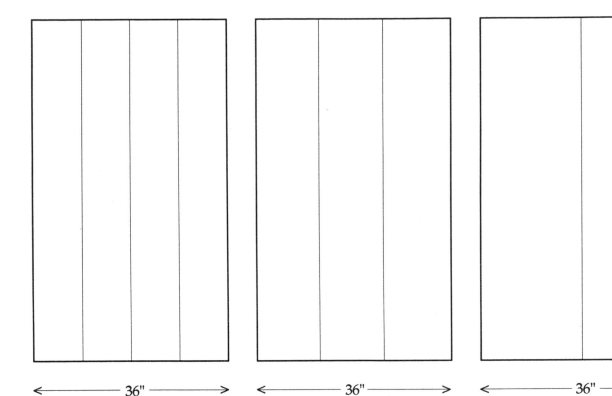

D. 3 ROWS

Plant first row on centerline and other rows 12 inches apart.

Distance between plants in row:

Beet—3 inches
Cabbage—12 inches
Carrot—2 inches
Garlic—3 inches
Kohlrabi—4 inches
Mustard—12 inches
Peanut—8 inches
Turnip—3 inches
Pea, Green—1.5 inches

E. 2 ROWS

Plant each row 9 inches off centerline.

Distance between plants in row:

Bean, Bush—3 inches
Bean, Pole*—6 inches
Broccoli—18 inches
Cauliflower—18 inches
Corn—8 inches
Cucumber—12 inches
Eggplant—18 inches
Kale—12 inches
Okra—18 inches
Pea, Southern—4 inches
Pepper—12 inches
Soybean—4 inches

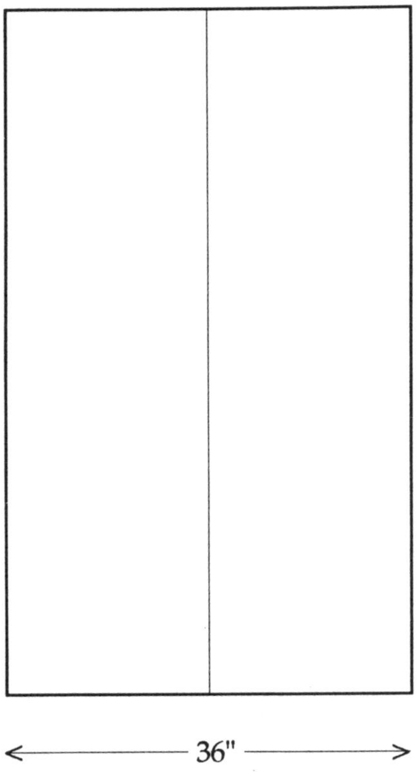

F. 1 ROW

Plant one row along or near centerline.

Distance between plants in row:

Squash, Bush—36 inches
Squash, Vine*—36 inches
Sweet Potato—12 inches
Tomato—36 inches

* = On trellis

APPENDIX F
The Large Food Garden

We have addressed this book largely to people without a great amount of outdoor gardening space—people who, instead, have a small backyard or perhaps just a kitchen counter for a sprout garden.

If you move to where you have a big backyard, you should keep your sprout garden but add to it by starting a new exciting game plan: the large, outdoor, PowerCharged food garden. Such a garden requires more of your time and more equipment, but it will much more than pay for itself. It will enable you to cut your grocery bills in half! You can do that with a medium-sized garden of only 500 square feet per person.

Even better for you might be the large-size garden of 1,000 square feet per person. For a family of four, that is approximately 4,000 square feet— only a tenth of an acre.

If you end up with a large food garden, you'll need the following items.

SMALL PICKUP TRUCK

An ideal vehicle is the mini-pickup truck such as the Chevy S-10 or Ford Ranger. The Japanese imports are not suitable, because they lack the vertical wells built into the bed to hold the upright stakes of sideboards. This is a must for hauling bulky organic materials, especially if you're using a mini-pickup with a smaller bed.

We plan to get a pickup truck, and it will be a temptation to put a camper on the back of it. But if we do that, then what about having an open bed for easy filling of bulky organic material or for dropping a skip-loader bucket full of compost or dairy manure in from the top? If you do consider a camper shell, be sure it is of the lightweight, plastic type that can easily be lifted off by two people. And you might want to use wing nuts for the fastening bolts so it will be easy and quick to put on or take off.

PLANTER

Another piece of equipment you will need is a push-type mechanical seed planter, available for less than $100. This is especially needed for plots of 4,000 or more square feet.

COMPOST SHREDDER

Still another piece of equipment you might find worthwhile is a compost shredder, especially one that works like a vacuum to suck up leaves, shred them, and blow the shredded material into a bag.

Handling leaves is a laborious, time-consuming activity. You have to rake them into piles, then put all that fluffy stuff into bags that don't like to stay open. The wind might act up while you are trying to get the leaves into the sack. Then you haul a few bags of fluffy leaves to your leaf pen. Ten bags of dry, fluffy leaves or six bags of wet leaves end up neatly as only one bag of shredded leaves. Whole leaves must go into a leaf pen to break down before being used as mulch or placed in the compost pile. Shredded leaves, however, can immediately be used as mulch or placed in the compost pile.

ROTOTILLER

The rototiller manufacturers won't like us for writing this, but we feel we must share this information with you, then let you decide whether you want to invest $1,200 to $2,000 for a good, heavy-duty, rear-tine tiller that cuts the standard 20-inch swath in one pass.

The question is whether to rent a tiller or to buy one, not whether to use one. We wouldn't be without the use of our rototiller, but we use it only once or twice a year, when making up beds. We have owned two rototillers and found that they stay parked most of the time. That is because rather than control weeds with cultivation, we control them with mulch, which is much better for your soil and your plants.

If you live within easy driving distance of a rental place, you can rent a tiller for probably less than $50 a year. Or look around for a good used one.

Gardeners with a quarter-acre mini-farm (10,000 square feet) can probably justify spending $2,000 or more for a good, heavy-duty rototiller, but the small-scale gardener will probably find his money better spent on a compost shredder.

DAIRY MANURE FOR FERTILIZER

For the medium- or large-size garden, you will need large amounts of mulch and organic fertilizer. The best source of good, inexpensive, wholesale lots of organic fertilizer is your nearest dairy. But you will need a pickup truck with the bed open so the manure can be loaded from the top with a mechanical loader. You will probably also need sideboards, since much of the organic materials you will haul are bulky.

Manure for Soil Fertility

If you have a large garden (1,000 square feet or more) and a pickup truck, your local dairy is the best, cheapest source of good organic fertilizer.

A good application rate is 20 tons per acre (2 cubic feet of fertilizer per 100 square feet of land), or about 1 cubic yard for a 1,000-square-foot garden, or 16 gallons per 100 square feet. Although that might sound like a lot of manure, when spread out evenly it produces only a thin layer, about a quarter of an inch. You should go straight to a dairy for that much manure rather than buy the bagged manure you see in garden centers. Locally produced dairy manure is much less expensive and has a much better quality. It is not diluted with sawdust or other fillers, and it is low in salt. The bags of manure from garden centers contain feedlot manure high in salt.

Salt, even table salt, is an environmental pollutant and for the most part should be left in the salt mines. But feedlot cattle operators have found that if they force-feed extra sodium chloride (table salt) to their fattening cattle it does the same thing to them as it does to us: it makes the animals terribly thirsty. The thirsty cattle drink water and more water, which makes them weigh more. But their bodies do not need all that salt for their nutrition, so the excess salt goes right through them and comes out in the manure.

When animals are allowed salt-free choices, pure cattle manure contains only a small amount of salt. (See Table A.1.) Both sodium and chlorine—the two components of table salt—are trace elements, or micronutrients, and are needed by plants, but only in minute amounts. (See Table A.2.)

A typical application of cattle manure is 10 tons (17 cubic yards) per acre. This basic application not only supplies large amounts of desirable nutrients such as nitrogen, phosphorus, and potassium, but large—and sufficient—amounts of sodium and chlorine.

An acre of top-yielding crops of vegetables needs about 693 pounds of the six major nutrient elements (nitrogen, phosphorus, potassium,

Table A.1

Pollution of Cattle Manure by Feeding Table Salt to Cattle

(Expressed on a Dry Weight Basis in Parts Per Million, or ppm)

Element/Compound	Pure Manure[1]	Dairy Manure[2]	Feedlot Manure[3]
Sodium (Na)	Less than 618 ppm	2,275 ppm	9,000 ppm
Chlorine[4] (Cl)	Less than 927 ppm	3,412 ppm	13,500 ppm
Table Salt (NaCl)	Less than 1,545 ppm	5,687 ppm	22,500 ppm

1. Pure manure taken fresh and oven-dried.
2. Dairy in Fort Stockton, Texas.
3. Feedlot in Pecos, Texas.
4. Sodium x 1.5 = chlorine.

calcium, magnesium, sulfur), which are hauled out of the field at harvest, but it needs only about one-tenth of a pound of sodium and chlorine. Any fertilizer application beyond that is in excess and becomes a pollutant—especially sodium, which tends to interfere with water penetration by sealing the pores of soils. Applying 10 tons of feedlot manure per acre pollutes the soil with about 148 pounds of sodium and 220 pounds of chlorine, which together equal 236 pounds of table salt, which is about 235 pounds more than the acre needs. (This data comes from the Texas Agricultural Extension Service, leaflet L-1220, "Fertilization of Crops With Feedlot Wastes.")

What about salt in dairy manure? It's there, but in much smaller amounts. Applying 10 tons of dairy manure per acre will add only about 30 pounds of salt. Applying 20 tons per acre (20 cubic feet per 1,000 square feet) adds only about 60 pounds of salt. You can easily get rid of this pollutant with a leaching irrigation or, if the average annual rainfall is more than 25 inches, with natural rain.

The secret with using dairy manure is to think of it in terms of volume (cubic feet or cubic yards) and to apply a moderate amount every year. Do not skip a year or two before applying more. For example, do not apply a large application every third year. Applying

Table A.2

Nutrient Removal by Crop Harvest*

(Listing of 8 of the 17 Nutrients Needed by Soil)

NUTRIENT ELEMENT	REMOVED PER ACRE Pounds	Percent
MAJOR NUTRIENTS		
Potassium (K)	271	39.0
Nitrogen (N)	212	30.0
Calcium (Ca)	94	13.5
Sulfur (S)	43	6.0
Magnesium (Mg)	39	5.6
Phosphorus (P)	34	4.8
TOTAL	693	98.9
MICRONUTRIENTS		
Sodium (Na)	0.1	0.0001
Chlorine (Cl)	0.01	0.00001

* = by top yields of six major vegetable crops.

SOURCE: *Knott's Handbook for Vegetable Growers.*

moderate rates every year results in nutrients being released at a steady level instead of in a yo-yo pattern. Experiment with rates.

Dr. Peavy did his Ph.D work on manure as a fertilizer, so he has a great deal of factual information on the subject. He has used manure for years for nearly all of his fertilizer needs, reaping huge yields of high-quality food. But he co-wrote this book mainly for apartment dwellers with no outdoor garden space and for home owners with only a small amount of backyard space. Most of those people do not have the pickup truck that is needed to haul manure, so he suggests they do their soil charging with an alternative, easy-to-haul organic fertilizer available at feed stores: cottonseed meal.

About the Authors

DR. WILLIAM PEAVY is one of the world's top authorities on the connection between fertile soil, nutritious food, and human health. His four degrees include a master's in horticulture from the University of California and a Ph.D. in horticultural science from Kansas State University.

His lifelong study of health began in the 1950s when he operated a health resort where he taught people how to lose weight and gain glowing health. From that time to the present, he has continued to research the scientific literature on the links between soil, nutritious food, and human health.

While working on his Ph.D. (1969–1972), he found that a great deal more research was needed to find ways of growing more nutrition into foods as soil deficiencies worsened and people's diets were not delivering the nutrients needed. He's always believed that natural foods, not pills, are the best answer to problems in diets.

He is one of the few people to have done university research on the use of organic fertilizers to improve the nutrition of food. He later began his own non-profit research organization, the American Institute for Abundant Living, and began a private research program to find ways of growing more nutrition into food. Part of his research has been completed and is reported for the first time in this book.

Dr. Peavy's first book, *Southern Gardeners Soil Handbook,* was published in 1979 by Gulf Publishing. He has had over 100 of his articles appear in national and state magazines, and he wrote a weekly column on home food growing for the *El Paso Times* for seven years.

As an extension horticulturist for Texas A&M University for thirteen years, he taught thousands how to grow healthy food. His classes and seminars and his numerous appearances on radio and television have educated the public about nutritious food, its effect on human health, and how to grow it. He currently hosts a weekly radio talk show in Albuquerque, New Mexico, and offers a horticultural consultant service. He is preparing a sequel to this book, entitled *Living Off the Land.*

WARREN PEARY is an investigative health journalist and Dr. Peavy's son. He has worked closely with Dr. Peavy in researching the current scientific literature on nutrition and health and using them as references in this book. He has spent over a thousand hours researching medical/nutritional journals and texts in the University of New Mexico Medical and Sciences Libraries, uncovering an astonishing array of up-to-date references on the effects of food on human health.

Backed up by authoritative sources, these two authors bring a lively and incisive clarity to the urgent health issues of the day, presenting individual solutions found in no other book.

Index